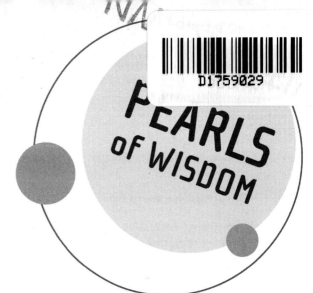

PEARLS OF WISDOM

Otolaryngology

BOARD REVIEW

Third Edition

Mary Talley Bowden, MD
Houston, Texas

Medical

New York   Chicago   San Francisco   Lisbon   London   Madrid   Mexico City   Milan
New Delhi   San Juan   Seoul   Singapore   Sydney   Toronto

Otolaryngology Board Review: Pearls of Wisdom, Third Edition

Copyright © 2012, 2006 by the McGraw-Hill Companies, Inc. All rights reserved. Printed in the United States of America. Except as permitted under the United States Copyright Act of 1976, no part of this publication may be reproduced or distributed in any form or by any means, or stored in a database or retrieval system, without the prior written permission of the publisher.

1 2 3 4 5 6 7 8 9 0 QDB/QDB 17 16 15 14 13 12

ISBN 978-0-07-176968-6
MHID 0-07-176968-4

Notice

Medicine is an ever-changing science. As new research and clinical experience broaden our knowledge, changes in treatment and drug therapy are required. The author and the publisher of this work have checked with sources believed to be reliable in their efforts to provide information that is complete and generally in accord with the standards accepted at the time of publication. However, in view of the possibility of human error or changes in medical sciences, neither the author nor the publisher nor any other party who has been involved in the preparation or publication of this work warrants that the information contained herein is in every respect accurate or complete, and they disclaim all responsibility for any errors or omissions or for the results obtained from use of the information contained in this work. Readers are encouraged to confirm the information contained herein with other sources. For example and in particular, readers are advised to check the product information sheet included in the package of each drug they plan to administer to be certain that the information contained in this work is accurate and that changes have not been made in the recommended dose or in the contraindications for administration. This recommendation is of particular importance in connection with new or infrequently used drugs.

This book was set in Adobe Garamond by Aptara®, Inc.
The editors were Kirsten Funk, Catherine A. Johnson, and Peter J. Boyle.
The production supervisor was Catherine H. Saggese.
Project management was provided by Samir Roy, Aptara, Inc.
Cover photo: Mark Thomas/Photo Researchers, Inc.
Quad/Graphics Dubuque was printer and binder.

This book is printed on acid-free paper.

Cataloging-in-publication data for this book is on file at the Library of Congress.

DEDICATION

To Peter, Jack, Charlie, and Thomas
for their love and support.

CONTENTS

SECTION I: ANATOMY AND BASIC SCIENCE

SECTION II: DIAGNOSTIC AND ASSESSMENT PROCEDURES

SECTION III: DISEASES, DISORDERS, AND CONDITIONS

SECTION IV: PHARMACOLOGY

SECTION V: BASIC SURGICAL CONCEPTS

SECTION VI: SPECIFIC SURGICAL PROCEDURES

SECTION VII: GENERAL TOPICS

PREFACE

Otolaryngology Board Review: Pearls of Wisdom is designed to help you prepare you for the In Service and Board Examination for Otolaryngology.

Since *Otolaryngology Board Review* is primarily intended as a study aid, the text is structured in a question and answer format. Most of the questions are short with short answers. This is to facilitate moving quickly through a large body of information. Such a format, while quite unlike the format used in the actual Board Examination, is useful to enable you to assess your strengths and weaknesses in a particular area. This allows you to concentrate further studies on areas of interest or weakness. Emphasis has been placed on distilling key facts that are easily overlooked, that are quickly forgotten, and that somehow seem to occur frequently on in-service or board examinations.

It must be emphasized that any question and answer book is most useful as a learning tool when used in conjunction with a subject-specific textbook. Truly assimilating these facts into a framework of knowledge absolutely requires further reading on the surrounding concepts. The more active the learning process, the better the understanding. **Use this book with your preferred source texts handy and open. When you encounter a question that you cannot recall the answer or that you find of particular interest, you are strongly encouraged to review the pertinent area in the textbook at hand.**

The third edition has been completely reorganized to to follow the format of the board exam as outlined by the American Board of Otolaryngology. New to this edition are high-yield images to test yourself on visual diagnosis. All aspects of otolaryngology are included, though some areas are covered more thoroughly than others. The questions within each chapter are randomly arranged to simulate board examinations and the way questions arise in real life. You may encounter several areas of redundancy. This is intentional – redundancy is a good thing when preparing for board examinations.

While great effort has been made to verify that the questions and answers are accurate, discrepancies and inaccuracies sometimes occur. Most often this is attributable to variance between original sources. We have tried to verify in several references the most accurate information. In addition, this book risks accuracy by aggressively pruning complex concepts down to the simplest level; the dynamic knowledge base and clinical practice of medicine is not like that. Furthermore, new research and current practice occasionally deviates from that which likely represents the correct answer for test purposes. Keep in mind that this book is designed to maximize your score on a test and answers may not be the ones you prefer. Refer to your most current sources of information and mentors for direction in daily practice.

We welcome your comments, suggestions, and criticism. Please make us aware of any errors you find. We hope to make continuous improvements and would greatly appreciate any input with regard to format, organization, content, presentation, or about specific questions.

Study hard and good luck on the Boards!

Mary Talley Bowden, M.D.

Section I

ANATOMY AND BASIC SCIENCE

CHAPTER 1 Ear

○ **What embryologic structures is the auricle developed from?**
The hillocks of His.

○ **How many hillocks are there and which branchial arches do they arise from?**
Six; the first three arise from the first arch and the last three arise from the second arch.

○ **What does each hillock become?**
1. Tragus.
2. Helical crus.
3. Helix.
4. Antihelix.
5. Antitragus.
6. Lobule and lower helix.

○ **How does a preauricular sinus tract form?**
From improper fusion of the 1st and 2nd branchial arches.

○ **When does development of the external auditory canal (EAC) begin?**
The canal begins to develop at 28 weeks gestation.

○ **At what month(s) gestation does the ear canal open?**
Seventh.

○ **At what age does the EAC reach adult size?**
Nine years.

○ **What is the significance of a congenitally malformed auricle?**
The auricle develops early, making malformations of the middle ear, mastoid, and VII more likely.

○ **What is the significance of a normal auricle with canal atresia?**
The EAC begins formation late (28th week), so the middle ear and ossicles are more likely to be normal.

○ **Which ossicles develop from the first branchial arch (Meckel's cartilage)?**

Head and neck of the malleus, body, and short process of the incus.

○ **Which ossicles develop from the second branchial arch (Reichert's cartilage)?**

Manubrium of the malleus, long process of the incus, and stapes (except footplate).

○ **What does the stapes footplate develop from?**

Otic mesenchyme.

○ **Which ossicular component develops from membranous bone?**

Anterior process of the malleus.

○ **Which ossicular components never completely ossify?**

Part of the manubrium and the vestibular portion of the stapes footplate.

○ **When do the ossicles reach adult size and shape?**

At the 16th week gestation, they are adult-sized, and by birth, they are adult-shaped.

○ **Why is the development of the bony otic capsule unique?**

It is formed from 14 centers of ossification that fuse and leave no suture lines; the centers are formed from cartilage, but retain no areas of chondral growth. The bone retains its fetal character, with Haversian canals.

○ **When does the otic capsule begin formation?**

At 8 weeks, the precursors of the otic capsule are present; at 15 weeks, the ossification centers are present.

○ **When does the otic capsule finish developing?**

By 21–24 weeks, it reaches adult size.

○ **What is the last part of the otic capsule to ossify?**

Fissula ante fenestrum.

○ **When does the fallopian canal begin developing?**

Fifth week gestation; its development is not complete until several years after birth.

○ **What is the last structure of the inner ear to develop?**

Endolymphatic sac.

○ **What does the eustachian tube (ET) develop from?**

From the 1st pouch, between the 2nd arch and the pharynx.

○ **Which branchial arch does the tensor tympani muscle arise from?**

First branchial arch.

○ **True/False: The tympanic membrane is derived from ectoderm.**

False; it is derived from ectoderm, mesoderm, and endoderm.

○ **At what age is the mastoid process completely pneumatized?**

Age 2.

○ **What is the sensory innervation of the auricle?**

Greater auricular nerve (C3), auriculotemporal nerve (V3), lesser occipital nerve (C2, 3), auricular branch of the vagus, and sensory branches of VII and IX.

○ **What is Arnold's nerve?**

Auricular branch of the vagus that innervates skin of the external auditory canal and auricle.

○ **What is the foramen of Huschke?**

An embryologic remnant that normally obliterates in the anteroinferior portion of the medial bony EAC.

○ **What is the clinical significance of the foramen of Huschke?**

Serves as a potential route for spread of tumor from the parotid gland to the temporal bone.

○ **Which wall of the EAC is shorter—the anteroinferior or posterosuperior?**

Posterosuperior (approximately 25 mm, whereas anteroinferior wall is 31 mm).

○ **How much of the EAC is cartilaginous?**

One-third.

○ **How much of the ET is cartilaginous?**

Two-thirds.

○ **Where is the tympanic notch of Rivinus?**

Superior portion of the tympanic ring (squamous portion of temporal bone).

○ **How does the composition of gas in the middle ear differ from that of room air?**

Lower oxygen level and higher carbon dioxide and nitrogen levels.

○ **What are the layers of the tympanic membrane?**

Squamous epithelium, radiating fibrous layer, circumferential fibrous layer, and mucosa.

○   **Which has greater sensory innervation—pars tensa or pars flaccida?**
Pars flaccida.

○   **What are the three nerves of the tympanic plexus?**
V3, IX (Jacobson's nerve), and X.

○   **Which part of the ossicular chain has the most tenuous blood supply and is most prone to necrosis?**
Long process of the incus.

○   **Which part of the malleus articulates with the incus?**
Head.

○   **Where in the ossicular chain does the tensor tympani muscle insert?**
Manubrium of the malleus.

○   **Which part of the malleus does the anterior ligament attach to?**
The neck, near the anterior process.

○   **Which part of the incus articulates with the stapes?**
Lenticular process (medial side of long process).

○   **What ligament supports the stapes?**
Annular ligament.

○   **Where does most of the movement of the stapes occur?**
Anterior–superior portion of the footplate.

○   **Where in the ossicular chain does the stapedius muscle insert?**
Posterior neck of the stapes.

○   **What is the scutum?**
Lateral wall of the epitympanum.

○   **What are the boundaries of the epitympanum?**
Superiorly, the tegmen; inferiorly, the fossa incudis; anteriorly, the zygomatic arch; posteriorly, the aditus; medially, the lateral semicircular canal (SCC) and VII; and laterally, the scutum.

○   **Which ossicles can be found in the epitympanic recess?**
Head of the malleus, body, and short process of the incus.

○ **What is the inferior boundary of the tympanic cavity?**

Jugular bulb.

○ **What structures are anterior to the tympanic cavity?**

The carotid artery, ET, and the canal for the tensor tympani muscle.

○ **What structures are posterior to the tympanic cavity?**

Aditus, posterior sinus, chorda tympani, fossa incudis, pyramidal prominence, and stapedial tendon.

○ **What is the promontory?**

Elevation of the medial wall of the tympanic cavity formed by the basal turn of the cochlea.

○ **Which three cranial nerves are found beneath the floor of the middle ear cavity?**

IX, X, and XI.

○ **Below is a diagram of a right middle ear showing its relationship with the inner ear. Name the structures.**

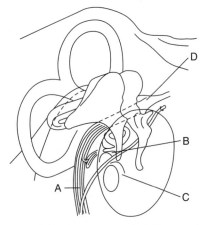

Reproduced, with permission, from Lalwani AK (ed.). *Current Diagnosis & Treatment in Otolaryngology—Head & Neck Surgery*, 3rd edn. New York: McGraw-Hill, 2012.

A—Facial nerve.
B—Ponticulus.
C—Subiculum.
D—Geniculate ganglion.

○ **What structure is located inferior to the subiculum and posteroinferior to the promontory?**

Round window.

○ **What structure lies between the subiculum and ponticulus?**

Sinus tympani.

○   **What structure lies superior to the ponticulus?**
Oval window.

○   **What structure lies between the prominence of SCC and the promontory/oval window?**
Prominence of the facial canal.

○   **The following diagram is of a right middle ear viewed from below. Name the structures.**

Reproduced, with permission, from Lalwani AK (ed.). *Current Diagnosis & Treatment in Otolaryngology—Head & Neck Surgery*, 3rd edn. New York: McGraw-Hill, 2012.

A—Facial recess.
B—Facial nerve.
C—Sinus tympani.

○   **What is the most anterior structure of the medial wall of the tympanic cavity?**
Cochleariform process.

○   **Cochleariform process: tensor tympani :: pyramidal process: _____?**
Stapedius.

○   **What structure is situated just medial to the tip of the cochleariform process?**
Geniculate ganglion of the facial nerve.

○   **Between which ossicles does the chorda tympani run?**
Manubrium of the malleus and long process of the incus.

○   **What is the function of the chorda tympani nerve?**
Parasympathetic innervation to the submandibular and sublingual glands, and taste to the anterior 2/3 of the tongue.

○ **Which planes are the oval and round windows oriented in?**

Oval window is in the sagittal plane; round window is in the transverse plane.

○ **What structure ends blindly at the round window?**

Scala tympani (lower compartment of the cochlea).

○ **What is the name of the central bony core of the cochlea through which nerves and vessels travel?**

Modiolus.

○ **What is the name of the area of communication between the scala vestibuli and the scala tympani?**

Helicotrema.

○ **What fluid surrounds the membranous labyrinth?**

Perilymph.

○ **How does perilymph differ from endolymph?**

Perilymph has a pH of 7.2, is high in sodium, low in potassium, and does not contain chloride; endolymph has a pH of 7.5, is low in sodium, and relatively high in potassium and chloride.

○ **True/False: The membranous labyrinth is a self-contained system.**

True.

○ **What are the main structures of the vestibular portion of the membranous labyrinth?**

Utricle, saccule, and SCCs.

○ **Which of these main structures receives the crura from the three SCCs?**

Utricle.

○ **What structures house the crista?**

Ampullae.

○ **What is the blood supply to the inner ear?**

Labyrinthine artery (branch of anterior inferior cerebellar artery).

○ **What structure produces endolymph?**

Stria vascularis.

○ **Where does most of the resorption of endolymph occur?**

Endolymphatic sac.

○   **What does the vestibular aqueduct carry?**
Endolymphatic duct and accompanying vein.

○   **Where is the primary auditory cortex?**
Brodmann's area 41 in the superficial portion of the temporal lobe.

○   **Which part of the vestibular labyrinth detects angular acceleration?**
SCCs.

○   **What do the utricle and saccule detect?**
Linear acceleration.

○   **Where are cupula found?**
SCCs.

○   **What three systems determine balance?**
Vestibular, vestibulo-ocular (visual), and vestibulospinal (proprioceptive) systems.

○   **Which part of the cochlea represents high-frequency sounds?**
The basal end.

○   **What range of frequencies can the human ear detect?**
20–20,000 Hz (greatest sensitivity is from 500 to 3000 Hz).

○   **What noise level begins to cause pain?**
140 dB.

○   **How many times louder is 60 dB than 0 dB?**
1,000,000 times.

○   **What are normal ear canal volumes in children and adults?**
0.5–1.0 cm^3 in children; 0.6–2.0 cm^3 in adults.

○   **Which cells emit otoacoustic emissions (OAEs)?**
Outer hair cells.

○   **What percent of normal ears emit spontaneous OAEs?**
35–60%.

○ **What are the four parts of the temporal bone?**

Squamous, tympanic, petrous, and mastoid.

○ **What are the four openings into the temporal bone?**

Internal auditory canal (IAC), vestibular and cochlear aqueducts, and subarcuate fossa.

○ **What is Hyrtl's fissure?**

Connection between the subarachnoid space near the IX ganglion and the hypotympanum that allows middle ear infections to spread to the brain; normally closes with maturation.

○ **What proportion of the population has a pneumatized petrous pyramid?**

One-third.

○ **What is Trautmann's triangle?**

Triangle between the external prominence of the lateral and posterior SCCs and the posterosuperior corner of the mastoid.

○ **What is Körner's septum?**

Otherwise known as the "false bottom," it represents the suture line between the petrous and squamous portions of the temporal bone.

○ **What is meant by a "diploic mastoid"?**

Occupied by bone marrow instead of air cells.

○ **What structure forms the arcuate eminence?**

Superior SCC.

○ **True/False: The position of the cochlear duct is always inferior to the lowest border of the stapes footplate.**

True.

○ **Besides the muscles of facial expression, what muscles does the facial nerve innervate?**

Posterior belly of the digastric, stylohyoid, and stapedius muscles.

○ **What does the facial nerve provide general sensation for?**

Part of the auricular concha, external auditory canal, and tympanic membrane.

○ **What is the function of the special visceral afferent fibers of the facial nerve?**

To provide taste to the anterior 2/3 of the tongue and palate (via the chorda tympani).

○ **Where are the cell bodies for these fibers?**

Geniculate ganglion.

○ **What is the function of the nervus intermedius?**

To carry visceral motor fibers to the lacrimal gland, minor salivary glands, and mucosal glands of the palate and nose (via the greater superficial petrosal nerve), and general sensory fibers from the auricular concha and external auditory canal.

○ **What are the six segments of the facial nerve?**

Intracranial, internal auditory canal, labyrinthine, tympanic, mastoid/vertical, and extratemporal.

○ **Where in the brainstem is the facial motor nucleus?**

Caudal pons.

○ **Where does the facial nerve leave the brainstem?**

Pontomedullary junction, close to the vestibulocochlear nerve.

○ **What are the limits of the tympanic segment of VII?**

Geniculate ganglion to the 2nd genu (adjacent to the pyramidal process).

○ **What are the limits of the mastoid segment of VII?**

Pyramidal process to the stylomastoid foramen.

○ **Which segment is shortest?**

Labyrinthine.

○ **Which segment has the narrowest passageway?**

Labyrinthine.

○ **What portion of the facial nerve is closest to the cochlea?**

Labyrinthine.

○ **What three branches of the facial nerve are given off in its course through the temporal bone?**

Greater superficial petrosal nerve, nerve to the stapedius muscle, and chorda tympani.

○ **What is the first branch of the facial nerve?**

Greater superficial petrosal nerve.

○ **Where along the course of the facial nerve does this nerve branch off?**

Geniculate ganglion.

○ **What is the blood supply to the geniculate ganglion?**

Greater superficial petrosal artery (branch of the middle meningeal artery).

○ **What is the function of the greater superficial petrosal nerve?**

Lacrimation, salivation from minor salivary glands, and mucosal secretions from nose and palate.

○ **Where do the preganglionic parasympathetic neurons of the greater superficial petrosal nerve synapse?**

Pterygopalatine ganglion.

○ **Branches of which nerve then carry the postganglionic parasympathetic neurons to the mucus-secreting glands in the nose, sinuses, and palate?**

Maxillary division of the trigeminal nerve.

○ **What is the facial hiatus?**

Dehiscence of variable size in petrous portion of the temporal bone in the floor of the middle cranial fossa, which marks the entrance of the greater superficial petrosal nerve into the middle cranial fossa.

○ **How is the facial hiatus clinically significant?**

The geniculate ganglion usually lies deep to the hiatus, but in 5–10% of patients, it lies under the dura within the hiatus and without a bony covering.

○ **What are the limits of the fallopian canal?**

Fundus of the IAC to the stylomastoid foramen.

○ **Describe the path of the facial nerve in the temporal bone.**

Enters the IAC; travels laterally for a short distance, then, just superior to the promontory, it makes a sharp turn to run posteriorly (at the *external/first genu* and the *geniculate ganglion*). Nerve continues posteriorly, with a slight inferolateral inclination (forming the prominence of the facial canal in the medial wall of tympanic cavity). Behind the base of the pyramidal eminence, the nerve makes a broad turn to descend vertically and somewhat laterally (2nd *genu*) through the mastoid cavity.

○ **What is the average diameter of the IAC?**

6.8 mm.

○ **What is the upper limit of normal diameter of the IAC?**

8 mm.

○ **What is the narrowest intratemporal portion of the fallopian canal?**

Entrance to the fallopian canal at the lateral aspect of the IAC (fundus).

○ **What structure bisects the IAC in the vertical direction and in the horizontal direction?**

Bill's bar; transverse/falciform crest.

○ **Below is a cross-sectional diagram of the IAC. Name the structures.**

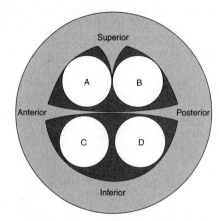

Reproduced, with permission, from Lalwani AK (ed.). *Current Diagnosis & Treatment in Otolaryngology—Head & Neck Surgery*, 3rd edn. New York: McGraw-Hill, 2012.

A—Facial nerve.
B—Superior branch of the vestibular nerve.
C—Cochlear nerve.
D—Inferior branch of the vestibular nerve.

○ **What does the superior vestibular nerve innervate?**

Superior and lateral SCCs, utricle, and saccule.

○ **What does the inferior vestibular nerve innervate?**

Posterior SCC and macula of the saccule.

○ **Where is the 2nd genu of the facial nerve?**

Just distal to the geniculate ganglion, at the sinus tympani between the tympanic and mastoid segments.

○ **What is the relationship of the 2nd genu of the facial nerve to the lateral SCC and short process of the incus?**

Inferior to the lateral SCC and medial to the short process of the incus.

○ **In its tympanic segment, between which structures does the facial nerve travel?**

Superiorly, the lateral SCC; inferiorly, the oval window.

○ **Where does the facial nerve lie in relation to the cochleariform process?** .

Posterosuperior.

○ **What is the cog?**

A ridge of bone that extends inferiorly from the tegmen epitympanum and partially separates the anterior epitympanic compartment from the mesoepitympanum.

○ **What is the relationship of the tympanic portion of VII to the cog?**

VII lies anterior to the cog in the floor of the anterior epitympanum.

○ **What percent of people have a dehiscence of the facial nerve in either the tympanic or mastoid segments?**

50–55%.

○ **Where is the most common site of dehiscence?**

Tympanic segment superior to the oval window.

○ **What is the last branch of the facial nerve before it passes through the stylomastoid foramen?**

Chorda tympani nerve.

○ **Where does the chorda tympani arise in relation to the stylomastoid foramen?**

Usually 4–7 mm superior.

○ **What artery accompanies the chorda tympani?**

Posterior tympanic artery.

○ **What is the name of the opening through which the chorda tympani nerve enters the infratemporal fossa?**

Petrotympanic fissure (canal of Huguier).

○ **Where are the cell bodies of the motor fibers of the chorda tympani nerve?**

Superior salivatory nucleus.

○ **What three motor branches does the facial nerve give off just after exiting the stylomastoid foramen?**

Nerve to posterior belly of the digastric, nerve to the stylohyoid, and nerve to the postauricular muscle.

○ **Where is the facial nerve trunk located in relation to the tympanomastoid suture line?**

6–8 mm anteroinferior (between the suture line and the styloid process).

○ **What is the name of the point at which the facial nerve divides into the upper and lower divisions?**

Pes anserinus.

○ **How far is the pes anserinus from the stylomastoid foramen?**

Approximately 1.3 cm.

○ **How does facial nerve innervation to the upper face differ from that to the lower face?**

Upper motor neurons sending information to the upper face cross twice in the pons; upper motor neurons sending information to the lower face cross only once in the pons. Therefore, lesions proximal to the nucleus only affect the lower face.

○ **True/False: There is a consistent topographic representation of fibers from a specific section of a nerve innervating certain parts of the face.**

False.

CHAPTER 2

Nose and Paranasal Sinuses

○ **When does aeration of the frontal sinus begin?**

Age 4–5 years, and continues into the late teens.

○ **What percent of the population has a unilateral frontal sinus?**

10%.

○ **At what age can the maxillary sinuses be visualized on a computed tomography (CT) scan?**

Age 4–5 months.

○ **The _____ is fully formed by the 5th week gestation and goes on to develop into the floor of the nose/palate.**

Oronasal membrane.

○ **What are the nasal anatomic subunits?**

Nasal dorsum, nasal sidewalls, nasal tip, alar lobules, and depressions of the supra-alar facets.

○ **Which muscles elevate the nose?**

Procerus, levator labii superioris alaeque nasi, and anomalous nasi muscles.

○ **Which muscles depress the nose?**

Alar nasalis and depressor septi nasi muscles.

○ **What are the other muscles of the nose (the compressor and dilators)?**

Transverse nasalis, compressor narium minor, and dilator naris anterior muscles.

○ **What is the narrowest portion of the nasal cavity?**

Nasal valve.

○   **What is the nasal valve?**

The angle between the caudal quadrangular cartilage and the distal upper lateral cartilages.

○   **What is the only septal component that is paired?**

The vomer, which may be bilaminar owing to its dual embryonic origin.

○   **What makes up the superior portion of the bony nasal septum?**

Perpendicular plate of the ethmoid.

○   **What are the major tip support mechanisms?**

Contour, size, and strength of the lateral crura; attachment of the medial crural footplate to the caudal septum; and attachment of the caudal edge of the upper lateral cartilages to the cephalic border of the alar cartilages.

○   **What are the minor tip support mechanisms?**

Nasal tip ligamentous aponeurosis; cartilaginous septum; nasal spine; strength and resilience of the medial crura; thickness of tip skin and subcutaneous tissue; and supportive strength of the alar sidewalls.

○   **What are the major anatomic features that determine tip projection?**

Thickness and character of tip skin; shape and strength of alar cartilages; length of infratip lobule and columella; anatomy of the quadrangular cartilage (especially the anterior septal angle); and size of the nasal spine and premaxilla.

○   **What type of epithelium lines the nasal cavity?**

Ciliated pseudostratified epithelium.

○   **What neuropeptide is thought to be a mediator of pain in the nose and paranasal sinuses?**

Substance P.

○   **What are odorous substances made of?**

Either gases or volatile liquids.

○   **How is the sensory epithelium of the olfactory system different from the surrounding respiratory epithelium?**

Both have cilia, but the cilia of the olfactory epithelium do not beat synchronously.

○   **What are Bowman's glands?**

They secrete mucus and yellow pigment in the olfactory epithelium; the odorant must dissolve in this layer of mucus to reach the sensory receptors.

○   **How are the receptor cells in the olfactory system different from those of the ear, eye, and tongue?**

They are bipolar nerve cells (others are specialized epithelial cells).

○ **Unlike the taste pathway to the cerebral cortex, the olfactory pathway does not relay in the _____. The olfactory nerve terminates in the _____ and sends axons via the olfactory tract to the piriform cortex, the periamygdaloid area, and the _____.**

Thalamus; olfactory bulb; olfactory tubercle.

○ **What is the most common cause of taste loss?**

Olfactory dysfunction.

○ **What is dysosmia?**

Perception of an unpleasant odor.

○ **What is phantosmia?**

Perception of an odor in the absence of a stimulus.

○ **What is parosmia?**

Distorted perception of an odor.

○ **Where does the nasolacrimal duct lie in relation to the ostium of the maxillary sinus?**

3–6 mm anteriorly.

○ **The majority of posterior ethmoid cells empty into which meatus?**

Superior meatus.

○ **What percent of the population has a supreme nasal concha?**

60%.

○ **What are the five basal or ground lamella of the paranasal sinuses?**

Uncinate process, bulla ethmoidalis, basal lamella of the middle turbinate, lamella of the superior turbinate, and lamella of the supreme turbinate (if present).

○ **What structure separates the anterior and posterior ethmoid complexes?**

Basal lamella of the middle turbinate.

○ **Where does the natural ostium of the maxillary sinus empty?**

Ethmoid infundibulum.

○ **What is the most posterior part of the middle turbinate attached to?**

Crista ethmoidalis of the perpendicular process of the palatine bone.

○ **Where does the anterior portion of the middle turbinate most often attach superiorly?**

Laterally onto the lamina papyracea (may also attach to the skull base).

○ **What is an agger nasi cell?**

Pneumatized area of the lateral nasal wall immediately anterior and superior to the insertion of the middle turbinate.

○ **What problem can an enlarged agger nasi cell cause?**

Narrowing of the frontal recess.

○ **What is the term for a persistent, nonpneumatized second basal lamella?**

Torus ethmoidalis/lateralis.

○ **What is the term for a pneumatized second basal lamella?**

Bulla ethmoidalis.

○ **What is the most posterior aspect of the anterior ethmoids?**

Retrobullar recess.

○ **When may the suprabullar recess extend into the retrobullar recess?**

If the posterior wall of the bulla lamella is not in contact with the basal lamella of the middle turbinate.

○ **What is another name for the retrobullar recess?**

Sinus lateralis.

○ **What does the retrobullar recess drain into?**

Hiatus semilunaris superior.

○ **What recess does the suprabullar recess open into?**

Frontal recess; anteriorly, it is separated from the recess by the bulla lamella.

○ **What are the borders of the ethmoid infundibulum?**

Medially, the uncinate process; laterally, the lamina papyracea and frontal process of the maxilla; and posteriorly, the ethmoid bulla.

○ **Into what does the ethmoid infundibulum drain posteriorly?**

Hiatus semilunaris inferior.

○ **Where does the maxillary sinus ostium lie in relation to the ethmoid infundibulum?**

At the floor and lateral aspect of the infundibulum, between its middle and posterior 1/3.

○ **Where is the anterior ethmoid artery found intranasally?**

Anterior to the vertical portion of basal lamella, immediately below the skull base, and posterior to the frontal recess.

○ **What is the distance from the posterior ethmoid artery to the optic foramen?**

5–10 mm.

○ **Which table of the frontal sinus is thinner?**

Posterior.

○ **Where is the natural ostium of the frontal sinus?**

The posteromedial aspect of the sinus floor.

○ **What is the frontal recess?**

The drainage pathway from the frontal sinus to the nasal cavity.

○ **What forms the anterior boundary of the frontal recess?**

The posterior wall of the agger nasi and frontoethmoid cells, if present.

○ **What structures form the posterior boundary of the frontal recess?**

The ethmoid bullae, suprabullar space, anterior skull base, and anterior ethmoid artery; frontal bulla cell.

○ **What structures can potentially compromise drainage of the frontal sinus?**

A frontal bulla cell, frontoethmoid cells, suprabullar cells, supraorbital cells, a prominent agger nasi, or an interfrontal septal cell.

○ **According to Kuhn, what is a type II frontoethmoid cell?**

Two or more cells above and directly behind the agger nasi.

○ **Which type of frontoethmoid cell is a single, large anterior ethmoid cell above the agger nasi cell, pneumatized and extending into the frontal sinus but not more than 50% of the height of the sinus?**

Type III.

○ **What is the difference between a type III frontoethmoid cell and a frontal bulla cell?**

The base of a frontal bulla cell is along the skull base, whereas the base of a type III frontoethmoid cell is along the agger nasi.

○ **Can a frontal bulla cell be distinguished from a type III frontoethmoid cell on a coronal CT scan?**

No, one must look at sagittal and axial views to distinguish the two.

○ **Which type of frontal recess pneumatization pattern is characterized by attachment of the superior uncinate process to the lamina papryacea?**

Recessus terminalis, a blind recess into which the ethmoid infundibulum terminates.

○ **Where does the frontal sinus drain when this is present?**

Directly into the middle meatus.

○ **What are the four possible configurations of the ethmoid roof described by Keros?**

1. *Type I*: Olfactory fossa 1–3 mm deep.
2. *Type II*: Olfactory fossa 4–7 mm deep.
3. *Type III*: Olfactory fossa 8–16 mm deep.
4. Asymmetric skull base.

○ **What are the nasal fontanelles?**

Bony dehiscences of the lateral nasal wall usually above the insertion of inferior turbinate where the nasal mucosa approximates the mucoperiosteum of the maxillary sinus.

○ **What is the thinnest bone of the anterior skull base?**

Lateral lamella of the cribriform plate, where the anterior ethmoid artery crosses from the medial orbital wall to the cribriform.

○ **What is a concha bullosa?**

Pneumatized middle or superior turbinate.

○ **Below is a coronal CT scan through the paranasal sinuses. What are the structures marked "A" and what are the arrowheads pointing to?**

Reproduced, with permission, from Lalwani AK (ed.). *Current Diagnosis & Treatment in Otolaryngology—Head & Neck Surgery*, 3rd edn. New York: McGraw-Hill, 2012.

A—Haller cells.
Arrowheads are pointing to the infundibula.

○ **What structures can a Haller cell potentially narrow?**

Maxillary sinus ostium or ethmoid infundibulum.

○ **What is the osteomeatal complex?**

Final common pathway for drainage and ventilation of the frontal, maxillary, and anterior ethmoid cells.

○ **What is the sphenoethmoid recess?**

Space between the superior (and supreme, if present) turbinate laterally, the cribriform plate superiorly, septum medially, anterior face of the sphenoid posteriorly, and inferior margin of the superior turbinate inferolaterally.

○ **What are sphenoethmoid or Onodi cells?**

Pneumatized posterior ethmoid cells superolateral to the sphenoid sinus.

○ **What percent of people have a sphenoethmoid cell?**

12%.

○ **What important structures may run through an Onodi cell?**

Optic nerve and carotid artery.

○ **Where does the sphenoid sinus lie in relation to the most posterior ethmoid cell?**

Inferior and medial.

○ **Where is the natural ostium of the sphenoid sinus in relation to the superior turbinate?**

Medial and within millimeters of its inferior border.

○ **What percent of patients have a bony dehiscence of the cavernous portion of the carotid canal?**

22%.

○ **What are the three types of sphenoid sinuses as described by Hamberger?**

1. *Sellar (67–76%)*: Sella turcia bulges into a well-developed sinus.
2. *Presellar (23–28%)*: Cancellous bone extends from under the sella to the anterior aspect of the floor.
3. *Conchal (0–5%)*: Sphenoid sinus is entirely filled with cancellous bone.

○ **True/False: Presence of a conchal sphenoid is an absolute contraindication to transsphenoidal hypophysectomy.**

False; the bone can be drilled out to permit access.

○ **What bony structure is found posterior to the sphenoid?**

Clivus.

○   **What structures are found within the cavernous sinus?**
Internal carotid artery, venous channels, III, IV, VI, V1, and V2.

○   **Which of these nerves is closely associated with the lateral wall of the internal carotid artery?**
VI.

○   **Where is the optic canal in relation to the sphenoid sinus?**
Anterolateral aspect of the sphenoid roof.

○   **From anterior to posterior, what structures comprise the medial orbital wall?**
Frontal process of the maxilla, lacrimal bone, lamina papyracea, and sphenoid bone to optic nerve foramen.

○   **Where does the sphenoid ostium lie in relation to the chonal bridge?**
1.5 cm above or 1/3 distance from chonae to the skull base.

○   **What is the normal angle of a line drawn from the nasal spine to the sphenoid ostium?**
30 degrees.

CHAPTER 3

Oral Cavity and Oropharynx

○ **What are the embryologic origins of the anterior 2/3 and posterior 1/3 of the tongue?**

The anterior 2/3 of the tongue develops from the 1st branchial arch and the posterior 1/3 of the tongue develops from the 3rd and 4th branchial arches.

○ **When does the primary palate develop?**

4–5 weeks gestation.

○ **When does the secondary palate develop?**

8–9 weeks gestation.

○ **How does the secondary palate develop?**

As a medial ingrowth of the lateral maxillae with fusion in the midline.

○ **How does the primary palate develop?**

As a mesodermal and ectodermal proliferation of the frontonasal and maxillary processes.

○ **True/False: At no time in the development of the normal primary palate is there a separation.**

True.

○ **True/False: A cleft lip is always associated with a cleft alveolus.**

False; a cleft alveolus is always associated with a cleft lip.

○ **During embryologic development, what causes a cleft lip?**

Lack of mesodermal proliferation results in an incomplete epithelial bridge.

○ **What divides the palate into the primary and secondary palates?**

Incisive foramen.

○   **What artery runs through the incisive foramen?**

Lesser palatine artery.

○   **What structures form the hard palate?**

Maxilla, horizontal process of the palatine bone, and the pterygoid plates.

○   **What muscles form the soft palate?**

Palatopharyngeus, salpingopharyngeus, levator and tensor veli palatini, muscular uvula, palatoglossus, and superior constrictor muscles.

○   **At which points is the normal vermillion the widest?**

At the peaks of Cupid's bow.

○   **What is the name of the space between the cheeks and the teeth?**

Vestibule.

○   **Why is the tongue a muscular hydrostat?**

It is a structure with incompressible muscles and no skeletal support that is capable of movement. Changes in the shape of the muscle do not change its volume.

○   **What are the four extrinsic muscles of the tongue?**

Genioglossus, hyoglossus, styloglossus, and palatoglossus.

○   **What is different about the palatoglossus compared to the other extrinsic tongue muscles?**

It is derived from the 4th branchial arch and its innervation comes from the nucleus ambiguous.

○   **What are the three groups of intrinsic muscles of the tongue?**

Vertical, transverse, and longitudinal.

○   **All the muscles participating in the oral phase of swallowing are striated muscles using _____ for neurotransmission via _____ receptors.**

Acetylcholine; nicotinic.

○   **What structure marks the boundary between the anterior 2/3 of the tongue and its posterior 1/3?**

Foramen cecum.

○   **What muscle functionally divides the oral cavity from the oropharynx?**

Palatopharyngeus.

○   **Which group of papillae on the tongue lacks taste buds?**

Filiform.

○   **Which three cranial nerves mediate taste?**

VII, IX, and X.

○   **What nerve mediates taste sensation from the circumvallate papillae?**

IX.

○   **Taste sensation is relayed by _____ fibers from the anterior 2/3 of the tongue via the _____ nerve, from the posterior 1/3 of the tongue via the _____ nerve, and from the epiglottis via the _____ nerve, with these fibers terminating in the _____.**

Special visceral afferent; chorda tympani; lingual; vagus; nucleus tractus solitarius.

○   **True/False: The four taste qualities can be perceived by all the taste buds.**

True.

○   **How long do taste sensory cells live?**

200–300 hours.

○   **How is the quality of taste determined?**

Via the central nervous system from the discharge pattern across all the sensory nerve fibers sensitive to the substance.

○   **How is the intensity of taste determined?**

Via the central nervous system from the frequency of discharge across all the sensory nerve fibers sensitive to the substance.

○   **A patient complains of not being able to taste. Upon further questioning, he admits to being able to taste salt crystals, sugar crystals, lemon juice and coffee but nothing else. What is the primary problem?**

Olfactory loss.

○   **At what age gestation can an infant suckle feed?**

34 weeks.

○   **How does infant swallowing differ from adult swallowing?**

The pharyngeal phase of swallowing in infants is faster and more frequent.

○   **What is the sequence of events during a normal swallow?**

1. *Oral phase*: Food is chewed and mixed with saliva.
2. *Oropharyngeal phase*: The food bolus is propelled posteriorly.
3. *Pharyngeal phase*: The soft palate elevates, glottis closes, pharyngeal constrictors contract, and the cricopharyngeus relaxes.
4. *Esophageal phase*: The bolus is propelled into the stomach by peristaltic waves.

○   **True/False: Boluses placed on the posterior tongue trigger swallowing at a lower volume than the anterior tongue.**

True.

○   **At what age should children be able to say multiword sentences?**

36 months.

○   **At what age should children be able to respond to their name and understand simple words?**

6–10 months.

○   **How many words should a child aged 24–36 months be able to say?**

Fifty.

○   **What is Gerlach's tonsil?**

Lymphoid tissue arising from the fossa of Rosenmüller that extends into the eustachian tube.

○   **Which muscles form the anterior and posterior tonsillar pillars?**

Palatoglossus and palatopharyngeus, respectively.

○   **What is the plica triangularis?**

Point at which the palatine and lingual tonsils meet.

○   **In what percent of the population does the carotid artery lie deep to the floor of the tonsillar fossa?**

1%.

○   **What immunoglobulin is produced by the tonsils?**

Antigen-specific secretory IgA.

○   **What artery provides most of the blood supply to the palatine tonsil?**

Tonsillar branch of the facial artery.

○   **What is the normal thickness of the soft palate in adults?**

About 12 mm; gets thinner laterally.

○   **What is the common insertion of the three pharyngeal constrictors?**

Median pharyngeal raphe.

CHAPTER 4 Salivary Glands

○ **With what other organs do the salivary glands share the same embryologic origin?**
Liver, gallbladder, and pancreas (all come from mesodermal buds of the foregut).

○ **When does the parotid gland encase the facial nerve?**
Third month gestation.

○ **What are the boundaries of the parotid compartment?**
Superiorly, the zygoma; posteriorly, the external auditory canal; anteriorly, the masseter muscle; inferiorly, the styloid process, carotid artery, jugular vessels, and styloid muscles.

○ **Where does Stenson's duct arise from in relation to the zygoma?**
1.5 cm inferior to the zygoma.

○ **What muscle does Stenson's duct pierce?**
Buccinator.

○ **Where does Stenson's duct open intraorally?**
Just opposite the 2nd upper molar.

○ **What branch of the facial nerve travels with Stenson's duct?**
Buccal.

○ **What membrane separates the parotid gland from the submandibular gland?**
Stylomandibular membrane.

○ **How does the saliva produced from the parotid gland differ from that of the sublingual gland?**
The saliva from the parotid gland is serous, high in enzymes, and low in mucin; that from the sublingual gland is primarily composed of mucin.

○ **What is the blood supply to the parotid gland?**

Transverse facial artery, a branch of the superficial temporal artery.

○ **What is the major venous drainage of the parotid gland?**

Posterior facial vein.

○ **What is unique about the lymphatic drainage of the parotid gland?**

The lymph nodes are contained within the gland, and it is the only salivary gland with two layers of lymph nodes.

○ **Which layer of lymph nodes has the most nodes (superficial or deep)?**

Superficial.

○ **Describe the pathway of parasympathetic innervation to the parotid gland.**

Preganglionic parasympathetic fibers leave the inferior salivatory nucleus via the glossopharyngeal nerve, pass through the jugular foramen, travel through the middle ear (as Jacobson's nerve), and then travel along the floor of the middle cranial fossa (as the lesser petrosal nerve) to the otic ganglion; postganglionic parasympathetic fibers leave the otic ganglion via the auriculotemporal branch of V3 and travel to the parotid gland.

○ **Where does the retromandibular vein lie in relation to the facial nerve?**

In most people, it courses deep to both trunks of the facial nerve. In up to 10% of people, the vein crosses either trunk laterally.

○ **Which lymph nodes drain tumors from the parotid gland?**

Nodes just inferior to the gland adjacent to the sternocleidomastoid muscle and the external jugular vein.

○ **What muscle separates the submandibular gland into a superficial and deep lobe?**

Mylohyoid.

○ **Where do the hypoglossal nerve and lingual nerve lie in relation to Wharton's duct as it exits the submandibular gland?**

Hypoglossal nerve lies inferiorly and lingual nerve lies superiorly.

○ **Which vein can be ligated and retracted superiorly during submandibular gland excision to protect the marginal mandibular branch of the facial nerve?**

Anterior facial vein.

○ **What duct(s) drain the sublingual gland?**

Typically there are about 10 ducts of Rivinus that drain the gland but occasionally several of these small ducts may join to form a larger sublingual/Bartholin's duct.

○ **What component of saliva agglutinates bacteria and activates autolysins?**

Lysozyme.

○   **What is the role of salivary peroxidase?**

Helps breakdown salivary thiocyanate into products that interfere with bacterial cell metabolism.

○   **What is the secretory potential?**

Hyperpolarization of acinar cells upon stimulation by the autonomic nervous system.

○   **What happens to the composition of saliva as it moves from the acinar cell (primary secretion) through the duct?**

It loses sodium, acquires potassium, and becomes increasingly hypotonic. The degree of modification depends on the salivary flow rate, with higher rates producing saliva closer in composition to the primary secretion.

○   **True/False: Only muscarinic acetylcholine receptors are involved in salivary gland stimulation.**

True.

○   **Which salivary glands contribute the highest % of resting/unstimulated saliva output?**

Submandibular glands.

○   **Which salivary glands contribute the highest % of stimulated saliva output?**

Parotid glands.

CHAPTER 5 Pharynx and Esophagus

○ **What are the three subsites of the hypopharynx?**

Pyriform sinus, postcricoid area, and posterior pharyngeal wall.

○ **Which structures separate the hypopharynx from the larynx?**

Aryepiglottic folds.

○ **What structure in the hypopharynx marks the location of the cricoarytenoid joint?**

Pyriform apex.

○ **What are the boundaries of the pyriform fossa?**

Superiorly, the inferior margin of the hyoid; anteriorly, the junction of the anterior and posterior halves of the thyroid cartilage; posteriorly, the posterior edge of the thyroid cartilage; apex, the cricoarytenoid joint.

○ **What are the layers of the posterior pharyngeal wall, from superficial to deep?**

Mucosa, constrictor muscles, longus colli, retropharyngeal space, prevertebral fascia.

○ **What are the boundaries of the parapharyngeal space?**

Inferior – Hyoid bone.
Superior – Petrous bone.
Medial – Soft palate, tonsils, and superior pharyngeal constrictor.
Lateral – Medial pterygoid muscle, ramus of the mandible, and posterior belly of the digastric.
Dorsal – Vertebral column and paravertebral muscles.
Ventral – Pterygomandibular raphe.

○ **What structures are found in the prestyloid compartment of the parapharyngeal space?**

Medial pterygoid muscle, fat, lymphatics, minor nerves, and vessels.

○ **What structures are found in the poststyloid compartment of the parapharyngeal space?**

Carotid sheath, IX, X, XII, and cervical sympathetic chain.

○   **What space does the parapharyngeal space communicate with dorsally?**

Retropharyngeal space.

○   **Where is the fossa of Rosenmüller?**

Just posterior–superior to the torus tubarius of the eustachian tube orifice.

○   **Which foramina of the skull lie in close proximity to the nasopharynx?**

Foramen lacerum, carotid canal, foramen spinosum, foramen ovale, foramen rotundum, hypoglossal canal, and jugular foramen.

○   **What is the relationship of the fossa of Rosenmüller to the parapharyngeal space?**

It lies at the convergence of the fascial planes that separate the parapharyngeal space into its three compartments (prestyloid, retrostyloid, and retropharyngeal).

○   **What kind of epithelium lines the nasopharynx?**

At birth, pseudostratified columnar epithelium; by age 10, the majority is replaced by stratified squamous epithelium. The lateral portion does not change, and the area where these two types meet is lined by transitional epithelium.

○   **By what age is the adenoid pad mostly atrophied?**

Age 7 or 8.

○   **What two structures pass between the superior and middle pharyngeal constrictors?**

Stylopharyngeus muscle and IX.

○   **What are the boundaries of the cervical esophagus?**

Cricopharyngeus muscle to sternal notch.

○   **What is the arterial supply to the cervical esophagus?**

Thyroid branch of the thyrocervical trunk.

○   **What is the venous drainage of the cervical esophagus?**

Inferior thyroid vein.

○   **What are the three areas of esophageal narrowing?**

Superiorly, from the cricopharyngeus; inferiorly, where the esophagus enters the cardia; and in the middle, where the left mainstem bronchus and the aorta cross anteriorly.

○   **True/False: At rest, the cricopharyngeus muscle is relaxed.**

False; the cricopharyngeus muscle has a resting pressure of 100 mm Hg in the anteriorposterior direction and 50 mm Hg in the right and left lateral direction.

○ **What is the average resting pressure of the remainder of the esophagus?**

−5 mm Hg for the body of the esophagus and 10–40 mm Hg for the lower esophageal sphincter.

○ **What effect do beta-adrenergic blockers have on lower esophageal sphincter pressure?**

Raise it.

○ **What effect does smoking have on lower esophageal sphincter pressure?**

Lowers it.

○ **How does the musculature of the upper 1/3 esophagus differ from the lower 2/3?**

Upper 1/3 is striated; lower 2/3 is smooth.

○ **Where is Auerbach's plexus in the esophagus?**

Between the longitudinal and circular muscle fibers.

○ **Where is Meissner's plexus in the esophagus?**

Submucosa.

○ **True/False: Unlike the rest of the gastrointestinal tract, the esophagus does not have a serosa.**

True.

○ **What are the three layers of the esophageal mucosa?**

Muscularis mucosa, lamina propria, and epithelium.

○ **Where are the left and right vagus nerves in relation to the esophagus?**

The left is anterior and the right is posterior.

○ **In what directions are the muscle fibers of the inferior constrictor oriented?**

Superiorly, in an oblique fashion; inferiorly, in a transverse fashion.

○ **Retained secretions in the hypopharynx that fail to clear with swallowing indicate a _____ disorder when thickened and mucoid and a _____ disorder when frothy or foamy.**

Neurological; structural.

○ **What are the six valves of the upper digestive tract that function during swallowing?**

Lips, tongue, velum to back of tongue (glossopalatal valve), velopharynx, larynx, and upper esophageal sphincter.

○ **What effect does chin tucking have on swallowing?**

It pushes the base of tongue and epiglottis anteriorly, causes the airway to narrow.

○   **True/False: Regardless of bolus volume, airway closure and cricopharyngeal opening always occur within 0.03 seconds of each other.**

True.

○   **True/False: Oral and pharyngeal transit times of the bolus are not affected by bolus volume or bolus viscosity.**

False; as volume and viscosity of the bolus increase, transit time increases.

○   **What effect does bolus volume have on the temporal relationship of the oral and pharyngeal stages of swallowing?**

With small volumes, the oral phase preceeds the pharyngeal stage, but with larger volumes (10 cc or more), the stages occur simultaneously.

CHAPTER 6 Larynx/Trachea

○ **True/False: Embryologically, the supraglottis and glottis are separate entities.**
True.

○ **Which branchial arches is the larynx derived from?**
III, IV, and VI.

○ **From which branchial arch does the stylohyoid muscle arise?**
II.

○ **What are the nine cartilages of the larynx?**
Three unpaired: thyroid, cricoid, and epiglottis.
Three paired: arytenoids, corniculates, and cuneiforms.

○ **What are the two branches of the superior laryngeal nerve?**
Internal and external.

○ **Which of these supplies sensation to the larynx above the glottis?**
Internal branch.

○ **What membrane must the internal branch penetrate?**
Thyrohyoid.

○ **What blood vessel travels with the internal branch?**
Superior laryngeal artery.

○ **What does the external branch innervate?**
Cricothyroid muscle.

○ **What is the function of the cricothyroid muscle?**
To lengthen the vocal fold and increase pitch.

○ **What separates the two valleculae associated with the tongue and the epiglottis?**
Median glosso-epiglottic fold.

○ **What nerve provides sensory innervation to the pyriform recess of the larynx?**
Internal laryngeal branch of the superior laryngeal nerve.

○ **What nerve provides sensory innervation to the infraglottic space?**
Recurrent laryngeal nerve.

○ **What is the name of the upper free margin of the conus elasticus?**
Vocal ligament.

○ **What is the name of the lower free margin of the quadrangular membrane?**
Vestibular fold.

○ **What is the vertebral level of the hyoid in adults?**
C3.

○ **What is the vertebral level of the cricoid in adults?**
C6.

○ **What is the vertebral level of the carina in adults?**
T4–T5.

○ **What muscle descends to insert upon the hyoid?**
Geniohyoid.

○ **What is the membrane between the cricoid cartilage and the first tracheal ring?**
Cricotracheal membrane.

○ **What part of the thyroid cartilage articulates with the cricoid cartilage?**
Inferior cornu.

○ **What is the only unpaired muscle of the larynx?**
Transverse arytenoid muscle.

○ **What is the only abductor of the vocal cords?**
Posterior cricoarytenoid muscle.

○ **What muscle adducts the false vocal cords and aryepiglottic folds?**

Thyroarytenoid muscle.

○ **Which muscles anchor and elevate the larynx?**

Omohyoid, sternohyoid, and sternothyroid muscles.

○ **Which muscles does the anterior branch of the recurrent laryngeal nerve innervate?**

Lateral cricoarytenoid, thyroarytenoid, and vocalis muscles.

○ **Where does the superior laryngeal artery lie in relation to the superior laryngeal nerve?**

Inferior.

○ **What is the angle of the thyroid cartilage at the anterior commissure in men and women?**

90 degrees in men; 120 degrees in women.

○ **How do the vocal folds move during quiet respiration?**

Adduct during expiration and abduct during inspiration.

○ **What are the layers of the vocal fold from superior to deep?**

Squamous epithelium, Reinke's space (superior layer of lamina propria), intermediate and deep layers of the lamina propria (comprising the vocal ligament), and thyroarytenoid muscle.

○ **What are the two types of squamous epithelium lining the true vocal cords?**

Pseudostratified columnar (superiorly and inferiorly) and stratified nonkeratinizing squamous (at the contact points of the TVCs).

○ **How does the position of the larynx differ between neonates and adults?**

In the neonate, the larynx is positioned more anterosuperiorly, lying at the level of C2–C3, with the cricoid lying at C3–C4. In the adult, the larynx lies at the level of C5 and the cricoid at C7.

○ **What is Broyles' tendon?**

Vocalis muscle tendon that inserts into the thyroid cartilage.

○ **What is its significance?**

Serves as a pathway for tumor extension into the thyroid cartilage.

○ **What anatomic structures inhibit malignant invasion by laryngeal cancers?**

Conus elasticus, quadrangular membrane, thyrohyoid membrane, cricothyroid membrane, and internal perichondrium of the thyroid lamina.

○ **What are the boundaries of the preepiglottic space?**
Epiglottic cartilage posteriorly, thyrohyoid membrane and hyoid bone anteriorly, and hyoepiglottic ligament superiorly.

○ **What anatomic feature of the epiglottis facilitates extension of carcinoma into the preepiglottic space?**
Fenestrations/dehiscences.

○ **Which portion of the larynx has sparse lymphatic drainage?**
Anterior glottis (epithelium of the TVC).

○ **What structures are considered part of the supraglottis?**
Epiglottis, false vocal cords, aryepiglottic folds, and arytenoids.

○ **What is the average tracheal wall mucosal capillary pressure?**
20–30 mm Hg.

○ **What is the only complete cartilage ring of the respiratory tract?**
Cricoid.

○ **What vessels are in direct contact with the anterior trachea?**
Brachiocephalic artery and the left brachiocephalic vein.

○ **What percent of the population has a thyroidea ima artery?**
3–10%.

○ **What is the significance of a thyroidea ima artery to a head and neck surgeon?**
It can cause excess bleeding while performing a tracheostomy.

○ **Which layers of the vocal cord are primarily responsible for TVC vibration?**
Epithelium and superficial layer of the lamina propria.

○ **What is the Bernoulli principle?**
A column of air flowing through a conduit produces a partial vacuum or negative pressure at the margins of the column that increases as the rate of flow increases.

○ **Which laryngeal muscle is primarly responsible for pitch elevation?**
Cricothyroid.

○ **What is the average fundamental frequency for a child? Adult female? Adult male?**
250 Hz; 200 Hz; 120 Hz.

○ **What is the average decibel level of the human voice?**
65–75 dB.

○ **What is the maximum range of fundamental frequency for the human voice?**
36–1760 Hz.

○ **What is the average maximum phonation time for an adult male? Adult female?**
17–35 seconds; 12–26 seconds.

○ **What is the Venturi effect?**
The acceleration of flow as a current of air or liquid enters a narrowed passage.

○ **What are the anatomic correlations to hoarseness and breathiness?**
Mucosal irregularity causes hoarseness; incomplete glottic closure causes breathiness.

○ **What are the three phases of speech?**
Pulmonary, laryngeal, and oral.

○ **True/False: Compared to the gag reflex, the cough reflex correlates better with a newborn's ability to eat safely.**
True.

○ **What percent of neonates less than 5 days old have a functioning cough reflex?**
25%.

○ **What prevents air from escaping through the glottis during the cough reflex?**
Adduction and turning down of the false vocal cords (FVC).

○ **What is the sequence of events during the glottic closure reflex?**
Closure of the true vocal cords (TVC), followed by closure of the FVC, followed by adduction of the aryepiglottic folds.

○ **What is laryngospasm?**
Maladaptive and exaggerated glottic closure reflex.

○ **Unlike the glottic closure reflex, laryngospasm is mediated solely by stimulation of what nerve?**
Superior laryngeal nerve.

CHAPTER 7

Thyroid and Parathyroid Glands

○ **What is the embryologic origin of the thyroid gland?**

The median downgrowth of the first and second pharyngeal pouches in the area of the foramen cecum.

○ **From which pharyngeal pouches are the inferior parathyroid glands derived?**

Third.

○ **What is the arterial blood supply to the thyroid gland?**

Superior thyroid branch of the external carotid artery and the inferior thyroid branch of the thyrocervical trunk.

○ **What is the venous drainage of the thyroid gland?**

Superior and middle thyroid veins, which drain into the anterior facial and internal jugular veins, and the inferior thyroid and thyroid ima veins which drain into the innominate veins.

○ **What is the predominant glycoprotein found in colloid?**

Thyroglobulin.

○ **What is the function of pendrin?**

Mediates exchange of iodide from the thyrocyte to the colloid, which is one of the first steps of thyroid hormone synthesis.

○ **What is the NIS?**

A Na^+/I^- symporter that serves to concentrate I^- into cells. It is found in the thyroid gland, salivary glands, gastric mucosa, placenta, ciliary body of the eye, the choroids plexus, the mammary glands, and certain cancers. Except for the thyroid gland, the NIS in these tissues does not respond to TSH.

○ **What are the three plasma proteins that bind thyroid hormonse?**

Albumin, transthyretin, and thyroxine-binding globulin (TBG).

○ **What are the functions of parathyroid hormone (PTH)?**

Stimulates osteolysis and release of calcium and phosphorus from the bone; increases reabsorption of calcium and magnesium and the excretion of phosphorus and bicarbonate in the kidney; enhances intestinal absorption of calcium by stimulating the activation of vitamin D in the kidney.

○ **What percent of the population has more than four parathyroid glands?**

10%.

○ **What percent of the population has only three parathyroid glands?**

3%.

○ **What percent of parathyroid glands are located in the mediastinum?**

2%.

○ **True/False: The inferior glands vary more in location than the superior glands.**

True.

○ **Where are the inferior parathyroids typically located?**

Inferior and anterior to the inferior thyroid artery.

○ **Where are the superior parathyroids typically located?**

Superior and posterior to the inferior thyroid artery and more likely to extend posteriorly and inferiorly or be found retroesophageally.

○ **What is the primary blood supply of the parathyroid glands?**

The superior and inferior parathyroid arteries, which are usually branches of the inferior thyroid artery.

○ **What are the three types of cells comprising the parathyroid glands?**

Chief cells, clear cells, and oxyphil cells.

○ **Which cells produce PTH?**

Chief cells.

○ **What percent of a parathyroid gland is composed of fat?**

20–30%.

○ **Which terminal of PTH is active?**

N-terminal.

CHAPTER 8 Face, Neck, Integument, and Muscles

○ **What are the five layers of the epidermis from deep to superficial?**
Stratum basale, stratum spinosum, stratum granulosum, stratum lucidum, and stratum corneum.

○ **The dermis primarily contains what type(s) of collagen?**
Type I (80%) and Type III (15%).

○ **What is the ratio of Type I to Type II collagen in the skin?**
8:1.

○ **Which type of collagen is a crucial component of the basement membrane?**
Type IV.

○ **What is the predominant type of collagen in scar tissue?**
Type I.

○ **What is the main difference between a keloid and a hypertrophic scar?**
Keloids extend beyond the boundary of the original tissue injury; hypertrophic scars do not.

○ **What lines are perpendicular to the line of force of the underlying muscle?**
Relaxed skin tension lines.

○ **How does the aging process alter facial proportions?**
The area from the subnasale to the menton decreases significantly in size compared to the other areas of the face.

○ **How does the skin differ between Asians and Caucasians?**
Asians have thicker skin with greater collagen density and are more prone to hypertrophic scarring and prolonged erythema.

○   **How does the skin age differently between Asians and Caucasians?**

Asians develop fewer fine rhytids but more pigmented lesions than Caucasians.

○   **What muscles draw the eyebrows medially?**

Corrugator supercilii muscles.

○   **What muscle draws the medial edge of the brow inferiorly?**

Procerus.

○   **What muscle creates vertical and oblique rhytids in the medial eyebrow region?**

Corrugator supercilii muscle.

○   **What is the SMAS?**

Tissue plane of the face composed of fibrous and/or muscle tissue that is continuous with the platysma and lacks direct bony insertion.

○   **What is the relationship of the SMAS to the parotid gland?**

Densely adherent to, yet distinct from, the parotid fascia.

○   **Where are the branches of the facial nerve in relation to the SMAS?**

Deep.

○   **What is the relationship of the SMAS to the zygomatic arch?**

It terminates 1 cm below the zygomatic arch.

○   **What is the relationship of the SMAS to the lower eyelid?**

It merges with the muscle fibers of the periorbital orbicularis oculi.

○   **What is the only location in the face where the SMAS is not covered by the fascial-fatty layer?**

Superior portion of the lower eyelid.

○   **What is the relationship of the frontal branch of VII to the temporoparietal fascia?**

Lies within it.

○   **What plane separates the temporoparietal fascia from the deep temporal fascia?**

Subaponeurotic plane of loose areolar tissue.

○   **What separates the superficial and deep layers of the deep temporal fascia?**

Superficial temporal fat pad.

○ **What fat pad separates the temporalis muscle from the deep temporal fascia and the zygomatic arch?**

The deep temporal fat pad, an extension of the buccal fat pad.

○ **What is the relationship of the frontal branch of VII to the zygomatic arch?**

Travels over it on the surface of the loose areolar layer and superficial layer of the deep temporal fascia.

○ **What are the only mimetic muscles that receive innervation from VII on their superficial surfaces?**

Buccinator, levator anguli oris, and mentalis muscles.

○ **Where are dense fibrous attachments between the superficial and deep facial fascias located?**

Along the zygomatic arch, overlying the parotid gland, along the anterior border of the masseter muscle.

○ **True/False: The buccal fat pad, parotid duct, facial artery and vein, and facial nerve lie in the same anatomic plane in the cheek.**

True.

○ **What nerve parallels the superficial temporal vessels?**

Auriculotemporal nerve.

○ **What is the function of the auriculotemporal nerve?**

Sensation of the scalp and auricle, and carries postganglionic parasympathetic nerves from the otic ganglion to the parotid gland to stimulate secretions.

○ **What are the two types of retaining ligaments that support the facial skin?**

Osteocutaneous ligaments and fusion of the superficial and deep fascias.

○ **What ligaments support the malar pad over the zygomatic eminence?**

Zygomatic ligaments.

○ **What ligaments support the soft tissue of the medial cheek?**

Masseteric cutaneous ligaments.

CHAPTER 9

Facial Skeleton and Skull Base

○ **What is the craniofacial ratio at birth?**
8:1.

○ **What is the craniofacial ratio in adulthood?**
2:1.

○ **Due to these differences, which facial fractures are more common in children than in adults?**
High facial fractures (orbital roof and temporal bone fractures).

○ **What is the foramen of Morgagni?**
Gap between superior constrictor muscle and skull base.

○ **What is the clinical significance of the foramen of Morgagni?**
Serves as a potential route for spread of nasopharyngeal tumors to the skull base and brain.

○ **Name the foramen through which the structure passes:**

Meningeal branch of V3	Foramen spinosum
Terminal branch of V2	Infraorbital foramen
V3 and accessory meningeal artery	Foramen ovale
Sphenopalatine artery	Sphenopalatine foramen
III, IV, VI, and V1	Superior orbital fissure
V2	Foramen rotundum

○ **What structure is found in Meckel's cave?**
Gasserian ganglion of V.

○ **Where is Dorello's canal and what nerve does it contain?**

Between the petrous tip and the sphenoid bone; contains VI and the inferior petrosal sinus.

○ **Does the foramen rotundum lie lateral or medial to the pterygoid canal?**

Lateral.

○ **What is the largest artery in the pterygopalatine fossa?**

Sphenopalatine.

○ **What opening in the medial wall of the pterygopalatine fossa permits the passage of neurovascular structures into the nasal passages?**

Sphenopalatine foramen.

○ **What is the name of the opening through which the maxillary artery passes after giving rise to infraorbital and posterior superior alveolar branches?**

Pterygomaxillary fissure.

○ **What is the name of the maxillary artery after it passes through the pterygomaxillary fissure?**

Sphenopalatine artery.

○ **What are the weakest areas of the mandible?**

Area around the 3rd molar, socket of the canine tooth, and the condyle.

○ **What structures pass through the mandibular foramen?**

Inferior alveolar artery and nerve.

○ **True/False: The medial pterygoid muscle elevates the mandible.**

True.

○ **What muscle protracts the mandible?**

Lateral pterygoid muscle.

○ **The pterygoid plates are part of which bone?**

Sphenoid.

○ **What type of joint is the temporomandibular joint (TMJ)?**

Ginglymoarthrodial (hinge/sliding) joint.

○ **What muscle inserts on the disk of the TMJ?**

Superior part of the lateral pterygoid muscle.

○ **What is normal interincisal opening?**

40–50 mm.

○ **Why is the midface inherently prone to deficient projection?**

It lacks good sagittal buttresses.

○ **What are the three paired vertical buttresses of the midface?**

Nasomaxillary, zygomaticomaxillary, and pterygomaxillary.

○ **What are the horizontal buttresses of the midface?**

Frontal bar and cranial base, zygomatic arch and temporal process of the zygoma, maxillary palate and alveolus, and the greater wing and pterygoid plates of the sphenoid.

○ **What are the horizontal buttresses of the nasoethmoidal region?**

Superiorly, the frontal bone and bilateral superior orbital rims; inferiorly, the bilateral inferior orbital rims.

○ **What are the vertical buttresses of the nasoethmoidal region?**

The paired "central fragments" arising from the frontal process of the maxilla and internal angular process of the frontal bone.

○ **What is the most prominent portion of the zygomaticomaxillary complex (ZMC)?**

Malar eminence.

○ **What are the four bony attachments to the skull radiating from the malar eminence?**

Superior attachment to the frontal bone (frontozygomatic suture); medial attachment to the maxilla (zygomaticomaxillary suture); lateral attachment to the temporal bone (zygomaticotemporal suture); and a deep attachment to the greater wing of the sphenoid (zygomaticosphenoidal suture).

○ **Which of these is strongest?**

Zygomaticofrontal buttress.

○ **What is the weakest part of the entire ZMC complex?**

Orbital floor.

○ **What is the normal inclination of the orbital floor?**

Inclines superiorly at a 30-degree angle from anterior to posterior and at a 45-degree angle from lateral to medial.

○ **What determines the projection of the upper face?**

The frontal bar (supraorbital rims and frontal sinuses).

CHAPTER 10

Nervous System Structures

○ **What is the terminal branch of V2?**
Infraorbital nerve.

○ **What is the only sensory nerve arising from the anterior division of V3?**
Buccal nerve.

○ **What nerve usually passes from lateral to medial over the optic nerve?**
Nasociliary.

○ **From what nerve do the anterior and posterior ethmoidal nerves arise?**
Nasociliary nerve.

○ **With one exception, all the muscles of the pharynx are innervated by what nerve?**
X.

○ **What are the nuclei of the vagus nerve?**
Nucleus ambiguus, dorsal motor nucleus, and the nucleus of the solitary tract.

○ **Which of these controls voluntary motor information?**
Nucleus ambiguus.

○ **Which of these receives sensory information?**
Nucleus of the solitary tract.

○ **What are the two ganglia of the vagus nerve?**
Superior (jugular) ganglion and inferior (nodose) ganglion.

○ **What information is relayed through the superior ganglion?**
Sensation from the external auditory canal and posterior auricle via Arnold's nerve.

○   **What information is relayed through the inferior ganglion?**

Sensation from the epiglottis and larynx.

○   **What is the function of the glossopharyngeal nerve?**

Motor to the stylopharyngeus; taste to posterior 1/3 tongue; parotid gland stimulation; sensation of postauricular skin, pharynx, soft palate, tympanic cavity, and eustachian tube.

○   **Which cranial nerve has the longest intracranial course?**

VI.

○   **What are the 4 ganglia associated with the cranial parasympathetic system?**

Ciliary, pterygopalatine, submandibular, and otic.

○   **Preganglionic parasympathetic cell bodies are associated with which nerves in the head and neck?**

Cranial nerves III, VII, IX, X and spinal nerves 2, 3, and 4.

○   **What is the stellate ganglion?**

Fusion of the of the first thoracic ganglion and the inferior cervical ganglion; it relays sympathetic input to the upper limbs.

CHAPTER 11 Orbit

○ **What is the average volume of the orbit?**

30 cm^3.

○ **What is the average depth of the orbit?**

40–50 mm.

○ **What are the layers of the eyelid from superficial to deep?**

Skin, subcutaneous tissue, voluntary muscle, orbital septum, tarsal plate, smooth muscle, and conjunctiva.

○ **What is unique about the anatomy of the Asian eyelid?**

Levator muscle lacks attachment to the pretarsal skin, resulting in an absent pretarsal fold.

○ **What structure divides the lacrimal gland into two lobes?**

Levator aponeurosis.

○ **What provides static support to the lower lid?**

Tarsal plate and its associated medial and lateral canthal tendons.

○ **What provides dynamic support to the lower lid?**

Adhesion of the pretarsal portion of the orbicularis to the tarsal plate.

○ **What structure in the lower lid is analogous to the levator aponeurosis of the upper lid?**

Capsulopalpebral fascia.

○ **What are the lower eyelid retractors?**

Capsulopalpebral fascia and the inferior tarsal muscle.

○ **What lines the posterior surface of the eyelid?**

Palpebral conjunctiva.

○ **What creates the gray line in the lid margin?**

The muscle of Riolan.

○ **What does the gray line divide?**

The anterior and posterior lamella.

○ **What structures make up the anterior lamella of the lid?**

Pretarsal orbicularis oculi muscle and the eyelid skin.

○ **What structures make up the posterior lamella of the lid?**

Conjunctiva and the tarsal plate.

○ **Periosteum and periorbita meet at the orbital margin and continue into the eyelids as what?**

Orbital septum.

○ **What is the origin of the superior tarsal muscle (of Muller)?**

Deep side of the levator palpebrae superioris.

○ **What structure forms the medial canthal tendon?**

The superficial head of the pretarsal fibers of the orbicularis oculi muscle.

○ **What are the three limbs of the medial canthal tendon?**

Anterior, superior, and posterior limbs.

○ **Which of these covers the lacrimal fossa?**

Superior limb.

○ **What is Whitnall's tubercle?**

Insertion site of the lateral canthal tendon.

○ **Which part of the lacrimal system is most vulnerable to injury?**

The inferior canaliculus near the medial canthal tendon.

○ **Where are the anterior and posterior ethmoid arteries and optic canal in relation to the anterior lacrimal crest?**

24–12–6 rule: Anterior ethmoid artery is approximately 24 mm posterior to the lacrimal crest; the posterior ethmoid artery is 12 mm posterior to the anterior ethmoid artery; the optic canal is 6 mm posterior to the posterior ethmoid artery.

○ **What does the medial epicanthal fold cover?**

Lacrimal lake.

○ **What is the function of the deep head of the orbicularis oculi?**

Inserts on the posterior lacrimal crest and provides structural support to the lid.

○ **What happens with disruption of the deep head?**

Lateral and anterior displacement of the medial canthal angle.

○ **Where does the lateral canthal tendon insert?**

Orbital tubercle located 5 mm posterior to the lateral orbital rim.

○ **What is the name of the fleshy, pink mound of tissue in the medial canthus?**

Lacrimal caruncle.

○ **What glands are contained within the tarsal plates?**

Tarsal glands (Meibomian).

○ **Which muscles are innervated by the superior division of III?**

Superior rectus and levator palpebrae superioris muscles.

○ **Which skeletal muscles are innervated by the inferior division of III?**

Inferior oblique, inferior rectus, and medial rectus muscles.

○ **What structures pass through the superior orbital fissure?**

III, IV, VI, V1, and superior ophthalmic vein.

○ **What is trichiasis?**

Abnormal direction of the eyelashes.

○ **What is Argyll Robertson pupil?**

Pupil reacts to accommodation but not light; often associated with syphlis.

○ **What test may elicit a Marcus Gunn pupil?**

Swinging flashlight test.

○ **What is the term for gross asymmetry of eye movement?**

Heterotropia.

CHAPTER 12 Basic Science

● ● ● IMMUNOLOGY/ALLERGY ● ● ●

○ **Coombs and Gell described 4 types of hypersensitivity reactions of the immune system; which of these is mediated primarily by T cells and macrophages?**

Type IV

○ **Inhalant allergy and anaphylaxis are examples of which type of Coombs and Gell hypersensitivity reaction?**

Type I, mediated by IgE.

○ **What is the mechanism of type II immune reactions?**

IgG and IgM antibodies form against the self.

○ **What is the mechanism of type III immune reactions?**

IgG and IgM complexes deposit in the basement membranes of blood vessels, resulting in outflow of plasma into the tissues, activation of complement, and influx of neutrophils.

○ **What is the mechanism of type IV or delayed-type hypersensitivity immune reactions?**

An overenthusiastic T-cell response to an environmental antigen where macrophages damage adjacent tissues.

○ **Rheumatoid arthritis is an example of which type of Coombs and Gel hypersensitivity reaction?**

Type III

○ **Myasthenia gravis is an example of which type of Coombs and Gel hypersensitivity reaction?**

Type II

○ **Which cells can serve as antigen-presenting cells?**

Monocytes, macrophages, dentritic cells, Langerhans cells and B cells.

○ **True/False: Class I MHC antigens appear on the surface of all nucleated cells in the body and have CD8 as their T-cell receptor.**

True.

○ **What type of T-cell receptor do Class II MHC antigens have?**

CD4

○ **Do helper T cells (TH) work with Class I or Class II MHC antigens?**

Class II

○ **Which subtype of TH cells requires IL-1 to proliferate in response to an antigen?**

TH2 cells.

○ **Which subtype off TH cells upregulate allergic inflammation?**

TH2 cells.

○ **Which type of T cells remove the body's own cells that have undergone change from a virus or malignancyin response to an antigen?**

Cytotoxic or "killer" T cells.

○ **True/false: The light chain determines the class of the immunoglobulin.**

False; the heavy chain determines the class.

○ **What is the only immunoglobulin that can cross the placenta?**

IgG.

○ **Which immunoglobulin plays an important role in the prevention of parasitic infections?**

IgE.

○ **Which immunologic cells display CD2, CD16, and CD56 markers and kill some types of tumor cells without depending on prior immunization?**

Natural killer cells.

○ **In which area of the inner ear are immunologically active structures most commonly found?**

Endolymphatic sac.

○ **What is the predominant immunoglobulin in the endolymphatic sac?**

IgA.

○ **What is the concentration of immunoglobulins in the perilymph compared to the serum?**

1/1000th.

○ **What is the predominant immunoglobulin in the perilymph?**

IgG.

○ **How do lymphocytes responding to antigenic stimulation in the inner ear enter from the systemic circulation?**

Via the spiral modiolar vein.

○ **What role does substance P play in the allergic response?**

Through VIP, it causes vasodilation of the blood vessels in the nose, and through acetylcholine, it causes mucus secretion.

● ● ● MICROBIOLOGY/VIROLOGY ● ● ●

○ **What are some ways to distinguish between true infection and contamination or colonzation?**

The presence of large numbers of epithelial cells suggests contamination and the growth of normal skin flora suggests colonization.

○ **How long does it take most acid-fast bacilli to grow?**

7–10 days.

○ **A single blood culture containing which organsisms suggests contamination?**

Staphylococcus epidermis, Staphylococcus hominis, Bacillis spp., *Corneybacterium diptheriae* (and other diptheroids).

○ **Darkfield examination is necessary for detection of which organism?**

Treponema pallidum.

○ **How does a virus replicate?**

Only through infecting a cell.

○ **Are bacteria eukaryotic or prokaryotic?**

Prokaryotic.

○ **Which infectious organisms are eukaryotics?**

Fungi and protozoa.

○ **Which cell type contains peptidoglycan in its cell wall?**

Prokaryotes.

○ **The ability of bacteria to take up extracellular DNA from their environment is known as what?**

Competence.

○ **Which are the four primary features of "competent" bacteria?**

Can self-aggregate, easily form protoplasts, are prone to autolysis, and have increased H^+ and Na^+ content that leads to increased glycolysis and ATP reserves.

○ **Which bacterial infection accounts for more deaths than any other vaccine-preventable bacterial disease?**

Streptococcal pneumoniae.

○ **What percent of the population is colonized in the nasopharynx with *Streptococcal pneumoniae*?**

40%.

○ **What are the five stages of biofilm development?**

Initial attachment, irreversible attachment, maturation I, maturation II, and dispersion.

● ● ● ENDOCRINOLOGY ● ● ●

○ **What are the three primary ways a cell reacts to a hormonal signal?**

Changing its metabolite or protein; generating an electric current; contracting.

○ **What are the two major classes of hormone receptors?**

Membrane receptors, binding peptides and catecholamines, and nuclear receptors, binding small molecules that can diffuse across a cell membrane.

○ **Steroid hormones and thyroid hormones use which type of receptor?**

Nuclear.

○ **Which hormone normally regulates protein synthesis and breakdown?**

Insulin.

○ **What is the half-life of T4?**

7 days.

○ **The thyroid hormones are stored as _____, the main component of colloid.**

Thyroglobulin.

○ **Most of the circulating thyroid hormone is bound by _____.**

Thyroxine-binding globulin.

○ **In patients treated for thyroid cancer, posttherapy thyroglobulin levels are less useful in the presence of elevated _____.**

Antithyroglobulin antibodies.

○ **What time of day does cortisol production peak?**

Early morning.

○ **What hormone receptors are present in juvenile nasopharyngeal angiomas?**

Dihydrotestosterone and testosterone.

○ **Which part of the pituitary gland is derived from Rathke's pouch?**

Anterior pituitary.

○ **Secretion of ADH from the posterior pituitary gland results in decreased or increased urine volume?**

Decreased.

○ **Secretion of TSH from the anterior pituitary gland results in increased or decreased colloid production in the thyroid gland?**

Decreased.

○ **What is the major inhibiting hormone of TSH?**

T3.

○ **When during the day does growth hormone production peak?**

2–3 hours into sleep (stage III or IV).

○ **What is the major inhibiting hormone to growth hormone?**

Somatostatin.

○ **What effect do exercise and stress have on growth hormone secretion?**

Stimulate secretion.

○ **What is the most common cause of diabetes insipidus?**

50% of cases are idiopathic.

○ **Pituitary microadenomas are smaller than _____ mm in diameter.**

10.

○ **What effect does PTH have on urine phosphorus?**

Increases urine phosphorus excretion.

○ **What hormone is produced by the parafollicular C cells of the thyroid?**

Calcitonin.

○ **What happens to PTH levels as people age?**

Rise.

○ **What will happen to reverse T3 and T3 levels during fasting, systemic illness, and acute psychiatric illness?**
Reverse T3 levels will increase and T3 levels will decrease.

○ **Which thyroid blood test correlates best with the metabolic state of the patient?**
Free thyroxine index (FT4I).

○ **The FT4I is the product of total T4 level and what?**
Thyroid hormone binding ratio (THBR).

• • • NEUROLOGY • • •

○ **How long does it take for 100% Wallerian degeneration to occur after complete nerve transection?**
3–5 days.

○ **How long does it take for 100% Wallerian degeneration to occur after a compressive conduction block?**
14–21 days.

○ **Between which days after injury is the degree of axonotmesis and neurotmesis unclear?**
6–14.

○ **What are the three types of nerve injury?**
Neuropraxia, axonotmesis, and neurotmesis.

○ **Which of these result in Wallerian degeneration?**
Axonotmesis and neurotmesis.

○ **Which of these has a more rapid rate of Wallerian degeneration?**
Neurotmesis.

○ **What is Sutherland's classification for nerve injury?**

1st degree	Reversible conduction block.
2nd degree	Wallerian degeneration occurs but endoneurium stays intact and recovery is usually complete.
3rd degree	Endoneurium is destroyed but perineurium stays intact and recovery is incomplete.
4th degree	All is destroyed except for the epineurium; recovery is poor.
5th degree	Complete nerve transection; untreated recovery is not expected.

○ **What produces CSF?**

Choroid plexus.

○ **What structures facilitate passage of CSF into the dural venous sinuses?**

Arachnoid villi.

○ **What substance is unique to CSF, perilymph, and vitreous humor?**

β-2-transferrin.

○ **Where in the brain is the "biological clock"?**

Suprachiasmatic nuclei.

○ **What is "clock-dependent alerting"?**

Internal signal from the biological clock that opposes the tendency to fall asleep.

○ **When is clock-dependent alerting most active?**

In the afternoon.

○ **Motor impulses are carried by the _____ root of the spinal cord and sensory impulses are carried by the _____ root of the spinal cord.**

Ventral; dorsal.

○ **How many cervical spinal nerves are there?**

Eight.

○ **Which of these sends motor and sensory fibers to the posterior and superior scalp as the greater occipital nerve?**

The second cervical nerve.

○ **The parasympathetic nervous system originates in the _____ segments of the spinal cord while the sympathetic nervous system originates in the _____ segments of the spinal cord.**

Craniosacral; thoracolumbar.

● ● ● **MOLECULAR BIOLOGY** ● ● ●

○ **What is the basic structure of DNA?**

A right-handed double helical structure composed of two antiparallel strands of unbranched polymeric deoxyribonucleotides (adenine, cytosine, guanine, and thymine) linked by phosphodiester bonds.

○ **Which deoxyribonucleotides always pair together?**

Adenine with thymine and cytosine with guanine.

○   **What are the four phases of a cell's cycle?**

G1 (1st gap phase before DNA synthesis), S (DNA synthesis), G2 (gap before mitosis), and M (mitosis).

○   **Extracellular signals primarily impact which phases of the cell cycle?**

G1 and G2.

○   **Cellular proliferation is goverened by which group of enzymes?**

Cyclin-dependent kinases (CDKs).

○   **Cellular apoptosis is goverened by which group of protienases?**

Capsases.

○   **What are the products of platelet degranulation?**

TGF-β and platelet-derived growth factor (PDGF).

○   **True/False: TGF-β stimulates cell proliferation.**

False; it inhibits it.

○   **What group of intracellular proteins does TGF-β stimulate to inihibit cell proliferation?**

SMAD proteins.

○   **What are the two primary classes of cancer genes?**

Oncogenes and tumor suppressor genes.

○   **What is the most common genetic alteration found in human cancers?**

An acquired mutation in p53, a tumor-suppressor gene.

○   **What is the role of p53?**

In the presence of cellular injury and DNA damage, p53 is upregulated, arresting the cell cycle at the G1/S checkpoint.

○   **What chromosome is p53 located on?**

17p.

○   **What is senescence?**

An irreversible arrest in G1 of the cell cycle.

○   **What is the role of retinoblastoma tumor-suppressor protein (pRB) in cell proliferation?**

In its hypophosphorylated state, it inhibits entry from G1 into the S phase of the cell cycle; loss of pRB enables cancer cells to enter a mitotic cycle without the normal input from external signals.

○ **What is the role of cyclin D1 in head and neck cancer?**

Cyclin D1 is a kinase that leads to phosphorylation of the RB protein (inactivating it) and has been shown to be amplified in up to 1/3 of head and neck cancers.

○ **What is the role of cyclooxygenase (COX-1 and COX-2) in head and neck cancer?**

Upregulation of cyclooxygenase has been shown to increase prostaglandins, decrease apoptosis, and increase angiogenesis via vascular endothelial growth factor in head and neck tumors.

○ **What is the role of HPV in head and neck cancer?**

More than 50% of tumors in the oropharynx harbor oncogenic HPV. Those associated with E6 and E7 proteins have better outcomes than HPV-negative tumors. HPV binds to pRB and inactivates it.

○ **What happens when epidermal growth factor receptor (EGFR) is bound by EGF or TGF-α?**

Intracellular tyrosine kinase is activated, leading to inhibition of apoptosis and activation of cell proliferation and angiogenesis.

○ **What is the role of EGFR and TGF-α in head and neck cancers?**

They are overexpressed in 80–90% of squamous cell carcinomas of the head and neck.

○ **What is the prognostic significance of EGFR expression?**

High levels of EGFR expression are correlated with poor prognosis and resistance to radiation therapy.

○ **What enzyme is responsible for the Warburg effect in tumor cells?**

Tumor M2-PK, a form of the pyruvate kinase enzyme.

○ **What is the Warburg effect?**

Tumor cells use the tumor M2-PK enzyme to consume glucose at an accelerated rate; tumor cells predominately produce energy by a high rate of anaerobic glycolysis followed by lactic acid fermentation in the cytosol, even in the presence of oxygen.

○ **What is the role of the MHC (major histocompatability complex) in the development of head and neck cancer?**

Tumor cells can escape early detection by the patient's immune system via decreased expression of class I MHC antigens.

● ● ● **GENETICS** ● ● ●

○ **What is the term for cell division in gametes?**

Meiosis.

○ **What are the most common numerical chromosome abnormalities in humans?**

Trisomies.

○ **True/False: All complete autosomal monosomies are lethal early in development.**

False; sex chromosome monosomy, such as Turner syndrome (45,X), can be viable.

○ **What does 47, XY+21 mean?**

A male with three copies of chromosome 21.

○ **What is mosaicism?**

The presence of two or more different chromosome constitutions in different cells in the same individual (i.e., may have some cells with 46 chromosomes and some with 47).

○ **Autosomal recessive conditions are frequently associated with _____ defects whereas autsosomal dominant conditions are frequently associated with _____ defects.**

Enzyme; protein structure.

○ **In autosomal recessive disorders, what is the risk of a child receiving a mutant gene from both parents and having the recessive trait?**

25%.

○ **What is the risk of the sibilings of affected persons being carriers?**

67%.

○ **In which type of genetic defect can the father not pass a mutation to any offspring?**

Mitochondrial defects.

○ **How could a person with an autosomal dominant disease have no affected family members?**

Due to a new mutation in the gene or nonpenetrance, where the gene lacks a phenotypic effect in a known carrier.

○ **Which type of inheritance pattern has a recurrence risk that varies with the number of affected family members?**

Polygenic inheritance.

○ **Hurler-Scheie syndrome is caused by which gene mutations with which inheritance pattern?**

This syndrome is inherited in an autosomal recessive pattern with the phenotype a product of two different mutations of the IDUA gene (compound heterozygotes.)

○ **What is a syndrome?**

Pattern of multiple anomalies pathogenetically related.

○ **What is a microdeletion syndrome?**

Variable phenotypic pattern resulting from duplication or deletion of a small segment of linked chromosome material/genes that are functionally unrelated.

○ **What syndrome is caused by a microdeletion in chromosome 17 and is associated with mental retardation, broad feet and hands, peripheral neuropathy, hearing loss and recurrent otitis media, disturbed sleep patterns, and inserting foreign objects into bodily orifices?**

Smith-Magenis syndrome.

○ **What is a sequence?**

Multiple defects arising from a single structural anomaly where the order of maldevelopment is understood.

○ **What is an association?**

Malformations occurring together more frequently than would be expected from chance alone.

○ **What is genetic anticipation?**

A phenomenon seen in disorders caused by unstable trinucleotide repeats where the age of onset of the disorder is younger and the phenotype becomes more severe with each succeeding generation.

○ **A classic example of genetic imprinting is seen with microdeletions of the region 15q11 to 15q13. A microdeletion of the paternal chromosome 15 causes _____ and microdeletion of the maternal chromosome 15 causes _____.**

Prader-Willi syndrome; Angelman syndrome.

● ● ● EPIDEMIOLOGY ● ● ●

○ **Tests with high sensitivity are useful to rule in or rule out disease?**

Rule out.

○ **What is a Type I error?**

A false-positive result.

○ **What is the beta level of a test?**

The likelihood of obtaining a type II error (false-negative).

○ **1 – beta = _____.**

The statistical power (likelihood of detecting a true difference between the groups).

○ **How is the required sample size affected if one decreases the acceptable type I error?**

Increases.

○ **What happens to the required sample size if the variability of the outcome diminishes?**

Decreases.

○ **Observational studies where the investigator determines the exposure status of the subjects and then follows them for subsequent outcomes are known as what?**

Cohort studies.

○ **A prospective cohort study where exposure to the risk factor and subsequent health outcomes are observed after the beginning of the study is also known as what?**

A longitudinal study.

○ **Observational studies where the subjects are sampled based on presence or absence of disease and then their prior exposure status is determined are known as what?**

Case-control studies.

○ **What are the advantages of case-control studies over cohort studies?**

Less expensive and time-consuming and easier for studying rare diseases.

○ **What is external validity?**

The extent to which the results of a study are applicable to other populations.

○ **What are the three primary forms of bias?**

Selection bias, information bias, and confounding.

Section II

DIAGNOSTIC AND ASSESSMENT PROCEDURES

CHAPTER 13 Face

○ **What is the ideal nasofrontal angle?**
125–135 degrees.

○ **What is the ideal nasolabial angle?**
90–120 degrees.

○ **What is the ideal nasofacial angle?**
36–40 degrees.

○ **What is the ideal alar-to-lobular ratio?**
1:1.

○ **How does the ideal supratip break differ between men and women?**
More pronounced in women.

○ **What is the single most important aesthetic quality of the nasal tip and base?**
Symmetry.

○ **What is the ideal configuration of the alar margin?**
S-shaped, exposing 2–3 mm of the caudal columella on lateral view.

○ **In a female, where should maximum brow elevation occur?**
At a line tangent and vertical to the lateral limbus of the eye.

○ **What is the ideal brow position in a woman?**
Medial segment club shaped and inferior to the lateral segment; peak of arch above the orbital rim at the lateral limbus; lid margin to brow distance >2 cm.

○ **What is the ideal brow position in a man?**
At the level of the supraorbital rim with a less pronounced arch.

○ **What is the ideal ratio of the length of the lower lip to the upper lip?**
2:1.

○ **What are the physical signs of aponeurosis disinsertion?**
Thin upper lid skin and high lid fold with good levator function (>10 mm).

○ **Define mild, moderate, and marked ptosis.**
Mild: 1–2 mm, moderate: 2–3 mm, marked: >4 mm.

○ **How is lower lid laxity defined?**
If >10 mm or >25% of the skin can be gathered without distortion of the rim.

○ **What is the significance of a "negative vector" profile?**
Describes patients with protuberant eyes and hypoplastic malar eminence—fat should not be removed from these patients during blepharoplasty.

○ **What measurement can be used to determine deficiency in the malar area?**
The distance from the malar prominence to the nasolabial groove on lateral projection (ideally >5 mm).

○ **What is Hering's law?**
Unilateral ptosis with contralateral lid retraction—if you cover the ptotic eye with a patch for 30–60 minutes, the retracted eye will settle into the normal position and the ptotic eye will reveal itself.

○ **What are two angles used to determine chin projection?**
Legan angle (normal 12 degrees +/− 4), Merrifield Z angle (normal 80 degrees +/− 5).

○ **Which of these uses the Frankfort horizontal line as a reference?**
Merrifield Z angle.

○ **Where should the chin lie in relation to a vertical line dropped from the lips?**
In men, the chin should meet the line; in women, the chin should lie 2–3 mm posterior.

○ **What is the difference between microgenia and micrognathia?**
Microgenia is a small mandible with normal occlusion; micrognathia is an underdeveloped mandible with class II occlusion.

○ **What is retrognathia?**
Normal sized mandible with class II occlusion.

○ **What is the normal position of the lower lip in relation to the upper lip and chin?**
The most anterior portion of the white roll should lie slightly posterior to the upper lip and lie in the same plane as the soft tissue chin point.

○ **What is the normal angle between the ear and the head?**

25–30 degrees.

○ **What is the normal incline of the vertical axis of the auricle?**

20 degrees.

○ **What is the normal superior limit of the auricle?**

The level of the brow.

○ **Skin that rarely burns and tans more than average is which Fitzpatrick's class?**

IV.

○ **How do adnexal carcinomas arising from hair follicles classically present?**

A tuft of white hair emerges from the central portion of the tumor.

○ **The pneumonic "AEIOU" is useful for which type of tumor?**

Merkel cell carcinoma; "A" is for asymptomatic/nontender (seen in 88% patients); "E" is for expanding rapidly (63% of patients); "I" is for immune suppressed (8% of patients); "O" is for over age 50; "U" is for ultraviolet light exposed site (81% of patients); 89% of patients with Merkel cell carcinoma will have three of these features at presentation.

○ **What is the most commonly used system to classify alopecia?**

Norwood's system.

○ **What is the significance of the presence of a cerebrospinal fluid (CSF) leak when assessing a patient with a frontal sinus fracture?**

Usually associated with a displaced posterior table fracture and a dural tear.

○ **On physical examination, the nose and the maxillary alveolar process are found to be free floating. What type of fracture has occurred?**

LeFort II.

○ **What is the "bowstring sign"?**

An obvious give that occurs with lateral tension on the lower lid, indicating disruption of the medial canthal tendon.

○ **What test is performed to evaluate for entrapment of the extraocular muscles?**

Forced duction test.

○ **What is the normal intercanthal width?**

30–35 mm in Caucasians or roughly the width of the alar base.

○ **On physical examination, digital pressure on the nasal tip causes prolapse of the distal nose into the pyriform aperture. Which type of nasoethmoidal fracture is this according to Gruss' classification of nasoethmoidal injuries?**

Type II

○ **What is the most sensitive test to detect optic nerve injury after facial trauma?**

Pupillary reaction to light.

○ **A 6-year-old boy presents with the following rash on his face. What is the most likely diagnosis?**

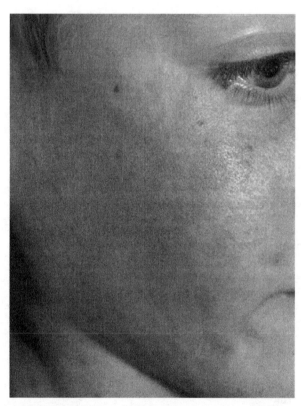

Reproduced, with permission, from Wolff K, Goldsmith LA, Katz SI, Gilchrest BA, Paller AS, Leffell DJ (eds). *Fitzpatrick's Dermatology in General Medicine*, 7th edn. New York: McGraw-Hill, 2008.

Erythema infectiosum, or Fifth disease. Usually the first sign of illness is the characteristic maculopapular rash on the cheeks that coalesces to give a "slapped-cheek" appearance.

○ **What physical exam findings are classic for measles?**

Rash, conjunctivitis, and Koplik's spots.

○ **A 3-year-old boy presents with a 10-day history of irritability, diarrhea, and malaise followed by a 5-day history of swollen, red lips, a polymorphous rash, fever, and peeling of the skin on his hands and feet. What is the diagnosis?**

Kawasaki disease or mucocutaneous lymph node syndrome.

CHAPTER 14 Ear

○ **What is Hitzelberger's sign?**

Hypoesthesia of the postauricular area associated with VIIth nerve compression secondary to an acoustic neuroma.

○ **How can one differentiate between relapsing polychondritis involving the ear and other causes of external otitis?**

Relapsing polychondritis spares the lobule.

○ **What is the likely diagnosis for someone who presents with vesicles on the pinna and external auditory canal (EAC), facial nerve weakness, and sensorineural hearing loss (SNHL)?**

Ramsey–Hunt syndrome.

○ **What is lobule colobomata?**

Bifid lobule.

○ **What is cryptotia?**

Absence of the retroauricular helix.

○ **What is cockleshell ear?**

Type III cup ear where the ear is malformed in all directions.

○ **Why is it particularly difficult to assess the auditory function in patients with bilateral aural atresia?**

Masking dilemma.

○ **What test should be used to assess auditory function in these patients?**

Auditory brainstem response (ABR).

○ **What finding on pneumatic otoscopy is most specific for otitis media?**

Immobility of the tympanic membrane.

○ **What is the Brown sign?**

Sign seen with glomus tympanicum tumors where the tympanic membrane blanches when pressure is applied from the pneumatic otoscope.

○ **What is the definition of auditory threshold?**

The lowest level at which the patient can detect a sound 50% of the time.

○ **Where is bone-conducted sound transmitted?**

Directly to the cochlea.

○ **Which part of the auditory system is assessed by air conduction tests?**

The entire auditory system.

○ **What is the significance of a negative Rinne at 256 Hz, 512 Hz, and 1024 Hz?**

At least a 15 dB conductive hearing loss (CHL), 25–30 dB CHL, and 35 dB CHL, respectively.

○ **What percent of the time will the Rinne test miss an air–bone gap <30 dB?**

50%.

○ **A patient has a negative Rinne at 256 Hz AS. At 512 and 1024 Hz, it is positive as it is at all three frequencies AD. The Weber test lateralizes to the left at all three frequencies. He hears a soft whisper AD and a soft to medium whisper AS. What is his hearing loss?**

15 dB CHL AS.

○ **What is the significance of the ability to hear a tuning fork placed on the teeth?**

Indicates that cochlear reserve is present and surgery may be beneficial.

○ **How are air and bone conduction thresholds measured?**

By first obtaining a positive response, then lowering the intensity by 10 dB increments until no response is obtained.

○ **What are the stimuli used to obtain a speech reception threshold (SRT)?**

Spondees.

○ **What is a spondee?**

A two-syllable word spoken with equal stress on both syllables.

○ **How is SRT measured?**

By starting at minimal intensity and ascending in 10 dB increments until the correct response is identified.

○ **What is the definition of SRT?**

The lowest hearing level at which half of the words are heard and repeated correctly, followed by at least two correct ascending steps.

○ **SRT should be within __ dB of pure tone average (PTA).**

10 dB.

○ **What is the speech detection threshold (SDT)?**

Hearing level at which 50% of the spondaic words are detected; usually 6–7 dB lower than the SRT.

○ **How is speech discrimination testing performed?**

Phonetically balanced monosyllabic word lists (50) are administered at 30–50 dB above threshold and the correct percentage is identified.

○ **What is a normal word recognition score?**

90–100%.

○ **What is the significance of speech discrimination scores?**

Patients with cochlear and retrocochlear pathology will have poor to very poor scores, respectively; those with only CHL will have normal scores when the intensity level is sufficiently loud.

○ **What is rollover?**

A decrease in speech discrimination scores when presented at higher intensities; suggestive of a retrocochlear lesion.

○ **A patient with an SRT of 55 dB HL and a speech discrimination score of 64% at 75 dB HL has what kind of hearing loss?**

Sensorineural.

○ **What is interaural attenuation?**

The reduction of sound when it crosses from one ear to another.

○ **What is normal interaural attenuation of air-conducted tones?**

40–80 dB depending on whether ear inserts or headphones are used and also on the frequency being tested.

○ **What is the normal interaural attenuation value for bone conduction?**

0 dB.

○ **When should masking be used?**

When the air conduction threshold of the test ear exceeds the bone conduction threshold of the nontest ear by a value greater than interaural attenuation.

○ **What is crossover?**

The attained responses represent the performance of the nontest ear rather than the test ear due to a large sensitivity difference between the ears.

○ **When does masking dilemma occur?**

Bilateral 50 dB or greater air–bone gaps.

○ **What is the Stenger's test?**

Test to see if the patient is malingering; appropriate to administer if there is >20 dB difference between ears in voluntary thresholds.

○ **Below is the audiogram of a 42-year-old professional singer. What is the likely etiology of his hearing loss?**

Reproduced, with permission, from Lalwani AK (ed.). *Current Diagnosis & Treatment in Otolaryngology—Head & Neck Surgery*, 3rd edn. New York: McGraw-Hill, 2012.

Noise-induced SNHL.

○ **Where is the peak pressure point in a normal tympanogram in an adult?**

Between −100 and +40 daPa.

○ **What would the tympanogram look like in an ear with an interrupted ossicular chain?**

Very steep amplitude, high peak (type A_d).

○ **What is the acoustic reflex threshold?**

The lowest stimulus level that elicits the stapedial reflex.

○ **In the normal ear, contraction of middle ear muscles occurs at which pure tones?**

65–95 dB HL.

○ **What are the neural pathways of the acoustic reflex?**

VIII to the ipsilateral ventral cochlear nucleus to the trapezoid body to the motor nucleus of VII to VII to the ipsilateral stapedius.

VIII to the ipsilateral ventral cochlear nucleus to the trapezoid body to the ipsilateral medial superior olive to the motor nucleus of VII to VII to the ipsilateral stapedius.

VIII to the ipsilateral ventral cochlear nucleus to the medial superior olive to the contralateral motor nucleus of VII to the contralateral VII to the contralateral stapedius.

○ **True/False: The acoustic reflex threshold is absent in patients with middle ear disease.**

True.

○ **What does the finding of elevated acoustic reflex in the presence of normal hearing or mild SNHL and a normal tympanogram suggest?**

Retrocochlear pathology.

○ **True/False: Brainstem lesions may abolish the acoustic reflex without affecting the pure tone thresholds.**

True.

○ **What does acoustic reflex delay measure?**

The ability of the stapedius muscle to maintain sustained contraction.

○ **How is this measured?**

A signal is presented 10 dB above the acoustic reflex threshold for 10 seconds; if the response decreases to one half or less of the original amplitude within 5 seconds, the response is considered abnormal and suggestive of retrocochlear pathology.

○ **What three audiometric test techniques are used to obtain behavioral response levels from a child?**

Behavioral observation audiometry (BOA), visual reinforcement audiometry (VRA), and conditioned play audiometry (CPA).

○ **What is the best audiometric method to use when assessing the hearing level of a 15-month-old child?**

BOA (observing reflexive/behavioral responses to sound stimuli at different frequencies) and VRA (employing lighted transparent toys to reinforced responses (head turn) to auditory stimuli.)

○ **What is the best audiometric method to use for a 4-year-old child?**

CPA where the child is trained to respond to auditory stimuli with a motor response (e.g., pointing to pictures).

○ **What stimulus is used to evoke the ABR?**

A simple acoustic click, between 2000 and 4000 Hz.

○ **What do the peaks of the ABR represent?**

Synchronous neural discharge at various locations along the auditory pathway.

○ **What does each wave represent?**

I—Eighth nerve.

II—Cochlear nucleus.

III—Superior olivary complex.

IV—Lateral lemniscus.

V—Inferior colliculus.

[Note: E. coli]

○ **Which of the waves is the largest and most consistent?**

V.

○ **True/False: The ABR is unaffected by state of sleep or medications.**

True.

○ **How is ABR most commonly used?**

To test newborns, difficult to test children, and malingerers.

○ **How is hearing threshold estimation performed using ABR?**

Wave V is tracked with decreasing sound intensity until it can no longer be observed.

○ **What does the interwave latency reflect?**

The time necessary for neural information to travel between places in the auditory pathway; any pathology that interferes with this transmission will prolong the latency.

○ **When is the interaural latency difference of wave V important?**

Used to document retrocochlear pathology when wave I is absent.

○ **When is wave I absent?**

When hearing loss exceeds 40–45 dB at higher frequencies.

○ **When determining interpeak latencies, which waves are compared?**

I–III, I–V.

○ **What is the difference in these interpeak latencies?**

Increased I–III intervals are almost always indicative of retrocochlear pathology, whereas increased I–V intervals is more likely associated with noise-induced SNHL.

○ **How will a retrocochlear lesion affect the ABR?**

Prolongation of absolute wave V latency, I–V latency, and interaural wave V latency.

○ **What are the three types of evoked OAEs?**

SFOAE (stimulus frequency).

TEAOE (transient evoked).

DPOAE (distortion product).

○ **Which of these is evoked by two pure tones?**

DPOAE.

○ **What are the typical objective auditory findings in patients with auditory neuropathy?**

Decreased or absent ABR, normal OAEs, absent auditory reflexes, very poor speech discrimination, mild-to-profound pure tone hearing loss.

○ **Why are OAEs useful as a screening tool in infants?**

Nearly 100% of people demonstrate evoked OAEs; testing is noninvasive and inexpensive; test time is short; cochlear hearing loss exceeding 30 dB can be detected.

○ **If otoacoustic emissions are present, can retrocochlear pathology be ruled out?**

No.

○ **What test can be use to exclude the absence of aidable hearing when the ABR is absent at maximum levels?**

ASSEP (auditory steady-state evoked potentials).

○ **True/False: ASSEP has little predictive value for hearing levels in children with auditory neuropathy.**

True.

○ **True/False: ASSEP cannot distinguish between cochlear and retrocochlear hearing loss.**

True.

○ **What are the indications for performing hearing screening in neonates if universal screening is not available?**

Family history of hereditary childhood SNHL.

Congenital perinatal infection (TORCH).

Head or neck malformation.

Birth weight <1500 g.

Hyperbilirubinemia requiring an exchange transfusion (>20).

Bacterial meningitis.

Apgar 0–4 at 1 minute or 0–6 at 5 minutes.

Prolonged ventilation (>5 days).

Ototoxic medications.

○ **What are the indications for performing hearing screening in infants 29 days to 2 years?**
Parent concern.
Developmental delay.
Bacterial meningitis.
Head trauma associated with loss of consciousness or skull fracture.
Ototoxic medications.
Recurrent or persistent otitis media with effusion for at least 3 months.

○ **What are the indications for hearing evaluation every 6 months until age 3?**
Family history of hereditary childhood hearing loss.
In utero infection (TORCH).
Neurodegenerative disorders.

○ **What does the audiogram typically look like in a child with SNHL secondary to rubella?**
Cookie-bite pattern.

○ **In the workup of congenital hearing loss, what test has the highest diagnostic yield?**
CT scan.

○ **What sort of hearing loss is most common in patients with Cogan's syndrome?**
Progressive to total deafness.

○ **In patients with chronic otitis media but no cholesteatoma, what level of hearing loss is associated with ossicular chain disruption or fixation?**
30 dB or more.

○ **What is the significance of hearing loss in the absence of middle ear effusion in patients with congenital cholesteatoma?**
Most lesions begin anterosuperiorly and extend posteriorly with growth. Hearing loss indicates posterior extension with involvement of the stapes superstructure and/or the lenticular process of the incus.

○ **What auditory tests are performed in tinnitus analysis?**
Pitch matching, loudness matching, minimum masking level (MML), and residual inhibition.

○ **How is the diagnosis of idiopathic intracranial hypertension (IIH) syndrome made?**
Exclusion of lesions producing intracranial hypertension, lumbar puncture with CSF pressure of more than 200 mm H_2O and normal CSF constituents.

○ **What proportion of patients with IIH will have an abnormal ABR?**
One-third.

○ **In patients with IIH, what is the usual pitch of the tinnitus?**

Low frequency.

○ **What maneuvers on physical exam will decrease or completely eliminate pulsatile tinnitus of venous origin?**

Light digital pressure over the ipsilateral internal jugular vein and head turning toward the ipsilateral side.

○ **What instrument is most helpful in examining nystagmus on physical exam?**

Frenzel goggles.

○ **What disorders are associated with down-beating nystagmus?**

Arnold–Chiari, cerebellar degeneration, multiple sclerosis, brainstem infarction, lithium intoxication, and magnesium and thiamine deficiency.

○ **What disorders are associated with up-beating nystagmus?**

Brainstem tumors, congenital abnormalities, multiple sclerosis, hemangiomas, vascular lesions, encephalitis, and brainstem abscess.

○ **What disorders are associated with bidirectional gaze-fixation nystagmus?**

Barbiturate, phenytoin, and alcohol intoxication.

○ **What findings on videonystagmography (VNG) are seen with central vestibular disorders?**

Disconjugate eye movements, skew deviation, vertical gaze palsy, inverted Bell's phenomenon, seesaw nystagmus, bidirectional nystagmus, periodic alternating nystagmus, and nystagmus that is greater with eyes open and fixed on a visual target than in darkness.

○ **What finding on VNG is pathognomonic for a lesion at the craniocervical junction?**

Spontaneous downbeat nystagmus with the eyes open, in the primary position that increases with lateral gaze or head extension.

○ **What is opsoclonus?**

Rapid, uncontrolled, mulitvectorial, conjugate eye movements, usually seen on physical exam and difficult to detect on VNG.

○ **What does computerized dynamic platform posturography specifically measure?**

Postural stability and sway.

○ **What are the clinical features of benign paroxysmal positional vertigo (BPPV)?**

10–20-second attacks of rotational vertigo, precipitated by head movements, with spontaneous resolution after several weeks to months in 80–90%.

○ **What are the physical exam findings in patients with BPPV?**

With the Dix–Hallpike maneuver, rotatory nystagmus toward the undermost ear accompanied by vertigo, both with a latent period of 5–30 seconds and duration <30 seconds.

○ **What features distinguish BPPV from vertigo due to CNS disease?**

CNS disease: no latent period, direction of nystagmus varies, nystagmus and vertigo are nonfatigable.

○ **What is measured in electrocochleography?**

Cochlear microphonic action potential (CM), action potential of VIII (AP), the summating potential (SP), and compound action potentials.

○ **Where are the recording electrodes placed?**

As close as possible to the cochlea and auditory nerve (promontory, tympanic membrane, EAC).

○ **When comparing the summating to the compound action potential, what value is considered abnormal?**

A ratio ≥ 0.45.

○ **What does an abnormal ratio suggest?**

Menière's disease.

○ **What technique can be used to differentiate the SP from the nerve potential of VIII (AP)?**

AP is a neural response that will respond to higher rates of stimulation. SP is a preneural response that is not affected by higher rates of stimulation. Therefore, increasing the click rate of the stimulus will affect the AP but not the SP.

○ **What is "Schwartze's sign"?**

Reddish hue on the promontory associated with otosclerosis.

○ **Is the acoustic reflex present in patients with otosclerosis?**

Usually it is absent bilaterally, even if the disease is unilateral.

○ **Is the acoustic reflex present in patients with superior semicircular canal dehiscence?**

Yes.

○ **What is Tullio's phenomenon?**

Vertigo with loud noise, commonly seen in patients with superior semicircular canal dehiscence.

○ **How does the hearing impairment from malleus ankylosis differ from that of otosclerosis?**

In patients with malleus ankylosis, hearing impairment is mostly unilateral (78%); the air–bone gap is smaller (majority less than 20 dB); SNHL is more frequent, particularly at 4 kHz; acoustic reflex is more likely to be present on the contralateral ear and absent on the impaired ear.

CHAPTER 15

Nose and Paranasal Sinuses

○ **What is stertor?**

Inspiratory low-pitched sound resulting from turbulent airflow through the nasal cavity and nasopharynx.

○ **What study confirms the diagnosis of primary ciliary dyskinesia?**

Electron microscopic study of cilia from nasal respiratory mucosa.

○ **What do the three valleys on acoustic rhinometry represent?**

1st valley—nasal valve; 2nd valley—anterior portion of the middle turbinate; 3rd valley—middle portion of the middle turbinate.

○ **Topical decongestants have a statistically significant different response between normal and allergic subjects are given a topical decongestant. For which valley on acoustic rhinometry will a statistically different response be seen?**

1st valley.

○ **Acoustic rhinometry showing decreased cross-sectional area and nasal volume that does not improve with a topical decongestant suggests what disorder?**

Septal deviation.

○ **What effect do nasal dilator strips have on nasal airflow as measured by spirometry?**

Increase peak inspiratory flow rates.

○ **What are the most common symptoms of chronic rhinosinusitis?**

Nasal congestion and obstruction.

○ **What is the most common symptom of isolated sphenoid disease?**

Headache.

○ **What is Sluder's syndrome?**

Sinonasal headaches secondary to irritation of the sphenopalatine ganglion.

○ **What are the diagnostic criteria for sarcoidosis of the sinuses?**

Radiographic evidence of sinusitis, histopathologic confirmation of noncaseating granulomas in the sinus tissue, negative serologic test for syphilis and c-ANCA, and negative stains for fungus and AFB.

○ **When is lumbar puncture indicated in patients with preseptal cellulitis?**

Age less than 2 months, meningeal or focal neurologic signs, clinical toxicity.

○ **A 30-year-old man presents with chronic sneezing, pruritus, rhinorrhea, and nasal congestion. His past medical history is significant for asthma. Comprehensive allergy testing and serum IgE are normal. What is the most likely diagnosis and what test should be ordered to confirm this?**

NARES (nonallergic rhinitis with eosinophilia syndrome); nasal smear will show marked eosinophilia (>25%).

○ **What signs on physical exam are suggestive of cerebrospinal fluid leak?**

Halo sign and reservoir sign.

○ **What is the reservoir sign?**

A rush of clear rhinorrhea occurs with sudden upright position.

○ **What is the most common presenting symptom of sinonasal neoplasms?**

Nasal obstruction (50%).

○ **What percent of patients with sinonasal tumors are asymptomatic at presentation?**

Approximately 10%.

○ **What three signs are classically present in patients with sinonasal neoplasms?**

Facial asymmetry, tumor bulge in the oral cavity, and nasal mass; the presence of all three is seen in about 50% of patients and is significant for advanced disease.

○ **What percent of patients with nasopharyngeal carcinoma will have a normal exam by fiberoptic endoscopy at the time of initial evaluation?**

6%.

CHAPTER 16 Oral Cavity

○ **What is lingua plicata?**

Scrotal tongue (seen in Melkersson–Rosenthal syndrome).

○ **What is the most common oral manifestation of AIDS?**

Candidiasis.

○ **What are the physical signs associated with submucous cleft palate?**

Bifid uvula, abnormal palatal motion, midline diastasis of the palatal muscles, V-shaped notch of the hard palate.

○ **When is a posttreatment culture indicated in a child with group A streptococcal pharyngitis?**

If the child is at an unusually high risk for rheumatic fever, remains symptomatic, or develops recurring symptoms.

○ **What are the typical presenting features of ankyloglossia?**

Infant has difficulty latching on during breast feeding and mother experiences prolonged nipple pain.

○ **What is class I occlusion?**

The mesiobuccal cusp of the maxillary 1st molar articulates with the mesiobuccal groove of the mandibular 1st molar.

○ **If the mesiobuccal cusp of the maxillary 1st molar lies anterior to the mesiobuccal groove of the mandibular 1st molar, what is the occlusion?**

Class II.

○ **What is the bite abnormality if the maxillary incisiors are lingual to the mandibular incisors?**

Anterior crossbite.

○ **What is an open bite?**

Lack of anterior incisal contact when the posterior teeth are in occlusion.

○   **What is the difference between overbite and overjet?**

Overbite occurs in the vertical plane, whereas overjet occurs in the horizontal plane.

○   **In an adult, what number is the left 3rd molar of the mandible?**

17.

○   **In an adult, what number is the right 3rd molar of the mandible?**

32.

○   **How many deciduous teeth are there?**

20.

○   **How are they numbered?**

A to T.

○   **Anterior open bite suggests which type of fracture?**

Bilateral condylar fractures.

○   **Contralateral open bite and ipsilateral chin deviation suggests what type of fracture?**

Unilateral condylar neck fracture.

○   **What substance can be applied to the mucosa of the oral cavity to help detect malignant and premalignant lesions?**

Toluidine blue.

CHAPTER 17 Hypopharynx/Larynx

○ **A 45-year-old woman presents with dysphonia and on exam is found to have left vocal cord paralysis in the paramedian position. Complete history and physical exam are otherwise unremarkable. CT scan of the neck and chest and laboratory findings, including electrolytes, RPR, and thyroid function tests, are normal. What are the next steps?**

Magnetic resonance imaging (MRI) of the neck and chest followed by laryngoscopy/bronchoscopy if necessary.

○ **A 78-year-old man presents with a weak, breathy voice and was recently treated for pneumonia. On exam, he was found to have left vocal paralysis in the intermediate position with a wide posterior gap that does not close with vocalization. What is the most appropriate test?**

MRI of the brain/skull base (his history and exam suggest a nerve lesion above the recurrent laryngeal nerve).

○ **What is the primary purpose of laryngeal electromyography (EMG) in patients with vocal cord paralysis?**

To distinguish paralysis from mechanical fixation.

○ **Which laryngeal muscles are typically analyzed with EMG?**

Thyroarytenoid and cricothyroid muscles.

○ **An EMG wave pattern of decreased frequency with normal amplitude suggests what sort of disorder?**

Neuropathy.

○ **An EMG wave pattern of decreased amplitude with normal frequency suggests what sort of disorder?**

Myopathy.

○ **What is the significance of a "picket fence" pattern on EMG?**

Indicates partial reinnervation (polyphasic action potentials).

○ **What are the features of a denervation pattern on EMG?**

Sharp waves or fibrillation potentials, complex repetitive discharges, and little or no electrical activity during attempts at voluntary contraction.

○ **What is the significance of a denervation pattern 1 year after injury?**

Spontaneous recovery is very unlikely.

○ **What disease does a fatiguing pattern on EMG suggest?**

Myasthenia gravis.

○ **How is the cricopharyngeus muscle identified with EMG?**

Electrical activity occurs at rest and diminishes or stops with swallowing.

○ **Stridor that increases in intensity with crying, agitation, or straining is characteristic of what disorders?**

Laryngomalacia and subglottic hemangioma.

○ **What is the test of choice for diagnosing laryngomalacia?**

Flexible fiberoptic laryngoscopy in the office.

○ **What are the indications for rigid bronchoscopy in children with laryngomalacia?**

Severe or atypical stridor, an abnormal high kilovolt cervical radiograph, or a high degree of suspicion for a synchronous airway lesion.

○ **What is the only clinical sign that is strongly associated with a synchronous airway lesion?**

Cyanosis.

○ **How can one diagnose exercise-induced laryngomalacia?**

With exercise flow-volume spirometry.

○ **What is the typical appearance of a type 1 posterior laryngeal cleft?**

A soft tissue defect in the interarytenoid musculature without a defect in the cricoid cartilage.

○ **What is the typical presentation of child with a laryngeal cleft type 2 or greater?**

History of aspiration, pneumonia, choking, coughing during feeds, and symptoms of airway obstruction.

○ **What common cause of congenital airway obstruction is characterized by inspiratory stridor at birth that decreases when placed on the side of the lesion?**

Unilateral vocal cord paralysis.

○ **What is the significance of vocal cord fixation in patients with laryngeal carcinoma?**

Invasion of the vocalis muscle has occurred, and lymph node metastasis is more likely.

○ **True/False: Any laryngeal tumor with vocal cord fixation is at least stage T3.**

True.

○ **What are the three most common presenting symptoms of hypopharyngeal cancer?**

Dysphagia, neck mass, and sore throat (in descending order of incidence).

○ **How does one assess for involvement of the prevertebral fascia from a hypopharyngeal tumor?**

Intraoperative evaluation is most accurate. During endoscopy, one can attempt to mobilize the posterior pharyngeal wall to assess for involvement. Video esophagography and CT scan are also helpful.

○ **What is Schaefer's classification system of laryngeal injuries?**

Group I: Minor hematomas or lacerations, no fractures, and minimal airway compromise.
Group II: Moderate edema, lacerations, mucosal disruption without exposed cartilage, nondisplaced fractures, and varying degrees of airway compromise.
Group III: Massive edema, mucosal disruption, displaced fractures, cord immobility, and varying degrees of airway compromise.
Group IV: Same as group III but with two or more fracture lines and/or skeletal instability or significant anterior commissure trauma.

○ **Which voice analysis test gives a three-dimensional representation of sound (time, intensity, and frequency)?**

Spectrogram.

○ **Which voice analysis test plots minimums and maximums of loudness at selected levels of fundamental frequency and reflects the patient's vocal capacity?**

Phonetogram.

○ **Which voice analysis test graphs multiple vocal parameters at once and is very useful for showing changes over time?**

Multidimensional voice profile.

○ **A patient complains of total aphonia yet generates sound with coughing. What is the likely diagnosis?**

Psychosomatic conversion dysphonia.

CHAPTER 18 Neck

○ **A supraclavicular stab wound is in which neck zone?**
I.

○ **True/False: Enlargement of the preauricular lymph nodes is indicative of parotid pathology.**
False: These nodes enlarge from inflammation or metastasizing tumors from the scalp.

○ **What is the most common head and neck manifestation of neuroblastoma?**
Cervical metastatic disease.

○ **What is the most common presentation of a parapharyngeal space tumor?**
Medial displacement of the lateral oropharyngeal wall or as a palpable mass beneath the angle of the mandible.

○ **What is the classic physical finding of carotid body tumors?**
Freely moveable in the lateral direction but fixed in the cephalic-caudal direction.

○ **How can one differentiate a vagal paraganglioma from a carotid body tumor?**
Vagal paragangliomas displace the internal and external carotid anteriorly and medially, whereas carotid body tumors displace the internal carotid artery posteriorly and the external carotid artery anteriorly.

○ **What is the risk of performing fine needle aspiration (FNA) on scrofula?**
May lead to a chronically draining cutaneous fistula.

○ **What percent of thyroid nodules are benign on FNA?**
70%.

○ **What is the incidence of a nondiagnostic or "suspicious" result on thyroid nodule FNAs?**
25%.

○ **What percent of thyroid nodules are malignant when FNA is suspicious?**
For papillary and Hürthle, the risk of malignancy is 57%. For follicular, the risk is 20–25%.

○ **What is the incidence of false positives and false negatives with FNA of thyroid nodules?**
4%; 4%.

○ **True/False: FNA should be performed on a 6-mm nodule if the ultrasound shows microcalcifications.**
True.

○ **What factors significantly increase the risk of sampling error from FNA?**
Very small (<1 cm) or very large (>4 cm) nodules, hemorrhagic nodules, or multinodular glands.

○ **Most false positive FNAs are due to what disease?**
Hashimoto's thyroiditis.

○ **Which thyroid tumors cannot be diagnosed as malignant with FNA?**
Follicular and Hürthle cell.

○ **What percentge of nodules with follicular or Hürthle cells on FNA are malignant?**
10–20%.

○ **What illness is characterized by a staccato cough?**
Chlamydial pneumonia.

○ **What diseases may present with hemoptysis in children?**
Bronchiectasis, cystic fibrosis, foreign body, pulmonary hemosiderosis, tuberculosis.

○ **What illness is characterized by a seal-like barking cough?**
Croup.

○ **What kind of stridor is heard in patients with tracheomalacia?**
Expiratory.

○ **What test has the highest yield for diagnosis of vascular rings?**
Direct laryngoscopy and bronchoscopy.

○ **What is the typical endoscopic appearance of innominate artery compression?**
Pulsatile compression of the anterior tracheal wall in the distal trachea.

○   **What is the "Waterson sign"?**

Obliteration of the right radial pulse by compressing the anterior tracheal indentation with the tip of the bronchoscope.

○   **What is the test of choice in the evaluation of caustic ingestion?**

Endoscopy.

○   **When is the ideal time to perform endoscopy after ingestion?**

24–48 hours postingestion.

○   **What information does esophageal manometry provide?**

Upper esophageal sphincter responsiveness and pharyngeal peristalsis.

○   **What is the sensitivity of the 24-hour pH probe for gastroesophageal reflux disease (GERD)?**

92–94%.

○   **What is the Euler–Byrne formula?**

$X + 4Y$, where X = number of episodes the pH is <4 and Y = number of episodes the pH is <4 for >5 minutes; a score of 50+ is clinically significant for GERD.

○   **What is the best test to distinguish obstructive from restrictive lung disease?**

Pulmonary function test (PFT).

○   **What would be the likely PFT results in a 75-year-old man with a 50-pack-year smoking history?**

Both FEV_1 and FEV_1/FVC would be decreased and RV and TLC would be increased.

○   **What would be the likely PFT results in a 44-year-old woman with pneumonia?**

Both FEV_1 and FVC would be decreased but FEV_1/FVC would be normal.

CHAPTER 19 Neurological

○ **When are all five divisions of the facial nerve present in the fetus?**

By the 8th week of gestation.

○ **How does the course of the facial nerve differ between adults and children?**

At birth, the nerve is located superficially within the poorly formed mastoid; with maturation, the nerve is displaced medially and inferiorly.

○ **When is myelination of individual axons of the facial nerve complete?**

Age 4.

○ **What prognostic information does electroneurography (EnoG) provide for facial nerve paralysis?**

Patients with 95% degeneration or greater have a 50% chance of unfavorable recovery; if at least 10% function is retained in the first 21 days of paralysis, 80–100% functional recovery is highly likely.

○ **When is ENoG evaluation meaningful?**

Between days 3 and 21 after complete loss of voluntary function.

○ **What is the next most accurate test when ENoG is unavailable?**

Maximal stimulation test.

○ **What test should be performed when 100% neural degeneration is recorded with ENoG?**

Voluntary electromyography (EMG) recording; regenerating nerve fibers conducting at different rates can result in an overestimation of neural degeneration on ENoG.

○ **What should be done if motor unit potentials are detected on EMG?**

No further therapy is indicated.

○ **What electrophysiologic test is more useful 3 weeks after the onset of complete facial paralysis?**

EMG.

○ **What test should be performed on Afro-Caribbean migrants with idiopathic facial nerve palsy?**

HTLV-1 antibody screen.

○ **What is the incidence of cranial nerve palsy at initial presentation in patients with nasopharyngeal carcinoma?**

12–18%.

○ **True/False: True diplopia should resolve with one eye closed.**

True.

○ **Small, irregular pupils that react irregularly to light but better to accommodation suggest what infectious disease?**

Neurosyphillis.

○ **What is the Myerson sign?**

Persistent blinking when the forehead is tapped repeatedly is an abnormal manifestation of the glabellar reflex, a primitive reflex seen in infants that may be a sign of frontal lobe disease in adults.

○ **Which cranial nerves are tested with the corneal reflex test?**

Tests V and VII on the side stimulated and VII consensually.

○ **When testing for dysarthria, problems with saying "Ka, Ka, Ka"; "La, La, La"; and "Me, Me, Me" indicate deficits in which nerves?**

IX and X; XII; and VII, respectively.

○ **Winging of the scapula is seen with deficits in which nerve?**

XI.

CHAPTER 20 Imaging Studies

○ **What is the imaging modality of choice for lymphatic malformations?**

Magnetic resonance imaging (MRI). Chest X-ray (CXR) should also be performed to rule out mediastinal extension or pleural effusion.

○ **What is the best radiographic test to evaluate swallowing?**

Videofluoroscopic barium swallow.

○ **Arteriography before surgery is recommended for stable injuries to which zones of the neck?**

I and III.

○ **What is the initial test of choice in patients with pulsatile tinnitus and normal otoscopy?**

Duplex carotid ultrasound and echocardiogram in patients suspected of carotid/coronary artery disease; otherwise, MRI/MRA/MRV brain and neck.

○ **What is the initial test of choice in patients with pulsatile tinnitus and a retrotympanic mass?**

CT scan of the temporal bones.

○ **A 45-year-old woman with type I diabetes comes into the emergency room with severe left otalgia. She has been on topical ciprofloxin eardrops for the past 2 weeks without improvement. On examination, she has significant swelling of the pinna and external auditory canal (EAC) and granulation tissue is seen in the lateral portion of the canal. What imaging studies should be ordered?**

CT scan with contrast and technetium-99m bone scan to evaluate for osteomyelitis of the temporal bone.

○ **A 54-year-old man presents with high fever, nausea, hypotension, and severe left-sided headache. Two weeks ago he was treated for left otitis media with azithromycin. On examination, he has severe edema and erythema over his left mastoid. Noncontrast CT scan of the brain shows the delta sign and contrast CT scan of the brain shows the reverse delta sign. What test should be ordered next?**

MRI with gadolinium and MRV brain to confirm sigmoid sinus thrombophlebitis.

○ **What tumor is shown below?**

Reproduced, with permission, from Lalwani AK (ed.). *Current Diagnosis & Treatment in Otolaryngology—Head & Neck Surgery*, 3rd edn. New York: McGraw-Hill, 2012.

Carotid body tumor. Angiogram shows splaying of the carotid bifurcation by a well-defined tumor blush ("lyre sign").

○ **A 72-year-old man presents with a 3-month history of worsening dysphagia. He was recently treated for pneumonia and reports frequently spitting up undigested food. His barium swallow is shown below:**

Reproduced, with permission, from Lalwani AK (ed.). *Current Diagnosis & Treatment in Otolaryngology—Head & Neck Surgery*, 3rd edn. New York: McGraw-Hill, 2012.

○ **What would be the likely findings if esophageal manometry were performed on this patient?**

Lack of coordination between the pharynx and cricopharyngeus muscle, hypertensive upper esophageal sphincter, hypotensive lower esophageal sphincter, and abnormal esophageal peristalsis.

● ● ● **PLAIN RADIOGRAPHS** ● ● ●

○ **What finding on barium swallow is classic for cricopharyngeal dysfunction?**

Cricopharyngeal bar.

○ **A 1-year-old child comes into the emergency room with a 3-day history of rhinorrhea and cough and now has stridor. Below are his AP neck films. What is the diagnosis?**

A

B

Reproduced, with permission, from Stone CK, Humphries RL (eds). *Current Diagnosis & Treatment: Emergency Medicine*, 7th edn. New York: McGraw-Hill, 2011.

Laryngotracheobronchitis (croup).

○ **A 6-month-old child comes into the emergency room with fever, dysphagia, and drooling. Below is his lateral neck film. What is the diagnosis?**

Reproduced, with permission, from Effron D (ed.). *Pediatric Photo and X-Ray Stimuli for Emergency Medicine*, Vol 2. Columbus, OH, Chapter of the American College of Emergency Physicians, 1997, case 27.

Retropharyngeal abscess; criteria for diagnosis on lateral neck film are 7 mm or greater thickness of the retropharynx at the level of C2 or 22 mm or greater thickness of the retropharynx at C6.

○ **How is atlantoaxial subluxation diagnosed?**

Neck pain and torticollis with an atlas–dens interval of >4 mm in children and >3 mm in adults.

○ **Which radiographic view on plain films of the face is best for visualizing the zygomatic arches?**

Submental vertex.

○ **What percent of cervical esophageal perforations will be missed with water-soluble contrast agents?**

50%.

○ **What percent of thoracic esophageal perforations will be missed with water-soluble contrast agents?**

25%.

○ **What is the sensitivity of barium in detecting esophageal perforations?**

80–90%.

○ **A 3-year-old boy presents to the emergency room with drooling but is breathing normally. Below is his chest radiograph. What is the diagnosis?**

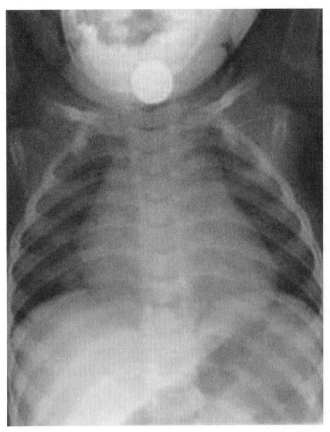

Reproduced, with permission, from Tintinalli JE (ed.). *Tintinalli's Emergency Medicine: A Comprehensive Study Guide*, 7th edn. New York: McGraw-Hill, 2011.

Retained coin in the esophagus.

○ **What is the sensitivity and specificity of inspiratory/expiratory and lateral decubitus films for foreign body aspiration?**

67% sensitive, 67% specific.

○   **Name the tumor based on findings from plain radiographs of the mandible.**

Sunburst appearance, radiating periosteal new bone	Osteosarcoma
Soft tissue mass with amorphous "popcorn" calcifications	Chondrosarcoma
Displaced surrounding structures, with multiple loculations and a honeycomb appearance	Ameloblastoma
Well-circumscribed lesion with a dense core and lucent rim; the core enlarges and rim diminishes with maturation	Cemento-ossifyling fibroma

● ● ● **COMPUTED TOMOGRAPHY** ● ● ●

○   **On CT imaging of the temporal bone, which ear structures are best seen on *axial* views?**
Body of the malleus and incus, incudostapedial joint, and the round window.

○   **On CT imaging of the temporal bone, which ear structures are best seen on *coronal* views?**
Stapes, oval window and the vestibule.

○   **On CT scan temporal bone with axial cuts, what structures are seen in the same plane as the porus acousticus?**
Head of the malleus, horizontal semicircular canal (SCC), and epitympanic recess.

○   **On CT scan temporal bone with axial cuts, what structures are seen in the same plane as the stapes?**
Sinus tympani, handle of the malleus, vestibule, cochlea, and pyramidal eminence.

○   **What is the most commonly identified inner ear malformation on temporal bone imaging studies?**
Isolated lateral SCC defects.

○   **What temporal bone malformation is classic for rubella?**
Scheibe malformation.

○   **In a patient with aural atresia and no evidence of sensorineural hearing loss, when should a CT scan of the temporal bones be obtained?**
Age 4 or 5.

○   **A 7-year-old boy is found on examination to have stenosis of his right EAC. CT scan shows ground glass appearance of the temporal bone. What is the likely diagnosis?**
Fibrous dysplasia.

○ **Below is the axial CT scan temporal bone of a patient with mild right SNHL. What advice should the patient receive in regard to preventing further hearing loss?**

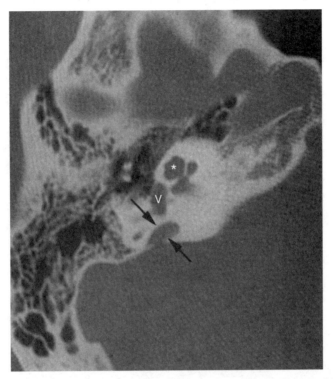

Reproduced, with permission, from Lalwani AK (ed.). *Current Diagnosis & Treatment: Otolaryngology—Head & Neck Surgery*, 3rd edn. New York: McGraw-Hill, 2012.

Avoid contact sports and wear head protection when possible; avoid roller coasters, weight lifting, scuba diving, and extreme/rigorous activities. (CT scan shows enlarged vestibular aqueduct.)

○ **CT scan of the temporal bones is performed on a 6-year-old boy with hearing loss. Findings include absence of the anterior 1 1/2 turns of the cochlea, a normally developed basal turn, wide vestibular aqueduct, plumb-deformed vestibule, and "empty cochlea." What is the likely diagnosis?**

Mondini malformation.

○ **How does otosclerosis appear on CT scan?**

Early on, areas of deossification, in particular, a double low attenuation ring paralleling the cochlear turns and lucencies along the margins of the oval window are present. As the disease progresses, foci of denser bone develop, eventually resulting in obliteration.

○ **What other diseases can mimic otosclerosis radiographically?**

Paget's disease and osteogenesis imperfecta.

○ **What distinguishes otosclerosis from Paget's disease radiographically?**

The radiographic changes are more extensive and pronounced with Paget's disease; they are also more likely to be bilateral and may include narrowing of the internal auditory canal (IAC).

○ **A 33-year-old woman complains of chronic disequilibrium and difficulty keeping her balance while jogging. Her physical examination is normal and complete audiometric examination shows unilateral low frequency conductive hearing loss (CHL) and normal acoustic reflexes. Below is a CT scan of her inner ear: What is the diagnosis?**

Reproduced, with permission, from Lalwani AK (ed.). *Current Diagnosis & Treatment: Otolaryngology—Head & Neck Surgery*, 3rd edn. New York: McGraw-Hill, 2012.

Superior SCC dehiscence.

○ **What is the differential diagnosis of a soft tissue mass on the promontory?**

Congenital cholesteatoma, paraganglioma, aberrant carotid artery, persistent stapedial artery, and glomus tympanicum.

○ **What is the accuracy of CT imaging in detecting bony erosion?**

85%.

○ **What is the main problem with using CT imaging to evaluate sinonasal tumors?**

Limited accuracy in differentiating soft tissue masses from secretions.

○ **A 16-year-old boy comes in with recurrent epistaxis. CT scan of the sinuses shows anterior bowing of the posterior wall of the maxillary antrum (Holman–Miller sign). What is the likely diagnosis?**

Juvenile nasopharyngeal angiofibroma.

○ **A 49-year-old woman comes in with headache and unilateral rhinorrhea. CT scan of the brain and sinuses shows an enlarged foramen cecum, crista galli erosion, increased interorbital distance, and a mixed soft tissue and fluid density mass. What is the likely diagnosis?**

Encephalocele.

○ A 23-year-old man comes in with chronic nasal congestion, sneezing, sinus pressure, and rhinorrhea. CT scan of the sinuses shows a peripheral rim of low-density edematous mucosa surrounding homogeneous, high-attenuation material in the maxillary and ethmoid sinuses bilaterally with scattered calcifications and sinus wall expansion. What is the likely diagnosis?

Allergic fungal sinusitis.

○ A limited coronal CT scan of the sinuses is least sensitive for detecting disease in which sinus?

Frontal sinus.

○ What percent of patients, asymptomatic with regard to their sinuses and undergoing CT scan of the head for other indications, have mucosal thickening of their sinuses?

24–39%.

○ How well do CT scan findings correlate with patient symptoms and endoscopic findings in patients with chronic rhinosinusitis?

Positive endoscopic findings correlate well with positive CT scans, but only 71% of patients with negative endoscopic findings will have a negative CT scan. CT scan findings correlate poorly with patient symptoms.

○ Where does mucosal thickening most often occur on CT scans of the sinuses?

Osteomeatal complex.

○ What is the incidence of incidental ethmoid mucosal thickening on CT scan in children?

30%.

○ Which plating material has been shown to have significantly less streak artifacts on CT scans?

Titanium (as compared with stainless steel and vitallium).

○ True/False: CT scan of the larynx underestimates the stage of laryngeal cancer.

True.

○ Why should radionuclide scanning precede CT scan imaging of the thyroid gland?

CT scan contrast will linger in the thyroid gland for up to 6 months and interfere with radionuclide scanning.

• • • MAGNETIC RESONANCE IMAGING • • •

○ What are the absolute contraindications to MRI?

Cardiac pacemaker, metallic intraocular foreign body, intracranial aneurysm clips.

○ What is a flow void?

Complete lack of signal after contrast due to moderate to high blood flow.

○ **How small of a lesion can MRI with gadolinium detect?**

2 mm.

○ **How small of a lesion can fast-spin echo MRI detect?**

4–5 mm.

○ **What should be applied when using fast-spin echo MRI?**

Fat saturation (otherwise fat will remain bright on T2 images with fast-spin echo).

○ **What is the signal intensity produced by fat on T1- and T2-weighted MRI?**

T1—high signal; T2—low signal.

○ **What is the signal intensity produced by water on T1- and T2-weighted MRI?**

T1—low signal; T2—high signal.

○ **Which temporal bone structures are best visualized with T1-weighted MRI?**

Nerves within the IAC.

○ **Which temporal bone structures are best visualized with T2-weighted MRI?**

Fluid-filled compartments.

○ **What problems can occur with MRI fat suppression at the skull base?**

Artifact, secondary to air meeting soft tissue, can obscure important anatomical details (i.e., foramina).

○ **An asymptomatic patient has an incidental finding of a high signal in the left petrous apex on T1-weighted images. What is the significance of this finding?**

Asymmetric pneumatization of the petrous tip is present in 4% of patients; the high signal is from the bone marrow.

○ **How does cholesterol granuloma appear on MRI?**

High signal on both T1- and T2-weighted images.

○ **How does a cholesteatoma appear on MRI?**

Intermediate signal on T1-weighted images and high signal on T2-weighted images.

○ **True/False: Cholesteatomas enhance with gadolinium.**

False.

○ **A 52-year-old man presents with a neck mass. Axial T1-weighted images of his neck show a round soft tissue mass with prominent flow voids at the level of the carotid bifurcation displacing the internal carotid artery posteriorly and the external carotid artery anteriorly. Postgadolinium, the mass enhances intensely. What is the likely diagnosis?**

Carotid body tumor.

○ **What are the typical findings of a meningioma on MRI?**

Broad based with "dural tail sign" on MRI with gadolinium.

○ **Using MRI, how can one distinguish inflammation from tumor in the sinuses?**

Tumor will be isointense on both T1- and T2-weighted images, while inflammation will be hyperintense on T2-weighted images.

○ **What are the typical MRI findings of hemangiomas?**

Serpentine high-volume flow voids surrounded by nonvascular soft tissue.

○ **A 62-year-old woman comes in for cerumen removal. Medial deviation of her soft palate is noted incidentally on examination and the rest of her physical examination is unremarkable. MRI of the neck is likely to show what?**

A deep-lobe parotid tumor with a "dumbbell" shape as it extends into the parapharyngeal space.

○ **What are the indications for MRI in a patient with tinnitus?**

Unilateral unexplained tinnitus with or without hearing loss; bilateral symmetrical or asymmetrical hearing loss suspicious for retrocochlear etiology (poor discrimination, absent acoustic reflexes, acoustic reflex decay, abnormal auditory brainstem response).

● ● ● ULTRASOUND ● ● ●

○ **What is the earliest gestational age that complete glottic atresia could be detected on ultrasound?**

22 weeks.

○ **What would the ultrasound show in a fetus with complete glottic atresia?**

Distension of the airway and lung parenchyma; flattening of the diaphragm; edema of the placenta; compression of the heart, great vessels, and thoracic duct.

○ **What are the advantages of ultrasound in the evaluation of thyroid nodules?**

Can detect nodules as small as 2–3 mm; can differentiate between solid, cystic, or mixed nodules with >90% accuracy; can detect the presence of lymph node enlargement.

○ **What findings on thyroid ultrasound are associated with an increased risk of malignancy?**

Irregular/indistinct margins, heterogeneous nodule echogenicity, intranodular vascular images, microcalcifications, complex cysts, and diameter >1 cm.

● ● ● NUCLEAR MEDICINE ● ● ●

○ **How does a PET/SPECT scan work?**

Radionuclide metabolic substrates are injected intravenously and detected by either production of positrons (PET) or by a directionally sensitive gamma camera (SPECT)—metabolically active tissues light up.

○   **What substrate is used in lymph node functioning imaging?**

Superparamagnetic iron oxide coated dextran.

○   **What is FDG?**

Fludeoxyglucose; a glucose analog with the radioactive isotope fluorine-18 substituted for one of the normal hydroxyl groups on the glucose molecule. It competes with glucose to enter into metabolically active cells. Like glucose, it is phosphorylated inside the cell, but unlike glucose-6-phosphate, FDG-6-phosphate cannot undergo further metabolism and becomes trapped.

○   **What is the half-life of FDG?**

20% is excreted quickly by the renal system; 80% remains in the tissues with a half-life of 110 minutes.

○   **What is the SUV?**

Standardized uptake value; ratio of FDG concentration in a region of interest to its concentration in the whole body.

○   **True/False: PET scans typically have minimal impact on T-staging following conventional assessment of head and neck tumors.**

True: PET scans are more valuable for providing additional information in relation to nodal and distant disease staging.

○   **Which type of tumors in the head and neck are less likely to be detected by FDG-PET?**

Salivary gland tumors and tumors with a large amount of necrosis.

○   **In patients with an unknown primary of the head and neck, how useful is a combined FDG-PET/CT scan in detecting the primary tumor site?**

Combined FDG-PET/CT scan will identify the primary in approximately 35% of cases of unknown primary.

○   **Which imaging device has the highest sensitivity and specificity for identifying and delineating residual and recurrent tumors of treated head and neck cancer?**

Combined FDG-PET/CT scan.

○   **What percentages of cold, warm/cool, and hot nodules on radioiodine scanning of the thyroid gland are malignant?**

17%, 13%, and 4%, respectively.

○   **What is the most useful application of thyroid scanning in patients with thyroid cancer?**

To detect residual thyroid tissue or occult distant metastases after thyroidectomy.

○   **Which cardiovascular medication will interfere with radioiodine scanning?**

Amiodarone.

○   **What is the optimal TSH value prior to radioiodine therapy?**
30 mU/L or higher.

○   **After ablation therapy, how often are repeat scans performed?**
6–12 months after ablation, then every 2 years.

○   **What is the most common long-term side effect from radioactive iodine therapy?**
Decreased saliva production.

○   **How long after ablation therapy should a woman avoid getting pregnant?**
One year.

○   **What study should be performed prior to reoperation for persistent or recurrent hyperparathyroidism?**
^{99}Tc sestamibi is 85% sensitive in experienced centers; accuracy is increased if the patient is placed on cytomel prior to the scan to suppress thyroid uptake.

○   **What imaging study is used to monitor the response to therapy for osteomyelitis?**
Gallium-67 scan.

○ 15-year-old boy presented with nasal obstruction and recurrent epistaxis. The polypoid mass shown below was resected and bled extensively. What is your diagnosis?

Juvenile nasopharyngeal angiofibroma. Histological features include an unencapsulated admixture of vascular tissue and fibrous stroma where the vessel walls lack elastic fibers and have decreased or no smooth muscle; mast cells are abundant in the stroma.

○ This firm, noncompressible nasal mass was resected from a young child. What is your diagnosis?

Glial heterotopia (nasal glioma).

○   **The tumor depicted below is most commonly found near the eyelid and in previously irradiated areas and is more common in patients with Muir–Torre syndrome. What is your diagnosis?**

Sebaceous carcinoma, characterized histologically by variously sized and irregularly shaped groups of sebaceous cells that contain lipid globules.

○   **What is the cell of origin of parotid gland squamous cell carcinoma?**

Excretory duct cell.

○   **The tumor shown below most commonly arises in the parotid gland of older males and is highly aggressive with a mean survival of 3 years. What is your diagnosis?**

Salivary duct adenocarcinoma.

○   **Following are three histopatholgical slides taken from parotid gland tumors. Name the type of tumor and their subtypes.**

A

B

C

Reproduced, with permission, from Wenig BM. *Atlas of Head and Neck Pathology.* Philadelphia: WB Saunders, 1993.

These are all adenoid cystic tumors.
"A" shows the cribriform pattern, which is the most common subtype (44%) and has a "Swiss cheese" appearance.
"B" shows the cribriform and tubular pattern, which is slightly less common (35%) and has the best prognosis.
"C" shows the solid pattern, which is the least common subtype (21%) and has the worst prognosis.

○   **The lesion below is also known as "papillary cystadenoma lymphomatosum," represents approximately 12% of benign tumors of the parotid gland, and is seen more commonly in smokers. What is the tumor?**

Warthin tumor, characterized histologically by papillary structures with lymphocytic infiltration, cystic areas, and double layers of granular eosinophilic cells.

○   **The low-grade malignant tumor shown below is most commonly found in the parotid gland, typically encased in a fibrous capsule, and is more common in females. What is your diagnosis?**

Reproduced, with permission, from Wenig BM. *Atlas of Head and Neck Pathology*. Philadelphia: WB Saunders, 1993.

Acinic cell carcinoma, characterized histologically by two cell types: serous acinar cells and cells with clear cytoplasm.

○   **The tumor below is the most common malignant tumor of the salivary glands and is more common in females. What is your diagnosis?**

Reproduced, with permission, from Wenig BM. *Atlas of Head and Neck Pathology*. Philadelphia: WB Saunders, 1993.

Mucoepidermoid carcinoma, showing the low-grade variant, which has a 5-year survival rate of 70% and 15-year disease-free survival rate of 50%.

○ **What feature distinguishes low-grade from high-grade mucoepidermoid carcinoma?**

The amount of mucin in the tumor.

○ **The tumor shown below is shown ultrastructurally to be composed of tumor cells filled with abundant mitochondria. It is most commonly found in the parotid gland but accounts for less than 1% of salivary gland tumors. What is your diagnosis?**

Oncocytoma.

○ **The benign tumor shown below accounts for 2% of salivary gland tumors, occurs most frequently in the parotid gland, is slightly more common in females, and shows a number of histologic patterns. What is your diagnosis?**

Basal cell adenoma.

○   **Which genus is responsible for the infection shown below, sometimes referred to as "lumpy jaw"?**

Patient with lumpy jaw

Actinomyces. Histopathology shows a sulfur granule.

○   **What are the histologic differences between a hemangioma and a vascular malformation?**
Cellular proliferation is characteristic of hemangiomas; vessel dilatation is characteristic of vascular malformations.

○   **What are the histologic features of vascular malformations?**
Dilated, ectatic vascular channels with a normal endothelial lining and areas of thrombosis.

○   **What are the typical histologic characteristics of lymphatic malformations?**
Multiple dilated lymphatic channels lined by a single layer of epithelium.

○   **What cells are unique to Hodgkin's lymphoma?**
Reed–Sternberg cells.

○   **What are the three main histologic types of rhabdomyosarcoma?**
Embryonal, alveolar, and pleomorphic.

○   **Which is most common in the head and neck?**
Embryonal.

○ **What are the characteristic histologic findings of recurrent respiratory papillomatosis?**

Exophytic papillary fronds of multilayered benign squamous epithelium containing fibrovascular cores; cytologic atypia, in particular, koilocytotic atypia, is not unusual.

○ **What test is used to diagnose invasive fungal sinusitis?**

Tissue biopsy.

○ **What are the histologic findings of invasive fungal sinusitis?**

Hyphae with tissue invasion and noncaseating granulomas.

○ **What feature seen on renal biopsy with electron microscopy is pathognomonic for Alport syndrome?**

Basket-weave configuration of the glomerular basement membrane.

○ **What other test can be useful in diagnosing Alport syndrome?**

Skin biopsy.

○ **What histologic finding distinguishes cholesteatoma from cholesterol granuloma?**

Squamous epithelium is present only in cholesteatomas.

○ **What cell patterns are characteristic of vestibular schwannomas?**

Antoni A (tightly arranged) and Antoni B (loosely arranged).

○ **In which pattern are Verocay's bodies found?**

Antoni A.

○ **True/False: Tumors with a high percentage of Antoni A cells relative to Antoni B cells have a better prognostic outcome.**

False: Outcome is independent of cell proportions.

○ **How does one differentiate between a benign and a malignant paraganglioma?**

There are no clear histologic characteristics of malignancy; malignant lesions are defined by the presence of metastases.

○ **What are the two primary cells of paragangliomas?**

Type I granule-storing chief cells and type II Schwann-like sustentacular cells (S-100 positive) arranged in a cluster called a Zellballen.

○ **What are the histologic features of basal cell carcinoma of the skin?**

Clefting, lack of intracellular bridges, nuclear palisading, and peritumoral lacunae.

○ **What histologic characteristic of recurrent basal cell cancers has negative prognostic significance?**

Irregularity in the peripheral palisade.

○ **What are the histologic features of squamous cell carcinoma of the skin?**

Keratin pearls in well-differentiated lesions; poorly differentiated lesions may require identification with a cytokeratin or vimentin.

○ **Which classification system for melanoma is based on histologic layers?**

Clark's.

○ **What are the levels defined in Clark's system?**

Level I: Epidermis.
Level II: Invasion of basal lamina into the papillary dermis.
Level III: Fill the papillary dermis.
Level IV: Invasion into the reticular dermis.
Level V: Invasion into subcutaneous fat.

○ **Which classification system is based on depth of invasion by millimeters?**

Breslow's.

○ **What are the histopathologic features of synovial sarcoma of the head and neck?**

Poorly differentiated, high-grade malignant neoplasms arising from pluripotential mesenchymal cells; biphasic cellular pattern containing spindle cells and epithelioid cells; microcalcifications in 30–60%; the existence of monophasic forms, containing either spindle or epithelioid cells, is controversial.

○ **What are the classifications of nasopharyngeal cancer designated by the WHO?**

Type I: Well-differentiated, keratinizing SCCA.
Type II: Poorly differentiated, nonkeratinizing SCCA.
Type III: Lymphoepithelioma or undifferentiated.

○ **Which of these is characterized by syncytia (fused multinuclear giant cells)?**

Type III.

○ **Which of these is most common in North America? Least common?**

Most common is type III (70%); least common is type II (10%).

○ **Which of these is not associated with positive Ebstein-Barr virus titers?**

Type I.

○ **What histological pattern is characteristic of an olfactory neuroblastoma?**

Homer–Wright rosettes.

○ **Which cells in the thyroid gland secrete calcitonin?**

Parafollicular or C cells.

○ **Name the thyroid tumor.**

Large polygonal thyroid follicular cells with abundant granular cytoplasm and numerous mitochondria	Hürthle cell thyroid cancer
Calcified laminated bodies called psammoma bodies; elongated, pale nuclei with a ground glass appearance (Orphan Annie eyes)	Papillary thyroid cancer
Nests of small, round cells; amyloid; dense, irregular areas of calcification	Medullary thyroid carcinoma
Cuboidal epithelial cells with large nuclei in a well-structured follicular pattern extending beyond the tumor's capsule	Follicular thyroid cancer

○ **What histological subtypes of thyroid tumors are associated with an increased risk of local recurrence and metastasis?**

Tall cell, columnar, insular, solid variant, and poorly differentiated.

CHAPTER 22 Laboratory Studies

○ **What are the only antigen-specific tests for syphilis?**

Fluorescent treponemal antibody-absorption (FTA-ABS) and microhemagglutination assay-treponema pallidum (MHA-TP) tests.

○ **What test is used to screen for syphilis?**

Venereal disease research laboratory (VDRL).

○ **True/False: FTA-ABS becomes negative once a patient has been adequately treated for syphilis.**

False.

○ **What are some common laboratory findings in patients with sarcoidosis?**

Hypergammaglobulinemia, elevated liver function tests, calcium, ESR, and angiotensin-converting enzyme (ACE).

○ **What is an abnormal Schirmer test?**

Less than 5 mm wetting after 5 minutes; less than 10 mm wetting after stimulation with 10% ammonia.

○ **What tests are use to diagnose Sjögren's syndrome?**

Minor salivary gland biopsy showing mononuclear cell infiltration, SS-A, SS-B, ANA, and RF.

○ **What laboratory test is associated with lymphoproliferative malignancy in patients with Sjögren's syndrome?**

Decreased level of serum IgM.

○ **What are the typical laboratory findings in patients with relapsing polychondritis?**

Elevated ESR, moderate leukocytosis, mild-to-moderate anemia.

○ **What lab test is most specific for Wegener's?**

c-ANCA.

○   **What is the significance of a rising c-ANCA titer in a patient with Wegener's?**
Usually indicates a relapse of active disease.

○   **HLA-DW4 antibodies are most commonly seen in which autoimmune disease?**
Rhuematoid arthritis.

○   **What autoantibody is present in 75% of patients with rheumatoid arthritis?**
Rheumatoid factor

○   **What is the most specific test for the diagnosis of autoimmune sensorineural hearing loss?**
Western blot assay for 68 kD inner ear antigen (Otoblot) (95% specific).

○   **The 68 kDa antigen is thought to represent what protein?**
Heat shock protein 70.

○   **What percent of patients with immune-mediated Menière's disease will have a positive anti-68-kD Western blot test?**
30–50%.

○   **What is the most specific test for the diagnosis of Cogan's syndrome?**
Western blot assay for 55 kD inner ear antigen.

○   **Patient with Cogan's syndrome usually have elevated titers to what organism?**
Chlamydia.

○   **What is the latency period for developing antibodies to hepatitis C?**
Up to 4 months.

○   **What is the latency period for seroconversion following exposure to the HIV virus?**
6–12 months.

○   **What adjunctive test should be performed in a female with suspected juvenile nasopharyngeal angiofibroma?**
Chromosome analysis.

○   **What test is used to diagnose pertussis?**
Culture from the nasopharynx using a Dacron or calcium alginate swab placed on a Regan–Lowe or Bordet–Gengou agar plate.

○   **What is the sensitivity of this test?**
80% (less if already on antibiotics).

○ **What tests confirm the diagnosis of infectious mononucleosis?**

Blood smear showing atypical mononuclear cells and a positive Paul–Bunnell test (elevated heterophile titer of Epstein–Barr virus).

○ **What is the most useful study of nontuberculous mycobacterial adenitis of the head and neck region in children?**

Culture.

○ **What test should be performed in a patient with suspected allergic fungal sinusitis who does not have classic findings on CT scan or positive middle meatal cultures?**

Aspergillus skin test and precipitins.

○ **How is congenital cytomegalovirus (CMV) diagnosed in the newborn?**

Identification of serum anti-CMV IgM, "owl eye" bodies in the urinary sediment, and intracerebral calcifications on radiographs.

○ **What is the most accurate method of determining if otorrhea is CSF?**

β-2-transferrin assay.

○ **What are the characteristics of CSF in the presence of meningitis?**

Elevated protein, WBC, and pressure; decreased glucose.

○ **What laboratory tests can be used to diagnose CSF leak?**

Measurement of glucose (nasal secretions are devoid of glucose), β-2-transferrin.

○ **What is the single best measure of nutritional status?**

Serum albumin level.

○ **What serum albumin level is associated with malnutrition?**

Less than 3 g/dL.

○ **Which serum proteins can be used to assess short-term nutritional status?**

Transferrin (half-life of 8–9 days), prealbumin (half-life of 2 days), and retinal-binding globulin (half-life of 12 hours).

○ **All patients with a paraganglioma should be tested for mutations in which gene?**

SDH (succinate dehydrogenase).

○ **What are the most common immunologic findings among patients with nasopharyngeal carcinoma (NPC)?**

Elevated IgA and IgG antibodies against the viral capsid antigen of EBV.

○ **What is the role of ascertaining EBV titers in patients with NPC?**

May be a valuable screening tool in high-risk populations and can help establish the diagnosis of NPC in the patient with an unknown primary. In patients with type I disease, EBV titers are not elevated and have no prognostic significance.

○ **What percent of patients with WHO types II and III tumors have abnormally increased titers to EBV VCA and NA?**

80–90%.

○ **What test provides prognostic information in patients with NPC?**

Antibody-dependent cellular cytotoxicity (ADCC) assay.

○ **How does this assay predict survival?**

Low levels are associated with worse prognosis.

○ **How do you test for multiple myeloma in a patient with extramedullary plasmacytoma?**

Measure serum M-protein and urine Bence Jones protein; bone survey; bone marrow biopsy.

○ **What test is used to distinguish a hypothalamic defect from a pituitary defect in a patient with hypothyroidism?**

The thyrotropin-releasing hormone (TRH) stimulation test.

○ **True/False: Thyroglobulin levels should be obtained prior to performing FNA on a thyroid nodule.**

True: FNA will falsely elevate thyroglobulin levels.

○ **What is the purpose of obtaining a thyroglobulin level prior to thyroidectomy?**

Thyroglobulin has been shown to correlate well with histologic tumor type and is useful as a marker for tumor recurrence.

○ **What test should be ordered in a patient with an elevated TSH?**

Antimicrosomal antibody (antithyroperoxidase level) to rule out Hashimoto's thyroiditis.

○ **What lab test should be obtained in patients with a family history of medullary thyroid cancer (MTC)?**

Calcitonin.

○ **What laboratory workup is necessary in patients with MTC?**

Basal and pentagastrin stimulated calcitonin levels, serum calcium, 24-hour urine catecholamines, VMA, and metanephrine, +/−CEA.

○ **What are the histochemical characteristics of MTC?**

Congo red dye positive, apple-green birefringence consistent with amyloid; immunohistochemistry positive for cytokeratins, CEA, and calcitonin.

○   **What is the false-negative rate of RET analysis?**

5%.

○   **What is the most accurate test for diagnosis of primary hyperparathyroidism?**

Measurement of intact PTH.

○   **Why is measurement of the C-terminal of PTH not accurate for diagnosis of secondary hyperparathyroidism?**

C-terminal fragments are cleared by the kidney; elevation may indicate either renal insufficiency or hyperparathyroidism.

○   **What is the difference in the Ca/Cr clearance ratio in someone with FHH and someone with primary hyperparathyroidism?**

Ca/Cr clearance <0.01 in FHH; >0.02 in primary hyperparathyroidism.

CHAPTER 23

Psychological, Social, and Occupational Assessment

○ **What is the primary limitation of the University of Washington Quality of Life Instrument, version 4?**

Does not assess psychological issues.

○ **In patients with head and neck cancer undergoing chemoradiation, when do quality of life scores rise above pretreatment QOL scores?**

6–12 months after treatment.

○ **What are the two most common residual symptoms after successful treatment of head and neck cancer with chemoradiation?**

Xerostomia and dysphagia.

○ **True/False: Laryngeal cancer patients who undergo chemoradiation with organ preservation have overall better quality of life than those who undergo total laryngectomy.**

True.

○ **What methods have been shown to help ameliorate the adverse effects of chemoradiation in head and neck cancer patients?**

Speech therapy, swallowing therapy, intensity-modulated radiation therapy, amifostine.

○ **What is the leading cause of years lost to disability in the world today?**

Major depression.

○ **A 16-year-old boy is suspended from school for cheating on an exam. He has several close friends. He occasionally has difficulty falling asleep but his mood is generally good. What would his GAF (global assessment of functioning) score be?**

70.

○ **What are the three most common psychiatric conditions encountered in patients seeking cosmetic surgery?**

Narcissistic and histrionic personality disorders and body dysmorphic disorder.

131

○ **What is the Occupational Safety and Health Administration's limit for noise exposure without hearing protection?**

140 dB.

○ **A patient with Menière's disease has been disabled for >1 year and is on disability. What functional level is he/she?**

6.

○ **A patient with a Karnovsky scale score between 50% and 70% is at what level of functioning?**

Not able to work but able to care for most of his/her personal needs and live at home.

Section III

DISEASES, DISORDERS, AND CONDITIONS

CHAPTER 24 Neoplastic

○ **What is the most common site of laryngeal cancer?**

Glottis.

○ **What are the seven different types of squamous cell aberrations occurring in the larynx?**

Benign hyperplasia, benign keratosis (no atypia), atypical hyperplasia, keratosis with atypia or dysplasia, intraepithelial carcinoma, microinvasive squamous cell carcinoma (SCCA), and invasive SCCA.

○ **What percent of patients with carcinoma in situ of the vocal cord will develop invasive SCCA after a single excisional biopsy?**

One in six (16.7%).

○ **What is "microinvasive" SCCA of the vocal cord?**

Invades through the basement membrane but not into the vocalis muscle.

○ **What is Ackerman's tumor?**

Verrucous carcinoma, thought to be less radiosensitive and less likely to metastasize than SCCA.

○ **What are the two most important factors predicting lymph node metastasis in laryngeal cancer?**

Tumor size and location.

○ **True/False: Once invasion of the laryngeal framework occurs, the ossified portions of cartilage have the least resistance to tumor spread.**

True.

○ **What percent of glottic tumors display perineural and vascular invasion?**

25%.

○ **What percent of patients with a primary laryngeal cancer will eventually develop a 2nd primary?**

10–20%.

○ **What is the stage of a transglottic tumor without vocal cord fixation, cartilage invasion, or extension beyond the larynx?**
T2.

○ **Which parts of the glottis are most difficult to treat with radiation?**
Anterior commissure, posterior 1/3 of the vocal cord.

○ **What percent of these tumors will metastasize to the cervical lymph nodes?**
25%.

○ **What are the two most common reasons for tumor recurrence after hemilaryngectomy?**
Inability to recognize the inferior tumor margin and spread of tumor through the cricothyroid membrane.

○ **What is the incidence of positive cervical nodes in patients with T3 glottic tumors?**
30–40%.

○ **Which type of laryngeal cancer is mostly likely to metastasize distally?**
Supraglottic.

○ **What is the most common site of distant metastasis from laryngeal carcinoma?**
Lungs.

○ **How does metastatic disease to the lungs normally present?**
Multiple small lesions less than 3 mm that are difficult to detect on X-ray.

○ **Where does supraglottic carcinoma most often begin?**
Junction of the epiglottis and false cords.

○ **What anatomic structure serves as a natural barrier to the inferior extension of supraglottic cancers?**
Ventricle (embryologic development is completely separate from the false cord).

○ **Which kinds of supraglottic cancers are more likely to extend inferiorly to the anterior commissure or ventricle—ulcerative or exophytic?**
Ulcerative lesions.

○ **True/False: Stage I lesions of the supraglottis can be controlled equally well with radiotherapy or surgery.**
True.

○ **What is the risk of cervical metastases in patients with T1, T2, T3, and T4 tumors of the supraglottis?**
Approximately 20%, 40%, 60%, and 80%, respectively.

○ **What percent of patients undergoing supraglottic laryngectomy and unilateral neck dissection will fail in the contralateral neck?**

16%, despite receiving radiation therapy to the area.

○ **What percent will fail if bilateral neck dissections are performed?**

9%.

○ **What percent of laryngeal tumors are primarily subglottic?**

5%.

○ **What are the differences between primary and secondary subglottic tumors?**

Primary tumors are less common, usually present with stridor or dyspnea and at a more advanced stage, and have a worse survival time than secondary tumors.

○ **What is the primary site of lymphatic drainage from subglottic tumors?**

Paratracheal nodes.

○ **Compared with supraglottic and glottic tumors, subglottic tumors are at a much higher risk for developing what?**

Stomal recurrence.

○ **What is the treatment of choice for primary subglottic cancer?**

Total laryngectomy, bilateral neck dissection, near total thyroidectomy, paratracheal node dissection, and postoperative radiation to the superior mediastinum and stoma; if the anterior cervical esophageal wall is involved, then laryngopharyngectomy with cervical esophagectomy instead of total laryngectomy.

○ **What was the first published randomized trial for organ preservation in head and neck cancer?**

The VA trial for SCCA of the larynx.

○ **What were the treatment arms?**

1. Surgery.
2. Two cycles of cisplatinum and 5-fluorouracil.
   a. Responders received a 3rd cycle followed by XRT.
   b. Nonresponders had surgery +/− postoperative XRT.

○ **What was the outcome of this study?**

No significant difference in survival among the three arms.

○ **What are the three major randomized studies on organ preservation as treatment for laryngeal cancer?**

VA, GETTEC, and EORTC.

○ **What conclusions can be made based on meta-analysis of these studies?**

The surgical patients had slightly higher (but not significant) survival advantage (6%). Among patients receiving chemotherapy, 58% were able to keep their larynx. Better outcomes were seen in patients with hypopharyngeal cancer who underwent chemotherapy than in those with laryngeal cancer.

○ **What is the best organ-sparing treatment for a patient with stage III SCCA of the supraglottis?**
Induction chemotherapy followed by radiation therapy.

○ **What are the indications for postoperative radiation after neck dissection?**
Multiple nodes or extracapsular spread.

○ **What is the significance of the number of pathologically positive nodes on prognosis?**
Greater than 3 pathologically positive nodes is a negative prognostic indicator.

○ **True/False: Chemosensitive tumors are usually radiosensitive.**
True.

○ **Which types of radiation beams are used for superficial tumors and why?**
Electron beams; their finite range spares deeper tissues.

○ **True/False: The dose of radiation necessary to kill hypoxic cells is 2.5–3.0 times greater than that required to kill well-oxygenated cells.**
True, as free radical formation requires oxygen.

○ **True/False: Cells undergoing DNA synthesis in the S phase are much more radiosensitive than cells in other phases of the cell cycle.**
False: They are much more radioresistant in the S phase.

○ **True/False: The cells responsible for acute radiation injuries are rapidly cycling.**
True.

○ **Which type of cancer is most sensitive to radiation therapy: exophytic, infiltrative, or ulcerated?**
Exophytic.

○ **When, after XRT or radiation therapy, is a positive biopsy a reliable indicator of persistent disease?**
3 months after treatment.

○ **How do XRT or radiation therapy failures differ from surgical failures in site of recurrence?**
XRT or radiation therapy failures often occur in the center of areas that were grossly involved with cancer initially, whereas surgical failures often occur at the periphery of the original tumor.

○ **What is conventional fractionated radiotherapy?**
1.8–2.5 Gy every day, five fractions every week, for 4–8 weeks (total dose 60–65 Gy for small tumors, 65–70 Gy for larger tumors).

○ **How is an altered fractionated schedule different?**

Lower dose per fraction, two or more fractions every day, decreased overall treatment time, with total dose same or higher.

○ **What are the two categories of altered fractionation?**

Accelerated and hyperfractionated.

○ **What is the difference between these?**

Accelerated: Total dose is the same as conventional treatment, but overall treatment time is decreased. Hyperfractionated: Overall treatment time is the same as conventional treatment, but total dose is increased, dose per fraction is decreased, and the number of fractions is increased.

○ **What impact does hyperfractionated therapy have on locoregional control and survival rates compared with conventional therapy?**

Significantly higher locoregional control and survival rates.

○ **What were the results from the EORTC 22851 study comparing accelerated split-course XRT with conventional XRT?**

The accelerated course resulted in significantly higher late side effects without significant locoregional control or survival advantage.

○ **What were the results from the RTOG 9003 study evaluating accelerated treatments with concomitant boost?**

This protocol resulted in significantly higher locoregional control and survival rates with somewhat higher rate of late side effects compared with conventional XRT.

○ **Radiation is not as effective for tumors with which characteristics?**

High volume, cartilage destroying, with bulky lymph node disease.

○ **What is the maximum dose of radiation to the spinal cord?**

45 Gy (increased risk of radiation myelitis above this level).

○ **What are the advantages of planned preoperative XRT or radiation therapy?**

Unresectable tumors may be made resectable; the extent of surgical resection may be diminished; the treatment portals preoperatively are usually smaller than those used postoperatively; microscopic disease is more radiosensitive preoperatively due to better blood supply; the viability of tumor cells that may be disseminated by surgical manipulation is diminished.

○ **What are the disadvantages of planned preoperative XRT or radiation therapy?**

Wound healing is more difficult, and the dose that can be safely delivered preoperatively is less than that which can be given postoperatively.

○ **What are the advantages of postoperative XRT or radiation therapy?**

The anatomic extent of the tumor can be determined surgically, making it easier to define the treatment portals required; a greater dose can be given postoperatively than preoperatively; the total dose to be given can be determined on the basis of residual tumor burden after surgery; surgical resection is easier and healing is better in nonirradiated tissue.

○ **True/False: XRT or radiation therapy should not be delayed in the presence of a fistula, open wound, or bony exposure.**

True: As long as the carotid artery is not exposed, radiation treatments should never be delayed.

○ **What is the primary role of concomitant chemoradiation in the treatment of head and neck cancer?**

To improve local and regional control in patients with unresectable disease.

○ **What is the primary problem with concomitant chemoradiation?**

Acute toxicities are markedly increased and result in patient noncompliance.

○ **Which patients are more likely to benefit from adjuvant chemotherapy?**

Those with high-risk tumors (extracapsular extension, carcinoma-in-situ, close surgical margins) and those with locally advanced nasopharyngeal cancer.

○ **What were the three treatment arms in the Head and Neck Intergroup R91-11 trial?**

Induction chemotherapy (cisplatin and 5-FU) versus radiation alone versus concomitant cisplatin and radiation therapy for the treatment of potentially resectable stage III and IV cancer of the larynx.

○ **Which arm had the best outcome?**

Concomitant cisplatinum and radiation therapy significantly increased the time to laryngectomy.

○ **What can be said of the presence of level V cervical metastases from SCCA of the upper aerodigestive tract?**

Uncommon (7%) and, if present, most likely to occur in the presence of level IV metastases.

○ **For SCCA of the tongue, invasion beyond __ is associated with a significantly higher incidence of lymph node metastasis.**

4 mm (30% vs. 7% if 4 mm or less invasion).

○ **True/False: Disease-free, but not overall, survival is improved in patients with early oral tongue cancer who undergo elective neck dissection.**

True.

○ **When SCCA grossly invades the adventitia of the carotid artery, how will resection of the artery affect survival?**

It will not improve long-term survival.

○ **True/False: Hypopharyngeal cancer has the worst prognosis of all head and neck cancers.**

True: 70% of patients present with advanced disease (stage III and IV) and the 5-year disease-specific survival is only 33%.

○ **What are the most common and least common sites of tumor involvement in the hypopharynx?**

Pyriform sinus is the most common site (75%); postcricoid area is the least common site (3–4%).

○ **How does the behavior of pyriform sinus tumors differ from postcricoid and posterior pharyngeal wall tumors?**

Tumors of the pyriform sinus tend to infiltrate deeply at early stages, whereas those of the postcricoid area and posterior pharyngeal wall tend to remain superficial until achieving an advanced stage.

○ **What features of hypopharyngeal tumors distinguish them from other head and neck tumors?**

Propensity for early submucosal spread and skip lesions.

○ **What significance do these features have on treatment?**

Wide surgical margins (4–6 cm inferior to gross, 2–3 cm superior to gross) and wide radiation therapy ports are necessary.

○ **What is the incidence of cervical metastases at the time of presentation of pyriform sinus tumors? What percent are bilateral or fixed?**

60%; 25%.

○ **True/False: The size of the primary lesion is related to the incidence of lymph node metastases in tumors of the hypopharynx.**

False.

○ **Where do posterior pharyngeal wall tumors metastasize?**

Bilaterally to level II cervical nodes, mediastinum, and superiorly to the nodes of Rouviere at the skull base.

○ **Which site of the hypopharynx drains bilaterally into levels IV and VI?**

Postcricoid area.

○ **True/False: The involvement of the medial (as opposed to lateral) wall of the pyriform sinus significantly increases the likelihood of *bilateral* cervical metastasis.**

True.

○ **True/False: Due to the high incidence of cervical metastases, treatment of the neck is necessary in all patients with hypopharyngeal cancer.**

True.

○ **What is the incidence of a 2nd primary at the time of diagnosis in patients with hypopharyngeal cancer?**
5–8%.

○ **What are the most common presenting symptoms in patients with tumor of the retromolar trigone?**
Referred otalgia and trismus.

○ **How many years does it take for a former smoker to have the same probability of developing an oral cavity cancer as a nonsmoker?**
16 years.

○ **What is the chance that a patient cured of an oral cavity cancer will develop a 2nd primary if they continue to smoke?**
40%.

○ **What is the incidence of cervical metastases from base of tongue, tonsil, and soft palate SCCA?**
70%, 60%, and 40%, respectively.

○ **What is the incidence of malignancy in adults with asymmetric tonsils with normal-appearing mucosa and no cervical lymphadenopathy?**
5%.

○ **What percent of T3/T4 tumors of the tonsil can be salvaged after failing primary XRT?**
50%.

○ **What are the risk factors for developing osteosarcoma in the mandible or maxilla?**
History of ionizing radiation, fibrous dysplasia, retinoblastoma, and prior exposure to thorium oxide (radioactive scanning agent).

○ **What chromosomal abnormality do osteosarcoma and retinoblastoma have in common?**
Deletion of the long arm of chromosome 13.

○ **True/False: There is a much lower risk of distant metastases with osteosarcoma of the head and neck than that of the long bones.**
True.

○ **What is the most common cause of death in osteosarcoma of the head and neck?**
Intracranial extension.

○ **What is the optimal treatment for osteosarcoma of the head and neck?**
Surgery and radiation therapy.

○   **True/False: A patient with T3N2aM0 SCCA of the base of tongue has a complete response to external-beam radiation therapy both at the primary site and the neck. A planned neck dissection should be done to increase the rate of regional control.**

True.

○   **What are the three most common odontogenic tumors?**

Ameloblastoma, cementoma, and odontoma.

○   **What are the three most common odontogenic cysts?**

Radicular cyst (65%), odontogenic keratocyst, and dentigerous cyst.

○   **What are odontomas composed of?**

Enamel, dentin, cementum, and pulp.

○   **Where does a radicular or periapical cyst occur?**

Along the root of a nonviable tooth, as the liquefied stage of a dental granuloma.

○   **Where do dentigerous cysts develop?**

Around the crown of an unerupted, impacted tooth.

○   **Multiple odontogenic keratocysts are a manifestation of what syndrome?**

Basal cell nevus syndrome.

○   **What is a Pindborg tumor?**

Calcified epithelial odontogenic tumor that is less aggressive than ameloblastoma and is associated with an impacted tooth.

○   **Which mandibular tumor or cyst produces white, keratin-containing fluid?**

Odontogenic keratocyst.

○   **What is the incidence of recurrence after excision of odontogenic keratocyst?**

62% in the first 5 years.

○   **What percent of parotid gland tumors are benign?**

75–80%.

○   **What is the most common site of a salivary gland neoplasm?**

Parotid gland (73%).

○   **What is the least common site of a salivary gland neoplasm?**

Submandibular gland (11%).

○ **What is the most common site of a *malignant* salivary gland neoplasm?**

Minor salivary glands (60%; of these, 40% occur on the palate).

○ **What is the least common site of a malignant salivary gland neoplasm?**

Parotid gland (32%).

○ **Which salivary gland has the best prognosis for malignant tumors?**

Parotid gland.

○ **Which salivary gland has the worst prognosis for malignant tumors?**

Submandibular gland.

○ **What is the most common tumor of the parotid gland?**

Pleomorphic adenoma in adults, hemangioma in children.

○ **How does metastasizing pleomorphic adenoma differ from carcinoma ex-pleomorphic adenoma?**

It is histologically benign, lacking malignant epithelial components.

○ **What is the most common malignant tumor of the parotid gland in adults?**

Mucoepidermoid carcinoma.

○ **What is the most important prognostic factor for malignant salivary gland neoplasms?**

Stage.

○ **Which five salivary gland tumors have the worst prognosis?**

High-grade mucoepidermoid, adenocarcinoma, squamous cell carcinoma, undifferentiated carcinoma, and carcinoma ex-pleomorphic adenoma.

○ **What are the indications for postoperative radiation after parotidectomy?**

High probability of residual microscopic disease; positive margins; advanced stage; high grade; deep lobe tumors; recurrent tumors; the presence of regional metastases; and angiolymphatic invasion.

○ **What factors are predictors of occult regional disease in parotid cancer?**

Extracapsular extension, preoperative facial paralysis, age >54 years, and perilymphatic invasion.

○ **What are the indications for neck dissection in the treatment of salivary gland malignancies?**

Clinical metastasis, submandibular tumor, SCCA, undifferentiated carcinoma, size >4 cm, and high-grade mucoepidermoid carcinoma.

○ **What is the most common site of distant metastasis for adenoid cystic carcinoma?**

Lung.

○ **What is the incidence of subclinical neck disease with adenoid cystic carcinoma of the parotid gland?**
Approximately 10%.

○ **What is the most common salivary gland malignancy following radiation?**
Mucoepidermoid.

○ **What is the most common malignancy of the submandibular and minor salivary glands?**
Adenoid cystic.

○ **What type of tumor comprises 50% of all lacrimal gland neoplasms?**
Adenoid cystic.

○ **What are the four types of growth patterns of adenoid cystic carcinoma and which is most common?**
Cribriform (most common—looks like Swiss cheese), tubular/ductular, trabecular, and solid.

○ **Which type of radiation therapy does adenoid cystic carcinoma respond best to?**
Neutron beam.

○ **What is the most common salivary gland malignancy to occur bilaterally?**
Acinic cell.

○ **What are the two most common malignant tumors of the parotid gland in children younger than 12?**
Mucoepidermoid is the most common, followed by acinic cell.

○ **What is the incidence of cervical metastasis of mucoepidermoid carcinomas?**
30–40%.

○ **Your patient has a mucoepidermoid carcinoma of the parotid gland. Histologic evaluation of the biopsy specimen reveals a scant amount of mucin. There is no clinical evidence of regional metastasis. Do you treat the neck?**
Yes.

○ **What is the second most common malignant tumor of the minor salivary glands?**
Adenocarcinoma.

○ **What are the four types of monomorphic adenomas?**
Basal cell, trabecular, canalicular, and tubular.

○ **Which salivary gland tumor is more common in women with a history of breast cancer?**
Mucoepidermoid carcinoma.

○   **What is the treatment of choice for metastatic cutaneous SCCA to the parotid?**
Total parotidectomy with preservation of VII (unless invaded by tumor) and postoperative radiation therapy to the parotid area and ipsilateral neck.

○   **What percent of malignant tumors of the parotid gland present with facial nerve weakness or paralysis?**
20%.

○   **Which salivary gland tumor has a high propensity for perineural invasion?**
Adenoid cystic carcinoma.

○   **What are the clinical features of salivary duct carcinomas?**
Most commonly involve the parotid gland and present as an asymptomatic mass; higher incidence in males; distant metastases are the most common cause of death.

○   **Parapharyngeal tumors arising from the deep lobe of the parotid will involve which compartment?**
Prestyloid compartment.

○   **What happens to the carotid sheath with deep lobe parotid tumors extending into the parapharyngeal space?**
It is displaced posteriorly.

○   **Which compartment are neurogenic tumors most likely to arise in?**
Poststyloid compartment.

○   **What is the most common tumor of the parapharyngeal space?**
Pleomorphic adenoma.

○   **What percent of head and neck paragangliomas are familial?**
7–10%.

○   **What is the most common paraganglioma of the head and neck?**
Carotid body tumor.

○   **What percent of carotid body tumors are multicentric?**
10% (30–40% in the hereditary form).

○   **What is the inheritance pattern of familial carotid body tumors?**
Autosomal dominant but only the genes passed from the paternal side are expressed (maternal genomic imprinting).

○   **What is a "nonchromaffin" paraganglioma?**
One that does not secrete significant amounts of catecholamines.

○ **What percent of cervical paragangliomas secrete catecholamines?**

5%.

○ **What percent of cervical paragangliomas are associated with an underlying germline mutation in the gene encoding succinate dehydrogenase (SDH)?**

40%.

○ **What is Shamblin's classification system for carotid body tumors?**

Group I: Small and easily excised.

Group II: Adherent to the vessels; resectable with careful subadventitial dissection.

Group III: Encase the carotid; require partial or complete vessel resection

○ **What are the two types of temporal bone paragangliomas?**

Glomus jugulare involving the adventitia of the jugular bulb and glomus tympanicum involving Jacobson's nerve (jugulotympanic glomus if unable to discern site of origin).

○ **How do glomus tumors differ clinically from carotid body tumors?**

More common in females, less likely to secrete catecholamines or metastasize, and are more radiosensitive.

○ **What is the primary advantage of stereotactic radiosurgery for treatment of recurrent glomus jugulare tumors compared with surgery and conventional radiation?**

Lower incidence of cranial nerve injury.

○ **When is stereotactic radiosurgery contraindicated in the treatment of recurrent glomus jugulare tumors?**

For larger tumors (>3.0–4.0 cm).

○ **How do most glomus jugulare tumors respond to external beam radiation?**

Less than 50% show tumor regression radiographically; lack of tumor growth is more common.

○ **After having a basal or squamous cell carcinoma of the skin, what are the chances of developing another one within 5 years?**

50%.

○ **What is basal cell-nevoid syndrome?**

Autosomal dominant disorder characterized by multiple basal cell carcinomas, odontogenic keratocysts, rib abnormalities, palmar and plantar pits, and calcification of the falx cerebri.

○ **What are some other genetic disorders that are associated with a high risk of cutaneous malignancies?**

Xeroderma pigmentosum, albinism, epidermodysplastic verruciformis, epidermolysis bullosa dystrophica, and dyskeratosis congenital.

○ **Which UV light is most responsible for acute actinic damage?**

B.

○ **Other than UV light and genetics, what are some other factors that increase the risk of cutaneous malignancy?**

Long-term immunosuppression after organ transplantation, long-term treatment of psoriasis with photosensitizing chemicals, chronic ulcers, and low-dose irradiation.

○ **What is Marjolin's ulcer?**

Burn or ulcer associated with the development of malignancy.

○ **What is the most common premalignant skin lesion of the head and neck?**

Actinic keratosis.

○ **What is the name of the skin lesion, most commonly located on the nose, characterized by rapid growth with a central area of ulceration followed by spontaneous involution?**

Keratoacanthoma.

○ **What is Bowen's disease?**

Squamous cell carcinoma in situ of the skin.

○ **True/False: Adnexal carcinomas of the skin are very aggressive and have a poor prognosis.**

True.

○ **Which adnexal skin carcinoma arises from a pluripotential basal cell within or around the hair cells?**

Merkel cell carcinoma.

○ **What virus is strongly associated with Merkel cell carcinoma that is known to cause cancer in animals?**

Merkel cell polyomavirus.

○ **What is the 5-year survival of patients with Merkel cell carcinoma?**

30%.

○ **What test should be ordered in the workup of Merkel cell carcinoma?**

Positron emission tomography scan.

○ **Should the N0 neck be treated in patients with Merkel cell carcinoma?**

Yes.

○ **What is the most common type of skin sarcoma?**

Malignant fibrous histiocytoma.

○ **What are the five main types of basal cell carcinomas?**
Nodular, cystic, superficial multicentric, morpheaform, and keratotic.

○ **Which of these is most common?**
Nodular.

○ **Which of these is more commonly found on the extremities or trunk?**
Superficial multicentric.

○ **Which of these is a variant of nodular basal cell carcinomas and produces pigment?**
Cystic.

○ **Which of these commonly resembles a scar?**
Morpheaform.

○ **Which of these is the most aggressive?**
Keratotic.

○ **What is unique about the path of growth of basal cell carcinomas?**
Follow the path of least resistance, which is typically along embryonic fusion planes.

○ **That being said, which areas of the face are most susceptible to basal cell carcinomas?**
Inner canthus, philtrum, mid-lower chin, nasolabial groove, preauricular area, and retroauricular sulcus.

○ **What proportion of incompletely excised basal cell cancers will recur?**
One-third.

○ **True/False: squamous cell carcinomas arising in sun-exposed areas tend to behave less aggressively than those arising de novo.**
True.

○ **What percent of squamous cell carcinoma arising in areas of actinic change metastasize?**
3–5%.

○ **What percent of squamous cell carcinoma arising de novo metastasize?**
8%.

○ **What percent of squamous cell carcinoma arising in areas of scar or chronic inflammation metastasize?**
10–30%.

○ **What are the five histopathologic types of squamous cell carcinoma?**
Generic, adenoid, bowenoid, verrucous, and spindle–pleomorphic.

○ **Which of these typically arises in areas of actinic change?**

Generic.

○ **Which of these is more common in the oral mucosa?**

Verrucous

○ **Which of these is the least common?**

Spindle–pleomorphic.

○ **What factors increase the likelihood of recurrence for squamous cell carcinoma?**

Tumors on the midface, diameter >2 cm or thickness >4 mm, perineural invasion, or regional metastases.

○ **What factors increase the likelihood of regional metastasis of squamous cell carcinoma?**

Tumors arising on the ear, diameter >2 cm or >4 mm thickness, poorly differentiated histology, and recurrent tumors.

○ **What are the four types of melanoma?**

Superficial spreading, lentigo maligna, acral lentiginous, and nodular sclerosing.

○ **Which is the most common?**

Superficial spreading.

○ **Which has the best prognosis?**

Superficial spreading.

○ **What is the most common form of hereditary cutaneous melanoma?**

Dysplastic nevus syndrome.

○ **Which type of melanoma occurs on palms, soles, nail beds, and mucous membranes?**

Acral lentiginous melanoma.

○ **What percent of melanomas occur in the head and neck?**

20%.

○ **What percent of tumors are not pigmented (amelanotic)?**

5%.

○ **What mutation has been found in more than half of malignant melanomas?**

BRAF somatic missense mutations; a single substitution (V599E) accounts for 80% of these.

○ **What cells are melanomas composed of?**

Melanocytes, which are derived from neural crest cells.

○ **What are the risk factors for developing melanoma?**

Family history, multiple atypical or dysplastic nevi, Hutchinson's freckle, presence of large congenital nevi, blond or red hair, marked freckling on upper back, history of three or more blistering sunburns prior to age 20, presence of actinic keratoses.

○ **What is the risk of melanomatous transformation of giant congenital nevi?**

14%.

○ **What percent of patients with xeroderma pigmentosa develop melanoma?**

3%.

○ **How should a lesion suspicious for melanoma be biopsied?**

A sample should be taken of the tumor and the underlying tissue so that depth can be ascertained; a shave biopsy should never be performed.

○ **What is the most important prognostic factor of melanomas?**

Depth of invasion.

○ **What is the incidence of nodal metastases if the depth of the tumor is >4.0 mm?**

>70%.

○ **What is the incidence of nodal metastases if the depth of the tumor is <1.5 mm?**

8%.

○ **True/False: Women with melanoma have a better prognosis than men regardless of tumor depth.**

True.

○ **What tumor factor, other than depth, influences regional metastasis in melanoma?**

Ulceration.

○ **Involvement of which areas of the body also increases the risk of metastases?**

BANS: back, arms, neck, and scalp.

○ **What is the chance that a patient with melanoma will develop a second melanoma?**

5%.

○ **Is melanoma radiosensitive?**

It may be sensitive to large dose fractions (600 cGy) but not to standard fractionation radiotherapy (180–200 cGy).

○ **What is the role of large-dose fraction radiotherapy in the management of melanoma?**
Decreases incidence of locoregional recurrence among N0 patients.

○ **What is the risk of developing esophageal cancer in patients who smoke and drink compared with those who do not?**
100 times higher.

○ **In which areas of the world is the incidence of esophageal cancer highest?**
Middle East, southern and eastern Africa, and northern China.

○ **What are the risk factors for developing esophageal cancer?**
Tobacco, alcohol, achalasia, Plummer–Vinson syndrome, prior head and neck cancer, tylosis, and Barrett's disease.

○ **What are the clinical features of Plummer–Vinson syndrome?**
Iron-deficiency anemia, upper esophageal web, hypothyroidism, glossitis/cheilitis, gastritis, and dysphagia.

○ **In patients with Plummer–Vinson syndrome, where is squamous cell carcinoma of the esophagus most likely to occur?**
Postcricoid area.

○ **Metaplasia of the distal esophagus is otherwise known as what?**
Barrett's esophagus.

○ **What percent of people with gastroesophageal reflux disease have Barrett's esophagus and what percent of these people will develop adenocarcinoma?**
5% and 5–10%, respectively.

○ **Cancer of the cervical esophagus is usually what type?**
Squamous cell carcinoma.

○ **What is the usual cause of death from esophageal cancer?**
Aspiration pneumonia.

○ **When do patients with synovial sarcoma usually present?**
Between ages 25 and 36.

○ **Where are most synovial sarcomas of the head and neck located?**
Hypopharynx and parapharyngeal space.

○ **What is the incidence of regional metastasis in synovial sarcomas of the head and neck?**
12.5%.

○ **What is the incidence of local recurrence?**

60–90%, usually within 2 years.

○ **What is the most common cause of death from synovial sarcoma of the head and neck?**

Lung metastases.

○ **What is the primary mode of treatment for synovial sarcoma of the head and neck?**

Wide surgical excision and postoperative radiation therapy.

○ **What is the 5-year survival rate?**

40–50%.

○ **What prognostic significance does the presence of microcalcifications have?**

Better prognosis.

○ **Nasopharyngeal cancer accounts for what percent of all cancers diagnosed in the Kwangtung province of southern China?**

20%.

○ **What is the incidence of nasopharyngeal cancer among native-born Chinese compared with that among Caucasians?**

118 times higher.

○ **What is the incidence of nasopharyngeal cancer among North American-born Chinese compared with that among Caucasians?**

Seven times higher.

○ **What EBV product is likely to play a role in malignant transformation of nasopharyngeal epithelium?**

Latent membrane protein (LMP-1).

○ **What environmental factor is most strongly linked to nasopharyngeal carcinoma?**

Frequent consumption of dried salted fish.

○ **What is the 5-year survival of patients with WHO II or III disease?**

70%.

○ **What is the 5-year survival of patients with WHO I disease?**

30%.

○ **What is the most common site of origin of nasopharyngeal cancer?**

Fossa of Rosenmüller.

○ **Which nodal groups does nasopharyngeal cancer spread to?**

Retropharyngeal nodes of Rouviere, jugulodigastric nodes, spinal accessory chain.

○ **In the staging system described by Ho, poorer prognosis is associated with cervical metastases to which area of the neck?**

Inferior to a plane spanning from the contralateral sternal head of the clavicle to the ipsilateral superior margin of the trapezius muscle.

○ **True/False: The presence of unilateral compared with bilateral nodal disease in patients with nasopharyngeal carcinoma has no prognostic significance.**

True.

○ **What is the incidence of skull base erosion in patients with nasopharyngeal carcinoma?**

25%.

○ **What is the most common site of distant metastases?**

Bones.

○ **Smooth, submucosal nasopharyngeal masses located in the midline are most often what?**

Embryologic remnants (Thornwaldt's cysts, pharyngeal bursa remnants).

○ **What factors, described by Ho and Neel, are regarded as important adverse prognostic indicators in patients with nasopharyngeal carcinoma?**

Length and symptomatology of disease, extension of tumor outside of the nasopharynx, presence of inferior cervical adenopathy, keratinizing histologic architecture, cranial nerve and skull base extension, presence of distant metastases, and low ADCC titers.

○ **Extension into which space is associated with the worst prognosis in patients with nasopharyngeal carcinoma?**

Anterior masticator space.

○ **What is the primary treatment modality for nasopharyngeal cancer?**

Radiation therapy to the nasopharynx (66–70 Gy) and neck (60 Gy).

○ **Why is the clinically negative neck treated?**

Studies have shown improved local control and disease-free survival for prophylactic irradiation of the clinically negative neck in patients with nasopharyngeal carcinoma.

○ **What are the complications from radiation overdosage in the treatment of nasopharyngeal carcinoma?**

Osteoradionecrosis, brain necrosis, transverse myelitis, hearing loss, hypopituitarism, hypothyroidism, and optic neuritis.

○ **What is the role of induction chemotherapy for treatment of nasopharyngeal carcinoma?**

No survival advantage has been proven.

○ **What is the standard treatment protocol for stage III and IV nasopharyngeal carcinoma?**

Concomitant cisplatin and XRT followed by adjuvant chemotherapy with cisplatin and 5-FU.

○ **How does treatment failure usually manifest in nasopharyngeal carcinoma?**

Disease at both the primary site and cervical lymph nodes.

○ **What is the most common site of recurrent/persistent nasopharyngeal carcinoma?**

Lateral wall of the nasopharynx.

○ **What are the treatment options for recurrent/persistent nasopharyngeal carcinoma at the primary site?**

Reirradiation with larger therapeutic dose than initial treatment; stereotactic radiotherapy; brachytherapy with split palate implantation of radioactive gold grains; surgical resection.

○ **What is the most common benign sinonasal neoplasm?**

Inverting papilloma.

○ **What is the most common malignant sinonasal neoplasm?**

Squamous cell carcinoma, comprising 80% of malignant sinonasal neoplasms.

○ **What is the 2nd most common malignant sinonasal neoplasm?**

Adenocarcinoma.

○ **What are the most common locations of sinonasal squamous cell carcinoma?**

Maxillary sinus, followed by the nasal cavity, then ethmoid sinuses.

○ **Are elective neck dissections warranted in patients with sinonasal squamous cell carcinoma?**

No, as the incidence of occult cervical metastases is 10%.

○ **What percentage of sinonasal tumors can be attributed to occupational exposures?**

Up to 44%.

○ **Where do these tumors most often originate?**

Lateral nasal wall, adjacent to the middle turbinate.

○ **Which substances are thought to predispose to sinonasal neoplasms?**

Nickel, chromium, isopropyl oils, volatile hydrocarbons, organic fibers from wood, shoe, and textile refineries.

○ **Which of these is classically associated with SCCA?**

Nickel.

○ **Which of these are classically associated with adenocarcinoma?**

Hardwood dusts and leather tanning substances.

○ **Which virus is thought to play a role in the etiology of sinonasal tumors?**

Human papilloma virus (HPV), particularly types 6 and 12.

○ **True/False: Smoking by itself is not a significant etiologic factor for sinonasal tumors.**

True.

○ **Which nasal masses should not be biopsied in the clinic?**

Masses in children or adolescents and masses suspicious for angiofibroma—some also recommend delaying biopsy of any nasal mass until after imaging has been obtained.

○ **What are the three subtypes of Schneiderian papillomas?**

Fungiform, inverting, and cylindrical.

○ **Where do inverting papillomas most commonly arise?**

Lateral nasal wall.

○ **What factor is most related to the chance of recurrence for inverting papilloma?**

Method of removal.

○ **What is the incidence of recurrence after resection of inverting papilloma via lateral rhinotomy/medial maxillectomy?**

13–15%.

○ **In patients who undergo resection of inverting papilloma via lateral rhinotomy/medial maxillectomy, what is the most important factor related to risk for recurrence?**

Mitotic index.

○ **What is the differential diagnosis of a small cell sinonasal tumor?**

Esthesioneuroblastoma, plasmacytoma, melanoma, lymphoma, sarcoma, poorly differentiated squamous cell carcinoma, Ewing's sarcoma, peripheral neuroectodermal tumor (PNET), and SNUC.

○ **What is a SNUC?**

Sinonasal undifferentiated carcinoma—a very aggressive small cell sinonasal tumor.

○ **What are the poor prognostic factors for SNUC tumors?**

Orbital involvement and neck metastases; tumors in the paranasal sinuses have a worse prognosis than those arising in the nasal cavity.

○ **SNUC tumors have antibodies to what substances?**

Cytokeratin, epithelial membrane antigen, and neuron-specific enolase.

○ **What is the treatment for SNUC?**

Preoperative chemoradiation, followed by surgical resection for those tumors without distant metastases or extensive intracranial involvement.

○ **In what age group is olfactory neuroblastoma typically seen?**

Bimodal distribution—people in their 20s and 50s.

○ **An olfactory neuroblastoma involving the ethmoid sinuses would be classified as what stage by the Kadish system?**

B.

○ **What are the three most common malignant bone tumors of the paranasal sinuses?**

Multiple myeloma, osteogenic sarcoma, chondrosarcoma.

○ **What is the pathophysiology of fibrous dysplasia?**

Normal medullary bone is replaced by collagen, fibroblasts, and osteoid.

○ **Where is it most commonly found in the head and neck?**

Maxilla.

○ **Where is adenoid cystic carcinoma of the head and neck most commonly found?**

Palate, followed by major salivary glands, then paranasal sinuses.

○ **Where is melanoma most commonly found in the nose and paranasal sinuses?**

Nasal septum.

○ **How does nasal melanoma differ from cutaneous melanoma?**

More aggressive with a worse prognosis and an unpredictable course—local recurrence is the most common cause of failure.

○ **What is the most common type of lymphoma of the nose and paranasal sinuses?**

Non-Hodgkin's lymphoma.

○   **What is Ohngren's line and how is it significant?**

Imaginary line from the medial canthus to the angle of the mandible; tumors below the line have a better prognosis than tumors above the line (with the palate as an exception).

○   **Name the tumor.**

Comprises only 3% of Schneiderian papillomas	Cylindrical papilloma
Most common type of Schneiderian papilloma, typically seen on the nasal septum	Fungiform papilloma
2–13% of these benign sinonasal tumors have malignant potential	Inverting papilloma
Has a predilection for the mandible and a sunray appearance on X-ray	Osteogenic sarcoma
More than 90% will have invaded through at least one wall of the involved sinus at presentation	SCCA
Benign tumor, most commonly seen in patients less than 20 years old and has a ground glass appearance on X-ray	Fibrous dysplasia
Benign tumor most commonly found in the frontal sinus	Osteoma
Encapsulated, benign tumor that arises from the surface of nerve fibers	Neurilemoma
Unencapsulated tumor that arises from within a nerve; 15% become malignant (when associated with von Recklinghausen's disease)	Neurofibroma
Second most common malignant sinonasal tumor; tend to be located superior to Ohngren's line	Adenocarcinoma
Arise from pericytes of Zimmerman and considered neither benign nor malignant	Hemangiopericytoma
Arise from stem cells of neural crest origin that differentiate into olfactory sensory cells; Homer Wright rosettes are characteristic	Olfactory neuroblastoma or esthesioneuroblastoma
May progress to multiple myeloma	Extramedullary plasmacytoma
Most common tumor to metastasize to the sinonasal area	Renal cell
Well-circumscribed, mobile, painless benign lesion most commonly found on the tongue that has malignant potential and histopathology shows polygonal cells with abundant eosinophils	Granular cell tumor
Metastasizes to the brain more frequently than any other soft-tissue sarcoma	Alveolar soft part sarcoma

○ **Which sinonasal neoplasms remodel rather than erode bone?**

Sarcomas, minor salivary gland carcinomas, hemangiopericytomas, extramedullary plasmacytomas, large cell lymphomas, and olfactory neuroblastomas.

○ **What is the primary modality of treatment for extramedullary plasmacytomas?**

Radiation.

○ **After benign lymphoid hyperplasia, what is the most common benign nasopharyngeal tumor?**

Juvenile nasopharyngeal angiofibroma (JNA).

○ **From which site in the nasopharynx does this tumor develop?**

Trifurcation of the palatine bone, horizontal ala of the vomer, and the root of the pterygoid process.

○ **What is the stage of a JNA eroding the skull base with minimal intracranial extension?**

IIIA.

○ **Where does the main blood supply to these tumors most often come from?**

Internal maxillary artery or the ascending pharyngeal artery.

○ **What is the second leading cause of death among children ages 1–14?**

Cancer.

○ **What is the most common solid malignant tumor in infants <1 year?**

Neuroblastoma.

○ **What are the precursor cells of neuroblastoma?**

Neural crest cells.

○ **What is the survival rate after complete excision of lesions in children <1?**

90%.

○ **What type of nystagmus is often seen in children with neuroblastoma?**

Opsoclonus.

○ **What is the most common head and neck tumor of children?**

Lymphoma.

○   **In what age groups is Hodgkin's lymphoma most common?**

Bimodal peak incidence, with one peak in the 15- to 34-year-old age group and another in later adulthood.

○   **What percent of Hodgkin's lymphoma cases are associated with EBV?**

40%.

○   **True/False: Axillary, inguinal, and Waldeyer's ring involvement is uncommon in patients with Hodgkin's lymphoma.**

True.

○   **Involvement of two or more lymph node sites on the same side of the diaphragm is designated as which stage according to the Ann Arbor system?**

Stage II.

○   **Which lymphoma accounts for 50% of childhood malignancies in equatorial Africa?**

Burkitt's lymphoma.

○   **What is the most common soft tissue sarcoma of the head and neck in children?**

Rhabdomyosarcoma.

○   **In what age groups is rhabdomyosarcoma most common?**

Ages 2–5 and 15–19.

○   **What is the treatment for rhabdomyosarcoma?**

Multimodality; primary chemoradiation followed by surgery for recurrent or residual disease.

○   **Involvement in which area of the head and neck by rhabdomyosarcoma has the best prognosis?**

Orbit.

○   **What is the most common type of well-differentiated thyroid carcinoma in children?**

Papillary.

○   **What is the most common benign neoplasm of the larynx in children?**

Papillomas.

○   **What percent of patients with recurrent respiratory papillomatosis (RRP) develop distal tracheal and pulmonary spread of papillomas?**

5%.

○ **High expression of which nuclear antigen is significantly associated with distal tracheobronchial spread and increased frequency of recurrences?**

Ki-67.

○ **What percent of patients with RRP require tracheostomy?**

15%.

○ **What percent of patients with distal spread have had a previous tracheostomy?**

95%.

○ **What is the incidence of stomal papilloma recurrence rate after tracheostomy for RRP?**

>50%.

○ **What are the most common subtypes of HPV isolated from RRP?**

6 and 11 (found in >95%).

○ **Which of these subtypes is associated with a more aggressive disease course?**

11.

○ **What are the most common respiratory complications of distal RRP?**

Pneumatocele, abscess, and tracheal stenosis.

○ **Why is aspergillus infection a risk factor for ear and temporal bone tumors?**

It produces aflatoxin B, a known carcinogen.

○ **What are other risk factors for development of ear and temporal bone tumors?**

History of radiation to the head and neck, chronic chromate burns secondary to using matchsticks to clean the ear canal.

○ **What is the most common site of ear and temporal bone tumors?**

External auditory canal (EAC).

○ **What is the most common route of spread of tumors in the cartilaginous portion of the EAC?**

Through the fissures of Santorini.

○ **What is the most common histologic type of tumor involving the EAC or middle ear?**

Squamous cell carcinoma.

○ **Where do most basal cell carcinomas of the EAC arise?**

Concha.

○ **What is the most common tumor of glandular origin to involve the EAC or middle ear?**
Adenoid cystic carcinoma.

○ **What are the most common types of sarcoma of the temporal bone?**
Rhabdomyosarcoma, chondrosarcoma, and osteosarcoma.

○ **What are the most common sites of origin of metastatic tumors of the temporal bone?**
Breast, lung, and kidney.

○ **Tumors that metastasize to the temporal bone hematogenously most often involve which area of the temporal bone?**
Petrous apex.

○ **Tumors that metastasize to the temporal bone via the meninges most often traverse what structure?**
Internal auditory canal.

○ **What is the most common presentation of tumors of the EAC?**
Unremitting pain and serosanguinous otorrhea.

○ **What percent of patients with a tumor in the EAC will present with cervical metastases?**
10%.

○ **What percent of patients with a tumor in the middle ear will present with facial nerve palsy?**
20–40%.

○ **What is the most common tumor of the cerebellopontine angle (CPA)?**
Vestibular schwannoma.

○ **What is the differential diagnosis of a CPA tumor?**
Schwannoma, meningioma, epidermoid, lipoma, arachnoid cyst, cholesterol granuloma.

○ **What is the incidence of patients with vestibular schwannomas who have normal hearing at presentation?**
5%.

○ **What is the nature of vertigo in the majority of patients with a vestibular schwannoma?**
Chronic disequilibrium with self-limiting episodes of vertigo.

○ **Below are axial MRI views of the CPA in an 18-year-old man with bilateral hearing loss. He has no skin lesions or subcutaneous nodules. What disease does he most likely have?**

Reproduced, with permission, from Ropper AH, Samuels MA. *Adams and Victor's Principles of Neurology*, 9th edn. New York: McGraw-Hill, 2009.

Neurofibromatosis type 2.

○ **What is the incidence of vestibular schwannoma in patients with unilateral SNHL?**
1–2%.

○ **What is the most common type of hearing loss in patients with a vestibular schwannoma?**
High-frequency unilateral SNHL.

○ **What is a typical word discrimination score in a patient with a vestibular schwannoma?**
0–30% in >50% of patients with an acoustic neuroma.

○ **Adenocarcinoma of the endolymphatic sac is more common in patients with what disease?**
Von Hippel–Lindau disease.

○ **What percent of thyroid cancers are well differentiated?**
>90%.

○ **What percent of thyroid nodules are malignant?**
<5%.

○   **What percent of thyroid nodules are malignant in patients with a history of radiation exposure?**
30–50%.

○   **What is the average lag time between radiation exposure and development of thyroid cancer?**
15–25 years.

○   **What is the most common thyroid nodule?**
Follicular adenoma.

○   **What is the significance of age with thyroid nodules?**
More likely to be malignant in women over 50 and men over 40 and in both men and women under 20.

○   **What percent of solitary thyroid nodules in children are malignant?**
50%.

○   **What is the significance of size with thyroid nodules?**
More likely to be malignant if >4 cm in diameter.

○   **What is the difference in incidence of malignancy between solitary and multiple nodules?**
Incidence of malignancy in solitary nodules is 5–12%; incidence is 3% in multiple nodules.

○   **What percent of malignant thyroid nodules are suppressible by exogenous TSH?**
16%.

○   **What percent of benign thyroid nodules are suppressible by exogenous TSH?**
21%.

○   **What are the three types of well-differentiated thyroid malignancies?**
Follicular, papillary, and Hürthle cell.

○   **Which of these is associated with iodine deficiency?**
Follicular.

○   **Which of these is more likely to be seen in a 30-year-old?**
Papillary.

○   **Which of these is more likely to be seen in a pregnant woman?**
Follicular.

○   **Which of these is the most common type of thyroid cancer?**
Papillary.

○ **Which of these has the best prognosis?**

Papillary.

○ **Which of these is relatively unresponsive to ablation with radioactive iodine?**

Hürthle cell.

○ **A 65-year-old woman presents with a cervical lymph node that is found to have well-differentiated thyroid tissue but the thyroid has no palpable abnormality. What is the next step in management?**

Total thyroidectomy and modified radical neck dissection.

○ **What factor best correlates with the presence of lymph node metastases in papillary carcinoma?**

Age.

○ **True/False: Microscopic lymph node involvement does not change the long-term survival in patients with papillary thyroid cancer.**

True.

○ **What is the incidence of multicentric disease on pathological examination of the entire thyroid in patients with papillary carcinoma (>1 cm)?**

70–80%.

○ **What histological subtypes of thyroid tumors are associated with an increased risk of local recurrence and metastasis?**

Tall cell, columnar, insular, solid variant, and poorly differentiated.

○ **A 36-year-old woman presents with a 3 cm papillary carcinoma and no clinical evidence of lymph node involvement, no intrathyroidal vascular invasion, and no gross or microscopic multifocal disease. She has no history of neck radiation and no family history of thyroid cancer. She was treated with a total thyroidectomy. Is radioiodine ablation therapy indicated?**

No.

○ **What is the most common site of metastasis from follicular thyroid cancer?**

Bone.

○ **How is the definitive diagnosis of follicular thyroid cancer made?**

By demonstration of capsular invasion at the interface of the tumor and the thyroid gland.

○ **What is the most important prognostic indicator of follicular thyroid cancer?**

Degree of angioinvasion.

○ **True/False: Follicular cell carcinoma is more aggressive than Hürthle cell.**

False.

○   **What is the incidence of patients with Hürthle cell carcinoma who present with distant metastases?**
15%.

○   **What are the three most well-known prognostic systems for well-differentiated thyroid cancer?**
GAMES, AMES, and AGES.

○   **What are the indications for adjuvant thyroid hormone in patients with well-differentiated thyroid carcinoma?**
All patients with well-differentiated carcinoma should be treated with thyroid hormone to suppress TSH for life, regardless of the extent of their surgery.

○   **In what four settings does medullary thyroid carcinoma (MTC) arise?**
Sporadic, familial, and in association with multiple endocrine neoplasia IIa or IIb.

○   **Which of these has the best prognosis?**
Familial.

○   **Which of these has the worst prognosis?**
Sporadic.

○   **Which of these tends to occur unilaterally?**
Sporadic.

○   **Which of these presents earliest?**
MEN IIb (mean age 19).

○   **What percentage of MTC occurs sporadically?**
70–80%.

○   **What are the characteristics of familial MTC?**
Autosomal dominant inheritance pattern; not associated with any other endocrinopathies.

○   **What other disorders are present in patients with MEN IIa?**
Pheochromocytoma, parathyroid hyperplasia.

○   **What is the mean age of presentation of MTC in patients with MEN IIa?**
27.

○   **True/False: All patients with MEN IIa will have MTC.**
True.

○ **What other disorders are present in patients with MEN IIb?**

Pheochromocytoma, multiple mucosal neuromas, marfanoid body habitus.

○ **What percent of MTCs secrete CEA?**

50%.

○ **What genetic mutation is associated with medullary thyroid cancer?**

Mutation of the RET proto-oncogene.

○ **When is prophylactic thyroidectomy recommended in patients with the RET mutation?**

By age 5 or 6.

○ **What is the surgical treatment for MTC?**

Total thyroidectomy with central node dissection, lateral cervical lymph node sampling of palpable nodes, and a modified radical neck dissection, if positive.

○ **What percent of patients have had well-differentiated cancer before developing anaplastic thyroid cancer?**

47%.

○ **What percent of patients have had benign thyroid disease before developing anaplastic cancer?**

53%.

○ **What are the two types of anaplastic thyroid cancer?**

Large cell and small cell.

○ **Which is more common?**

Large cell.

○ **Which of these is usually responsive to radiation therapy?**

Small cell.

○ **What is the appropriate management for a patient with an anaplastic thyroid carcinoma?**

Debulking and tracheostomy may be performed for palliation of airway obstruction.

○ **What is the best treatment for primary non-Hodgkin's lymphoma of the thyroid gland?**

Chemoradiation.

○ **A 44-year-old man presents with a 5 cm thyroid nodule. FNA returns fluid, the nodule disappears, and the cytology is benign. What is the next step in management?**

Total thyroid lobectomy with isthmusectomy should be considered because there is an increased chance of malignancy in large cysts.

○ **A 56-year-old man with no risk factors presents with a thyroid nodule. The FNA is nondiagnostic. What is the treatment of choice?**

Total thyroid lobectomy with isthmusectomy.

○ **What are the indications for postoperative radioiodine ablation therapy?**

Known distant metastases, gross extrathyroidal extension of tumor, tumors larger than 4 cm, tumors 1–4 cm when T and N status, age, and histological features predict an intermediate to high rate of recurrence.

○ **True/False: Multifocal well-differentiated thyroid tumors less than 1 cm without high-risk features do not require postoperative radioiodine ablation therapy.**

True.

○ **Which medication improves quality of life when preparing patients for radioiodine scanning and ablation therapy?**

Recombinant TSH stimulation (rTSH).

○ **How are patients with MTC managed postoperatively?**

Receive L-thyroxine and 2 weeks of calcium and vitamin D supplementation; serial measurements of calcitonin and CEA.

○ **Severe cerebellar symptoms with a normal MRI suggests what condition?**

Paraneoplastic cerebellar degeneration.

○ **What are the two primary subtypes of paraneoplastic cerebellar degeneration?**

Vestibulocerebellar syndrome and opsoclonus-myoclonus syndrome.

○ **Which malignancies most commonly cause paraneoplastic cerebellar degeneration?**

In adults, ovarian, uterine, breast, and small cell lung cancer. In children, neuroblastoma.

CHAPTER 25 Trauma and Foreign Bodies

○ **True/False: The incidence of foreign body aspiration is equal between the right and left bronchus in children.**
True: The left bronchus is not as obliquely angled in children as in adults.

○ **True/False: Airway foreign bodies are more common than esophageal foreign bodies.**
False.

○ **What is the most common esophageal foreign body in children <5?**
Coins.

○ **What is the most common diagnosis inappropriately given to a child with an airway foreign body?**
Asthma.

○ **What are the two types of nontraumatic cerebrospinal fluid (CSF) leaks?**
High pressure and normal pressure.

○ **What is the most common cause of CSF leak?**
Nonsurgical trauma.

○ **What percent of CSF leaks are from nontraumatic causes?**
3–4%.

○ **What percent of basilar skull fractures result in CSF leak?**
10–30%.

○ **What percent of patients with CSF leak secondary to nonsurgical trauma will develop meningitis?**
10–25%.

○ **What is the mortality rate of patients who develop meningitis with a traumatic CSF leak?**
10%.

○   **What percent of CSF leaks are cranionasal?**
80%.

○   **True/False: Cranio-aural CSF leaks are more likely to spontaneously close than cranionasal CSF leaks.**
True.

○   **What is the medical management of CSF leak?**
Elevation of the head of bed, antitussives, laxatives, antihypertensives, analgesics, bed rest, lumbar drain.

○   **What is a serious complication of lumbar drainage?**
Tension pneumocephalus.

○   **What percent of skull fractures involve the temporal bone?**
Approximately 20%.

○   **What are the three types of temporal bone fractures?**
Longitudinal, transverse, and mixed.

○   **Which of these is most common?**
Longitudinal (80–90%).

○   **Which of these is associated with conductive hearing loss (CHL)?**
Longitudinal.

○   **What is the most common mechanism of CHL in longitudinal fractures?**
Incudostapedial joint dislocation.

○   **Which of these fractures is most likely to result in facial nerve paralysis?**
Transverse.

○   **What is the incidence of facial nerve injury after transverse fracture of the temporal bone?**
40–50%.

○   **Which of these accounts for the majority of facial nerve injuries?**
Longitudinal.

○   **What is the incidence of facial nerve paralysis in patients with longitudinal temporal bone fractures?**
20–25%.

○   **What are the most common etiologies of nerve dysfunction after longitudinal temporal bone fracture?**
Edema and intraneural hemorrhage.

○ **What is the most common area of facial nerve injury following trauma?**

Perigenicular area.

○ **What is the strongest predictor of poor recovery of facial nerve function following temporal bone trauma?**

Immediate onset of facial paralysis in a patient with a closed head injury.

○ **Which type of temporal bone fracture is most likely to occur from a blow to the occiput?**

Transverse.

○ **What is the typical course of the fracture line in transverse temporal bone fractures?**

Foramen magnum across the petrous apex, across the internal auditory canal and otic capsule, to the foramen spinosum or lacerum.

○ **Where are the laceration and bony disruption in the external auditory canal most often found after longitudinal temporal bone fracture?**

Along the tympanosquamous suture line (posterior and superior).

○ **Where does the fracture line typically course in relation to the otic capsule?**

Anterior to the otic capsule.

○ **What is the most common etiology of dizziness after longitudinal temporal bone fracture?**

BPPV.

○ **When should middle ear exploration and ossicular reconstruction be performed after temporal bone fracture?**

At least 3 months after injury.

○ **What is the most common type of temporal bone fracture in children?**

Obliquely oriented fractures.

○ **Which of the LeFort fractures involves the infraorbital rim?**

LeFort II.

○ **What are the sequelae of untreated maxillary fractures?**

Midface retrusion, facial elongation, and anterior open bite deformity.

○ **What are the sequelae of untreated lateral zygomatic arch fractures?**

Increased midfacial width and malar flattening.

○ **What is a type I NOE fracture?**

Single, noncomminuted central segment fracture.

○   **What is a type II NOE fracture?**

Comminuted, but identifiable, central fragment.

○   **What is a type III NOE fracture?**

Severely comminuted fracture with disruption of the medial canthal tendon or too small of a central fragment to be repaired directly.

○   **How do type I, II, and III NOE fractures differ in terms of management?**

Type I fractures usually can be repaired with microplates; type II fractures usually require transnasal wires in addition to plate fixation; type III fractures usually require at least two sets of transnasal wires and may require bone grafting.

○   **What is a type A zygomaticomaxillary complex fracture (ZMC) fracture?**

Isolated to one component of the tetrapod structure (zygomatic arch, lateral orbital wall, or inferior orbital rim).

○   **What is a type B ZMC fracture?**

Injury to each of the four supporting structures.

○   **What is a type C ZMC fracture?**

Complex fracture with comminution of the zygomatic bone.

○   **Which of these is least common?**

Type A.

○   **What is a class I mandible fracture?**

Fracture between two teeth.

○   **What is a class II mandible fracture?**

Teeth are present on only one side of the fracture.

○   **What is a class III mandible fracture?**

Fracture in an edentulous area.

○   **Which parts of the mandible are most commonly fractured?**

Condyle (36%), body (21%), and angle (20%).

○   **What are favorable fractures?**

Fractures where the muscles tend to draw the fragments together.

○   **What is the most likely mechanism of injury for bilateral condylar fractures?**

Anterior blow to the chin.

○ **What percent of mandible fractures are associated with other injuries?**

40–60%.

○ **In patients with mandible fractures, what mechanisms of injury are most predictive of an associated cervical spine injury?**

Penetrating high-velocity gunshot injury; high-velocity MVA.

○ **What is the optimal treatment for a nondisplaced condylar fracture?**

If occlusion is normal, soft diet and close observation; bilateral fractures or unilateral fractures with malocclusion should be treated with MMF for 3 weeks, then elastics for 2 weeks.

○ **What are the absolute indications for open reduction of a condylar fracture?**

Displacement of the fractured fragments into the middle cranial fossa, inadequate reduction with MMF, lateral extracapsular displacement of the condyle, and foreign body (i.e., bullet) embedded in the joint.

○ **What are the relative indications for open reduction of a condylar fracture?**

Bilateral condylar fractures in an edentulous patient when MMF is impossible, condylar fractures when MMF is not recommended for medical reasons, and bilateral condylar fractures associated with midface fractures.

○ **What is the appropriate management for a deep puncture wound from a dog or cat bite?**

Postexposure rabies prophylaxis should be considered for all bites. If the animal is healthy, it should be quarantined for 10 days to exclude rabies. If the animal is unavailable or suspected rabid, immediate vaccination and immunoglobulin therapy should be administered. In addition, antibiotic coverage to include *Pasteurella multocida* should be initiated.

○ **What sort of neurologic sequelae usually result from isolated unilateral vertebral artery injury?**

None.

○ **After carotid artery injury, when is it too late to attempt revascularization?**

When coma has occurred beyond 3 hours, if an anemic infarction has occurred, or if no vascular back flow is present.

○ **What is the strongest predictor of negative outcome in trauma patients?**

Arterial hypotension <90 mm Hg.

○ **Transcatheter arterial embolization is most useful in the management of what type of neck injury?**

Gunshot wound to zone III of the neck.

○ **What is the major advantage of immediate aggressive reconstruction after a high-energy gunshot wound to the face?**

Less soft tissue scarring and contracture.

○ **What are the most common injuries associated with facial trauma in children?**

Dental injuries.

○ **Which part of the mandible is most commonly fractured in children?**

Condyle.

○ **What are the three types of condylar fractures?**

Intracapsular crush fractures of the condylar head, high condylar fractures through the neck above the sigmoid notch, and low subcondylar fractures.

○ **Which of these is most common?**

Low subcondylar fracture (often incomplete or "greenstick" injury).

○ **What is the usual treatment of condylar fractures in children?**

Soft diet.

○ **What are the indications for open reduction of condylar fractures in children?**

When the fractured condyle directly interferes with jaw movement; when the fracture reduces the height of the ramus and results in an open-bite deformity; when the condyle is dislocated into the middle cranial fossa.

○ **True/False: A mandible fracture in a child is much more likely to be associated with other injuries than in an adult.**

True.

○ **Among children, which mandible fractures result in the highest incidence of dentofacial abnormalities?**

Intracapsular crush fractures of the condyle.

○ **What is the difference in tooth viability when comparing plates versus wires for fixation of mandible fractures?**

There is a significant increase in the nonviability of teeth in the line and adjacent to fractures of the mandible treated by plates compared with those treated with wires.

○ **What is the best way to treat mandible fractures in infants <2 years of age?**

Acrylic splints x 2–3 weeks.

○ **What are the treatment options for children between 2 and 5 years of age?**

Interdental eyelet wiring, arch bars, cap splints, or soft diet.

○ **Which teeth can be used in children between the ages of 5 and 8 for immobilization?**

Deciduous molars.

○ **Which teeth can be used in children between the ages of 7 and 11 for immobilization?**

Primary molars and incisors.

○ **How long should immobilization typically be maintained in children?**

2–3 weeks.

○ **In a child, what is the treatment for an incomplete monocortical crack of the mandibular body with normal occlusion and movement?**

Soft diet.

○ **When can bicortical plates be used in children?**

When permanent dentition is present.

○ **What structure is most likely to be fractured after blunt trauma to the anterior neck?**

Thyroid cartilage.

○ **Which types of laryngeal injuries are best managed medically?**

Edema; small hematoma with intact mucosa; small glottic or supraglottic lacerations not involving the free margin of the vocal cords or the anterior commissure and without cartilage exposure; single nondisplaced thyroid cartilage fractures.

○ **What does medical management of laryngeal injuries consist of?**

24 hours or more of airway observation, voice rest, elevation of the head, humidified air, H2 blockers, steroids; antibiotics if lacerations are present.

○ **Which types of laryngeal injuries require open exploration and repair?**

Lacerations involving the free margin of the vocal cord or anterior commissure; large mucosal lacerations with exposed cartilage; multiple displaced cartilage fractures; avulsed or dislocated arytenoids; vocal cord immobility.

○ **When should open exploration be performed after injury?**

Within 24 hours.

○ **What injuries are more commonly associated with laryngotracheal separation than with other laryngeal injuries?**

Subglottic stenosis and bilateral recurrent laryngeal nerve injury.

○ **Which types of laryngeal injuries are more common in children than in adults?**

Soft tissue injury with edema, arytenoid dislocation, and recurrent laryngeal nerve injury; telescoping injuries where the cricoid becomes displaced under the thyroid.

○ **In what age groups is caustic ingestion most common?**

18–24 months, 20–30 years.

○   **What are the three stages of injury after caustic ingestion?**

1. Necrosis, bacterial invasion, sloughing of the mucosa.
2. Granulation tissue and reepithelialization (day 5–several weeks).
3. Scar formation and contraction.

○   **How does the injury differ after ingestion of acidic substances versus ingestion of basic substances?**

Acidic substances cause coagulation necrosis; the eschar limits the depth of injury. Basic substances cause liquefaction necrosis and are likely to cause deeper injury.

○   **Where is the most likely site of injury after ingestion of an acidic caustic agent?**

Stomach.

○   **After caustic ingestion, what sign is most likely to signal the development of a complication?**

Drooling.

○   **What is the most likely consequence of ingesting hair relaxer?**

No long-term sequelae.

○   **What percent of patients without oropharyngeal burn will have evidence of esophageal injury?**

8–20%.

○   **Once the ABCs have been stabilized, what is the acute management of caustic ingestion injury?**

Prevent ongoing injury with irrigation of eyes, skin, and mouth, +/− flushing of the esophagus and stomach with water or milk <15 mL/kg (nasogastric tube placement is controversial). Surgical exploration is indicated for perforation, mediastinitis, or peritonitis.

○   **What should be done for the patient who has ingested a battery?**

If the battery is still in the esophagus (confirmed by radiographs), immediate esophagoscopy is indicated. If it has passed into the stomach, it can be allowed to pass.

○   **True/False: Inducing emesis and activated charcoal are contraindicated in the management of caustic ingestion.**

True.

○   **What is the management of patients with evidence of grade 1 injury (superficial) on endoscopic exam?**

No intervention; schedule for esophagogram in 3 weeks.

○   **What is the management of patients with evidence of grade 2 or 3 injury (transmucosal or transmural) on endoscopic exam?**

Esophageal rest (NPO), reflux precautions, +/− steroids, +/− antibiotics, +/− lathyrogens, +/− subcutaneous heparin, +/− nasogastric tube, +/− prophylactic bougienage.

○ **What are the contraindications to steroid use?**

Grade 3 burns, esophageal or gastric perforation.

○ **What percent of children with esophageal burns will develop esophageal stricture?**

7–15%.

○ **Why should all patients with history of caustic ingestion be followed for life with repeated esophagograms and endoscopy?**

Risk of SCCA of the esophagus is 1000 times that of the general population.

○ **What percent of patients with esophageal stricture will develop esophageal cancer?**

1–4%.

○ **What are the typical features of esophageal cancer occurring after esophageal stricture from burn injury?**

Usually SCCA, with onset 25–70 years postinjury, occurring within the scar tissue, with a lower incidence of distant metastases and higher chance of cure with surgical resection.

CHAPTER 26 Idiopathic

○ **What condition would cause a tense sounding voice, vocal fatigue, and a prolonged closed phase with reduced vibratory and mucosal wave amplitude during videostroboscopy?**

Glottic hyperabduction dysphonia.

○ **What kind of dystonia is spasmodic dysphonia (SD)?**

Focal.

○ **What are the characteristics of focal dystonias?**

Inappropriate and excessive efferent activity of motor neurons in small areas.

○ **What are the two types of SD?**

Adductor and abductor.

○ **Which is more common?**

Adductor SD.

○ **Which of these is characterized by a harsh, strained voice with inappropriate pitch breaks, breathiness, and glottal fry?**

Adductor SD.

○ **What are the typical features of abductor SD?**

Breathy, effortful hypnotic voice with abnormal whispered segments of speech.

○ **The inability to sustain vowels during speech is suggestive of what disorder?**

Adductor SD.

○ **Voiceless consonant is suggestive of what disorder?**

Abductor SD.

○   **What percent of cases of SD are familial?**

12%.

○   **Which muscles are responsible for adductor SD?**

Thyroarytenoid and lateral cricoarytenoid muscles.

○   **Which muscle is responsible for abductor SD?**

Posterior cricoarytenoid muscle.

○   **What is the preferred method of treatment for SD?**

Chemical denervation with botulinum toxin.

○   **What are the two ways to deliver botulinum toxin to the posterior cricoarytenoid muscle?**

Transcricoid and retrograde (rotating the larynx away from the side of injection).

○   **How can one confirm placement of the needle in the posterior cricoarytenoid muscle?**

Using EMG guidance, have the patient sniff.

○   **What can be done if symptoms persist after complete paralysis of the posterior cricoarytenoid?**

Inject the contralateral posterior cricoarytenoid muscle with very small increments of toxin or inject the cricothyroid muscle.

○   **How is injection into the cricothyroid muscle accomplished, and how is proper placement confirmed?**

Peroral route; confirm by having the patient sing an ascending scale and observing an increase in EMG activity as the pitch increases.

○   **What are the adverse effects of posterior cricoarytenoid injections?**

Stridor (particularly with exertion), airway compromise, dysphagia, and aspiration.

○   **What is adductor laryngeal breathing dystonia?**

Paradoxical adduction of the vocal folds during inspiration, causing inspiratory stridor that worsens with exertion and disappears during sleep.

○   **What effect does adductor laryngeal breathing dystonia have on the voice?**

None.

○   **What syndrome is associated with blepharospasm?**

Meige's syndrome.

○   **Which muscles are involved in blepharospasm?**

Orbicularis oculi, procerus, and corrugator supercilii.

○ **What causes hemifacial spasm?**

A vascular loop, most commonly of the anterior or posterior inferior cerebellar artery, impinging on the root of VII.

○ **What is the initial treatment for hemifacial spasm?**

Baclofen.

○ **What is the procedure of choice for patients with hemifacial spasm?**

Microvascular decompression.

○ **Which muscles are injected when using botulinum toxin to treat hemifacial spasm?**

Zygomaticus major and minor, levator anguli oris, and risorius.

○ **What muscles are injected when using botulinum toxin to treat oromandibular dystonia?**

Masseter, temporalis, and medial and lateral pterygoid muscles.

○ **What percent of patients with unilateral tinnitus have retrocochlear pathology?**

11%.

○ **What is the most common cause of venous pulsatile tinnitus?**

Idiopathic intracranial hypertension syndrome (pseudotumor cerebri, benign intracranial hypertension).

○ **What is the most common cause of pulsatile tinnitus in young female patients?**

Idiopathic intracranial hypertension (IIH) syndrome.

○ **What are five other venous etiologies of pulsatile tinnitus?**

Jugular bulb abnormalities; hydrocephalus associated with stenosis of the Sylvian aqueduct; increased intracranial pressure associated with Arnold–Chiari syndrome; abnormal condylar and mastoid emissary veins; and idiopathic or essential tinnitus.

○ **What is the treatment for IIH?**

Weight reduction and acetazolamide (250 mg TID) or furosemide (20 mg BID); lumbar-peritoneal shunt for patients with visual deterioration, persistent headaches, or disabling tinnitus.

○ **What is the definition of sudden sensorineural hearing loss?**

>20 dB hearing loss over at least three contiguous frequencies occurring within 3 days.

○ **In what percent of these cases can a definite cause be determined?**

10%.

○ **What percent of these cases will turn out to have a vestibular schwannoma?**

Up to 4%.

○ **What are the two common theories on the etiology of idiopathic sudden sensorineural hearing loss (ISSNHL)?**

Circulatory disturbance and inflammatory reaction (usually viral).

○ **What is the current standard of care for the workup and treatment of ISSNHL?**

Otologic exam, audiogram, and rule-out retrocochlear pathology—treatment with steroids, $+/-$ antivirals, $+/-$ diuretics.

○ **What laboratory studies are useful in the workup?**

Coagulation profile (CBC, PT, PTT), viral studies, ESR.

○ **What is the prognosis of ISSNHL?**

Overall recovery to functional hearing levels in 65–69%; no conclusive evidence that outcome is improved by medical treatment.

○ **When is spontaneous recovery of hearing more likely?**

If patient is without vestibular symptoms and suffers only partial hearing loss, particularly low frequency (better prognosis if apex of the cochlea is involved).

○ **What treatments are used to try to optimize cochlear blood flow?**

Vasodilators (histamine, papaverine, verapamil, carbon dioxide) and blood thinners (defibrinogenation therapy, dextran, papaverine).

○ **What evidence supports the use of carbon dioxide for ISSNHL?**

Fisch et al. (1983) compared carbogen (95% oxygen and 5% carbon dioxide) inhalation therapy daily for 5 days with papaverine and low-molecular-weight dextran for 5 days and found a statistically significant improvement in hearing levels with carbogen therapy. These findings have not been replicated.

○ **What evidence supports the use of corticosteroids for ISSNHL?**

Steroid therapy is among the few treatment methods in ISSNHL to have single modality, randomized, prospective studies demonstrating effectiveness.

○ **What evidence supports the use of antivirals for ISSNHL?**

No randomized, prospective studies have demonstrated this therapy to be effective.

○ **What factors lead to the best rate of recovery after ISSNHL?**

Patients treated with steroids and vasodilators, with worse initial PTA and SDS, younger age, and greater number of treatments are most likely to improve.

○ **When is a middle ear exploration indicated?**

If the loss occurs in an only-hearing ear—to rule out a fistula.

○   **What are the two types of bony growths in the external auditory canal?**

Diffuse exostoses and osteomata.

○   **Which is more common?**

Exostoses.

○   **Which is usually attached to the tympanosquamous suture line?**

Osteomata.

○   **Which has a male predilection?**

Both.

○   **Which is more likely to be bilateral?**

Exostoses.

○   **Which is more likely to be seen in surfers?**

Exostoses.

○   **What are the indications for removal of exostoses?**

Less than 1 mm aperture, recurrent otitis externa, and water trapping.

○   **What are the symptoms of patulous eustachian tube?**

Aural fullness, autophony, tympanophonia that improve when the head is placed down between the legs; onset often occurs with weight loss or after irradiation to the nasopharynx.

○   **What is tympanophonia?**

Audition of one's own breath sounds.

○   **What are some treatments for patulous eustachian tube?**

Reassurance, weight gain, SSKI (10 gtt in juice po TID), Premarin nasal spray (25 mg in 30 cc NS, 3 gtt per nose TID), occlusion of the ET, and myringotomy and tympanostomy tube placement.

CHAPTER 27 Congenital

○ **What is the most common facial cleft?**
A cleft uvula.

○ **Which ethnic group has the highest incidence of cleft lip?**
Native Americans.

○ **Which ethnic group has the highest incidence of isolated cleft palate?**
Equal incidence among racial groups.

○ **What is the male:female ratio for cleft lip, with or without cleft palate?**
2:1.

○ **What is the male:female ratio for isolated cleft palate?**
1:2.

○ **What is the incidence of cleft lip, with or without cleft palate, in term newborns?**
1 in 1000.

○ **What is the incidence of isolated cleft palate in term newborns?**
1 in 2000.

○ **What is the incidence of submucous cleft palate in term newborns?**
1 in 1200.

○ **What is the chance of producing a cleft-lipped child when one parent is affected?**
4%.

○ **What is the most common single gene transmission error causing clefts?**
Trisomy 21.

○ **What are the most common environmental causes for clefts?**

Poorly controlled maternal diabetes and amniotic band syndrome.

○ **What is the characteristic nasal deformity in a child with a unilateral cleft lip?**

Inferior and posterior displacement of the alar cartilage on the cleft side.

○ **What happens to the orbicularis oris muscle in a complete cleft lip?**

Muscle fibers follow the cleft margins and terminate at the alar base.

○ **What happens to the orbicularis oris muscle in an incomplete cleft lip?**

Muscle fibers remain continuous but are hypoplastic across the cleft.

○ **What is Simonart's band?**

The bridge of tissue connecting the central and lateral lip in an incomplete cleft lip.

○ **What is the difference between a complete cleft of the primary palate and that of the secondary palate?**

A complete cleft of the primary palate extends into the nose, is always associated with a cleft lip, and does not expose the vomer. A complete cleft of the secondary palate involves both the hard and soft palates, extends into the nose, and exposes the vomer.

○ **What is an incomplete cleft?**

A varying amount of midline mucosal attachment is preserved with an underlying muscular deficiency.

○ **What type of cleft is a submucous cleft palate?**

Incomplete cleft of the secondary palate.

○ **What happens to the soft palate muscles in a secondary cleft palate?**

Muscle fibers follow the cleft margins and insert into the posterior edge of the remaining soft palate.

○ **What are the boundaries of a unilateral cleft of the primary palate?**

From the incisive foramen anteriorly, between the canine and adjacent incisor to the lip.

○ **What are the two most commonly used classification systems for clefts?**

Veau and Iowa classifications.

○ **Feeding difficulties are most severe with which type of cleft?**

Secondary palate clefts (either isolated or in combination with clefts of the lip and primary palate).

○ **What strategies can be used to assist feeding with a cleft palate?**

Specialized nipples, upright feeding to minimize nasal regurgitation, palatal plates.

○ **What percent of children with cleft palate do not require tympanostomy tubes?**

8–10%.

○ **What further facial deformities often occur as a child with a cleft palate grows?**

Collapse of the alveolar arch, midface retrusion, and malocclusion.

○ **What is the role of palatal plates in the treatment of cleft palates?**

A palatal plate, when worn for 3 months prior to surgery and adjusted weekly to bring the palate and alveolus into a more normal shape, has been shown to lessen closure tension during surgery.

○ **Which sounds are most difficult for patients with cleft palate?**

Consonants, as they require full palatal lift.

○ **What disorder should be suspected in children with cleft palate who fall below the 5th percentile in growth?**

Growth hormone deficiency, as it is 40 times more common in this population.

○ **What are the clinical differences between a hemangioma and a vascular malformation?**

Vascular malformations are present at birth, grow proportionately with the child, and are associated with distortion or destruction of surrounding bone or cartilage; hemangiomas generally emerge after birth, proliferate and then regress, and do not affect surrounding bone or cartilage.

○ **What are the typical clinical features of venous malformations?**

Soft, compressible, nonpulsatile masses most commonly found on the lip or cheek within the head and neck; also can be found within the masseter muscle or mandible.

○ **What are the clinical features of arteriovenous malformations?**

Brightly erythematous lesions of the skin with an associated thrill and bruit.

○ **What percent of infants have a hemangioma by age 1?**

12%.

○ **What is the incidence of hemangiomas in premature infants weighing less than 1000 g?**

23%.

○ **Between what ages do hemangiomas grow most rapidly?**

8–18 months.

○ **What percent of hemangiomas regress by age 7?**

70%.

○ **Where exactly are most subglottic hemangiomas located?**

Posterolaterally and submucosally.

○ **What percent of patients with a subglottic hemangioma have an associated cutaneous hemangioma?**

50%.

○ **What is the most common treatment for hemangiomas?**

Observation, parental reassurance.

○ **When is intervention warranted?**

For massive, ulcerative, disfiguring lesions; for those that produce hematologic, cardiovascular, or upper aerodigestive tract compromise; and for large periorbital lesions that obstruct vision.

○ **What syndrome is characterized by profound thrombocytopenia associated with a hemangioma?**

Kasabach–Merritt syndrome.

○ **What are the four main types of vascular malformations?**

Capillary, venous, lymphatic, and arteriovenous malformations.

○ **What is the most common vascular malformation?**

Port wine stain.

○ **Which type of vascular malformation is a port wine stain?**

Capillary.

○ **What syndrome is characterized by capillary hemangiomas along the distribution of V1 with concomitant capillary, venous, and arteriovenous malformations of the leptomeninges?**

Sturge–Weber syndrome.

○ **What is the optimal treatment for port wine stains?**

Argon laser in darker-skinned adults; flashlamp pulsed tunable dye laser in children and lighter-skinned adults.

○ **Which lesions respond best to pulsed dye laser?**

Lesions less than 20 cm^2 in children <1 year of age.

○ **What are the four categories of lymphatic malformations?**

Capillary, cavernous, cystic (hygroma), and lymphangiohemangioma.

○ **Which of these is associated with episodic bleeding?**

Lymphangiohemangioma.

○ **Which of these is most commonly found on the tongue or floor of mouth?**

Capillary.

○ **Which of these is associated with location in the posterior triangle of the neck?**

Cystic hygroma.

○ **Which of these is more likely to rapidly enlarge during an upper respiratory tract infection?**

Lymphangiohemangioma.

○ **An infant has a left-sided suprahyoid lymphatic malformation. Using the DeSerres classification system, which class is this?**

II.

○ **What are the indications for definitive treatment of lymphatic malformations?**

When vital structures are endangered, when episodic hemorrhage occurs, or if macroglossia is present.

○ **Which lesions are less likely to respond to sclerosis with OK-432 (Picibanil)?**

Microcystic, previously operated on, and those with massive craniofacial involvement.

○ **What condition is seen in adolescent patients with severe, frequently recurring epistaxis and pulmonary arteriovenous malformations?**

Hereditary hemorrhagic telangiectasia (HHT).

○ **What are the advantages of using argon plasma coagulation for the treatment of HHT?**

Noncontact application, limited and controlled tissue penetration with low risk of septal perforation, no safety measures required (i.e., for lasers), low thermal damage to adjacent tissue, and inexpensive.

○ **What are the three most common causes of stridor in children?**

Laryngomalacia, vocal cord paralysis, and congenital subglottic stenosis.

○ **What are the three modes of supraglottic obstruction causing laryngomalacia?**

Prolapse of the mucosa overlying the arytenoids, foreshortened aryepiglottic folds, and posterior displacement of the epiglottis.

○ **What is the incidence of synchronous airway lesions in children with laryngomalacia?**

18–20%.

○ **What percent of these require surgical intervention?**

<5%.

○ **What percent of infants with laryngomalacia require surgical treatment?**

10%.

○ **What are the indications for surgical treatment of laryngomalacia?**

Dyspnea at rest or during effort, feeding difficulties, and failure to thrive.

○ **What is the relationship between laryngomalacia and gastroesophageal reflux disease (GERD)?**

Essentially all children with laryngomalacia have GERD.

○   **What percent of children with choanal atresia have other congenital anomalies?**
50%.

○   **What percent of cases of choanal atresia are bilateral?**
40%.

○   **Persistence of what membrane results in choanal atresia?**
Buccopharyngeal.

○   **What percent of cases of choanal atresia involve only a mucosal diaphragm or membrane?**
10%.

○   **What percent of cases of congenital vocal cord paralysis are bilateral?**
20%.

○   **What percent of theses patients require tracheotomy?**
90%.

○   **What is the most common neurologic condition causing vocal cord paralysis in children?**
Arnold–Chiari malformation.

○   **What effect does the timing of treatment for Arnold–Chiari have on the outcome of vocal cord paralysis?**
If the ICP is normalized within 24 hours, vocal cord function will recover within 2 weeks in most patients.

○   **What is the recovery rate for idiopathic vocal cord paralysis in children?**
20%.

○   **Birth trauma accounts for what percent of vocal cord paralysis in children?**
20% (associated with forceps use and C-section).

○   **Where do most laryngeal webs occur?**
At the anterior glottis (75%).

○   **When is the typical onset of symptoms in patients with subglottic hemangioma?**
Usually asymptomatic at birth and symptomatic by 6 months of age.

○   **What is the most common vascular ring?**
Innominate artery compression.

○ **What is the most common anomaly associated with congenital tracheal stenosis?**

Aberrant left pulmonary artery (pulmonary artery sling complex).

○ **What syndrome is characterized by hypernasal speech, cardiac malformations, cleft palate, and medial displacement of the carotid arteries?**

Velocardiofacial syndrome (VCFS).

○ **What syndrome, characterized by deletion of band 11 on the long arm of chromosome 22, is a contraindication to adenoidectomy?**

VCFS.

○ **What is platybasia?**

Phenotypic characteristic of VCFS where the cranial base is angled obtusely, resulting in expanded velopharyngeal volume and incomplete velopharyngeal closure.

○ **What is the differential diagnosis of a midline neck mass in a child?**

Thyroglossal duct cyst (TGDC), dermoid cyst, ectopic thyroid tissue, lymphadenopathy, lipoma, hemangioma, and fibroma.

○ **Which of these is most common?**

TGDC.

○ **What is the etiology of TGDC?**

Persistence of the connection between the base of tongue (foramen cecum) and the descended thyroid gland.

○ **Why do some people recommend radioisotope scanning or ultrasound of the thyroid gland prior to removal of a TGDC?**

To prevent inadvertent removal of the only functioning thyroid tissue.

○ **What percent of TGDC contains thyroid tissue?**

20%.

○ **What is the incidence of carcinoma arising in a TGDC?**

<1%.

○ **What is the etiology of a preauricular pit?**

Failure of fusion between Hillocks of His 1 and 2.

○ **What percent of preauricular pits are bilateral?**

20%.

○ **What is the etiology of a type 1 first branchial cleft cyst?**

Duplication error of the ectodermal elements of the EAC.

○ **What is the etiology of a type 2 first branchial cleft cyst?**

Duplication error of the ectodermal and mesodermal elements of the EAC.

○ **Where are most type 1 cysts located?**

In the periauricular region, lateral to VII, connecting the skin to the EAC.

○ **Where are most type 2 cysts located?**

Just inferior or posterior to the angle of the mandible with variable relationship to VII.

○ **Where are most 2nd branchial cleft cysts located?**

Below the angle of the mandible and anterior to the sternocleidomastoid muscle.

○ **What is the typical course of the tract of 2nd branchial cleft cysts?**

Pass superiorly and laterally to IX, XII; turn medially to pass between the internal and external carotid arteries; terminate close to the middle constrictor muscle or may open into the tonsillar fossa.

○ **What is the typical course of the tract of 3rd branchial cleft cysts?**

Ascend lateral to the common carotid artery, pass posterior to the internal carotid artery, superior to XII, and inferior to IX; course medially to pierce the thyrohyoid membrane superior to the internal branch of the superior laryngeal nerve.

○ **What is the typical course of the tract of left-sided 4th branchial cleft cysts?**

Begin at the apex of the pyriform sinus, descend lateral to the recurrent laryngeal nerve into the thorax, loop around the aortic arch, ascend to the neck posterior to the common carotid artery, cross XII, descend to open into the skin at the anterior-inferior aspect of the sternocleidomastoid muscle.

○ **What is the typical course of the tract of right-sided 4th branchial cleft cysts?**

As above, except they loop around the subclavian artery instead of the aorta.

○ **What inflammatory disease is associated with 3rd and 4th branchial anomalies in children?**

Recurrent acute suppurative thyroiditis.

○ **What organisms are most commonly cultured from this disorder?**

Escherichia coli, Klebsiella, Proteus, and *Clostridium.*

○ **What are the four types of germ cell tumors?**

Dermoid cyst, teratoid cyst, teratoma, and epignathus.

○ **Which of these are composed only of mesoderm and ectoderm?**

Dermoid cysts.

○ **Where are dermoid cysts most commonly found in the head and neck?**

Submental area.

○ **How can one differentiate a dermoid cyst from a TGDC?**

Dermoid cyst will not elevate with tongue protrusion.

○ **What is the characteristic feature of a teratoid cyst?**

Very poor differentiation of all three germ layers.

○ **What differentiates a teratoid cyst from a teratoma?**

The germ layers are well differentiated in teratomas such that recognizable organs may be found within the masses.

○ **What percent of teratomas become malignant?**

20%.

○ **What prenatal condition is associated with a higher incidence of cervical teratomas?**

Maternal polyhydramnios.

○ **Which branchial pouch is the thymus derived from?**

3rd.

○ **What is the term for the connection of the 3rd branchial pouch to the thymus gland as the gland descends into the thorax?**

Thymopharyngeal duct.

○ **What is the etiology of cervical thymic cysts?**

Persistence of the thymopharyngeal duct.

○ **What is a Thornwaldt's cyst?**

Cyst in the nasopharyngeal bursa secondary to persistent embryonic communication between the anterior tip of the notochord and the nasopharyngeal epithelium.

○ **What are the three most common congenital midline nasal masses?**

Encephaloceles, gliomas, and dermoid cysts.

○ **Which of these has an intracerebral connection?**
Encephaloceles.

○ **What percent of gliomas have a fibrous tract connecting to the subarachnoid space?**
15%.

○ **Which chromosome carries the gene responsible for cystic fibrosis?**
Long arm of chromosome 7.

○ **True/False: Frontal sinus hypoplasia is common in patients with cystic fibrosis.**
True.

○ **What percent of Caucasians carry the gene defect for cystic fibrosis?**
5%.

○ **What is the incidence of congenital hearing loss?**
1:1000.

○ **What percent of these are hereditary?**
>60%.

○ **What percent of the hereditary cases are syndromic?**
30%.

○ **What is the typical inheritance pattern of syndromic hearing loss?**
Autosomal dominant (AD).

○ **What are the typical inheritance patterns of nonsyndromic hearing loss?**
10–20% AD, 75% autosomal recessive (AR), 2–3% X-linked, <1% mitochondrial.

○ **What genetic mutation is thought to be responsible for 50–80% of all AR hearing loss?**
Mutation of the DFNB1 gene on chromosome 13q encoding for connexin 26.

○ **What percent of sporadic cases of congenital hearing loss are caused by this mutation?**
27%.

○ **True/False: 1 in 31 people are carriers for the connexin 26 mutation.**
True.

○ **What is the function of connexin 26?**

Formation of gap junctions in the stria vascularis, basement membrane, limbus, and spiral prominence of the cochlea.

○ **What is the typical severity and pattern of AD hearing loss?**

Less severe, delayed onset, high-frequency hearing loss.

○ **What is the typical severity and pattern of X-linked hearing loss?**

Prelingual and more clinically diverse hearing loss.

○ **What is the term for complete agenesis of the petrous portion of the temporal bone?**

Michel aplasia.

○ **What is the term for a developmentally deformed cochlea where only the basal coil can be identified?**

Mondini aplasia.

○ **What is the most common form of inner ear aplasia?**

Scheibe aplasia (cochleosaccular dysplasia or pars inferior dysplasia).

○ **Which inner ear aplasia is characterized by high-frequency hearing loss with normal low-frequency hearing?**

Alexander.

○ **Which inner ear aplasia will not allow cochlear implant or amplification aids?**

Michel aplasia.

○ **Mutation of what gene is associated with enlarged vestibular aqueduct?**

Pendrin on chromosome 7q31.

○ **What inner ear malformation is associated with early onset sensorineural hearing loss, usually bilateral and progressive, and vertigo?**

Enlarged vestibular aqueduct.

○ **Which semicircular canal (SCC) forms first? Last?**

Superior canal forms first; lateral canal forms last.

○ **True/False: Superior SCC deformities are always accompanied by lateral SCC deformities.**

True.

○ **What syndrome accounts for the most common form of hereditary congenital deafness?**

Waardenburg's syndrome.

○ **What is the incidence of Waardenburg's syndrome?**

1 in 4,000 births.

○ **What are the four clinical subtypes of Waardenburg's syndrome?**

1. SNHL (20%), heterochromia irides, pigment anomalies, dystopia canthorum.

2. As above, without dystopia canthorum (SNHL in >50%).

3. Klein–Waardenburg's syndrome: microcephaly, mental retardation, limb and skeletal abnormalities, in addition to signs of #1.

4. Shah-Waardenburg's syndrome: #2 + Hirschsprung's disease

○ **What genetic mutation is responsible for most cases of types 1 and 3 of Waardenburg's syndrome?**

Mutation of the PAX3 gene on chromosome 2q37.

○ **What is dystopia canthorum?**

Shortened and fused medial eyelids resulting in small medial sclera, lateral displacement of the inferior puncta, and hypertelorism.

○ **What syndrome is characterized by cleft palate, micrognathia, severe myopia, retinal detachments, cataracts, marfanoid habitus, and hearing loss?**

Stickler.

○ **What genetic mutations are responsible for most cases of Stickler syndrome?**

Mutations in the COL2A1 gene on chromosome 12 or the COLIIA2 gene on chromosome 6.

○ **What syndrome is characterized by SNHL and retinitis pigmentosa?**

Usher's syndrome.

○ **What are the three clinical subtypes of Usher's syndrome?**

I—Severe–profound hearing loss, absent vestibular function, prepubertal retinitis pigmentosa.
II—Moderate–severe hearing loss, normal vestibular function, postpubertal retinitis pigmentosa.
III—Progressive hearing loss.

○ **What is the most common syndromic cause of hearing loss?**

Pendred syndrome, accounting for 10% of cases.

○ **What inner ear malformations are more common in patients with Pendred syndrome?**

Mondini aplasia and enlarged vestibular aqueduct.

○ **What gene is associated with both Pendred syndrome and enlarged vestibular aqueduct?**

PDS gene, encoding for pendrin protein, on chromosome 7q31.

○ **What are the clinical features of Alport syndrome?**
SNHL and renal failure (presenting as hematuria).

○ **What is the basic defect causing Alport syndrome?**
Mutation of the COL4A5 gene producing the alpha chain of type IV collagen in basement membranes.

○ **What syndrome is characterized by hearing loss, renal defects, and cervical fistula?**
Branchiootorenal.

○ **What is the inheritance pattern of branchiootorenal syndrome?**
Autosomal dominant.

○ **What percent of these patients have hearing loss?**
80% (50% mixed, 30% conductive, 20% sensorineural).

○ **What gene is responsible for this syndrome?**
EYA1 on chromosome 8q13.3.

○ **What are the clinical features of Jervell and Lange-Nielsen's syndrome?**
Prolonged QT interval, syncope, sudden death, and hearing loss.

○ **What is the basic defect causing this syndrome?**
Abnormal potassium channels.

○ **What percent of patients with neurofibromatosis type 1 have acoustic neuromas?**
5% and usually unilateral.

○ **What percent of patients with neurofibromatosis type 2 have acoustic neuromas?**
95% and usually bilateral.

○ **Which type of neurofibromatosis is characterized by cutaneous neurofibromas?**
Type 1.

○ **What genetic mutation is responsible for neurofibromatosis type 1?**
Mutation of the NF1 gene (nerve growth factor gene) on chromosome 17q11.2.

○ **What genetic mutation is responsible for neurofibromatosis type 2?**
Mutation of the NF2 gene (tumor suppressor gene) on chromosome 22q12.2.

○ **What is the name for the subtype of osteogenesis imperfecta in which progressive hearing loss begins in early childhood?**

Van der Hoeve's syndrome.

○ **What genetic mutations are thought to be responsible for osteogenesis imperfecta?**

Mutations of the COLIA1 gene on chromosome 17q and the COLIA2 gene on chromosome 7q.

○ **What disease is characterized by cranial synostosis, exophthalmos, parrot-beaked nose, and hypoplastic mandible?**

Crouzon's disease.

○ **What is the basic defect of this disease?**

Abnormal fibroblast growth factor receptors.

○ **What is Norrie syndrome?**

X-linked disease characterized by blindness, progressive mental retardation, and hearing loss.

○ **What syndrome is characterized by hypertelorism, short stature, broad fingers and toes, cleft palate, and conductive hearing loss?**

Otopalatodigital syndrome.

○ **What X-linked syndrome is associated with the Klippel–Feil syndrome, SNHL, and cranial nerve VI paralysis?**

Wildervanck syndrome.

○ **What disease is characterized by lower lid colobomas, downward slanting palpebral fissures, hypoplastic mandible, malformations of the external ear, cleft palate, and hearing loss?**

Treacher–Collins.

○ **What is the inheritance pattern of this disease?**

Autosomal dominant.

○ **What genetic mutation is responsible for Treacher–Collins syndrome?**

Mutation of TCOF1 on chromosome 5q.

○ **What protein does this gene produce?**

Treacle.

○ **What do Keams–Sayre, MELAS, MERRF, and Leber's hereditary optic neuropathy all have in common?**

They are all mitochondrial disorders with varying degrees of hearing loss.

○   **What organism is most commonly associated with virus-induced congenital deafness?**
Cytomegalovirus (CMV).

○   **What percent of children with congenital CMV have hearing loss?**
10% are born with hearing loss, 10–15% eventually develop hearing loss.

○   **What manifestation of congenital syphilis is most commonly related to SNHL?**
Interstitial keratitis.

○   **What are the three classic findings of congenital rubella syndrome?**
SNHL, cataracts, heart malformations.

○   **If one parent and one sibling are deaf, what is the risk of hearing loss for subsequent offspring?**
40% risk.

○   **What percent of infants with significant congenital hearing loss will not have risk factors?**
50%.

○   **What is the incidence of congenital aural atresia?**
1:10,000–20,000.

○   **What percent of these are bilateral?**
33%.

○   **What does stenosis of the EAC predispose to?**
Canal cholesteatoma.

○   **Which portion of the ossicular chain is least likely to be malformed in patients with congenital aural atresia?**
Stapes footplate.

○   **What is the incidence of facial nerve displacement in congenital aural atresia?**
25–30%.

○   **What is a congenital cholesteatoma?**
Embryonal inclusion of undifferentiated squamous epithelium in the middle ear behind an intact TM, usually with no history of otitis media.

○   **Other than the middle ear, where else may congenital cholesteatomas arise?**
Petrous apex, cerebellopontine angle, mastoid, EAC.

○   **What percent of congenital cholesteatomas are bilateral?**
3%.

○   **What is the mean age of presentation for congenital cholesteatoma?**
4.5 years.

○   **True/False: The mastoid bones of patients with congenital cholesteatoma are most often well aerated.**
True.

○   **What is thought to cause congenital malleus ankylosis?**
Poor development of the epitympanic space leaves the head of the incus and malleus in close contact with the tegmen; a bony bridge can result between the epitympanum and the head of the malleus.

○   **True/False: Histologically, the bony structures are normal, without evidence of otosclerosis, in cases of malleus ankylosis.**
True.

○   **What is the optimal treatment of malleus fixation?**
Removal of the head of the malleus and interposition of the incus between the manubrium and the stapes head.

○   **What genetic defect results in either Jansen's chondrodystrophy or Blomstrand's chondrodystrophy?**
Mutation of the type 1 parathyroid hormone receptor.

○   **Which of these is lethal prenatally?**
Blomstrand's chondrodystrophy.

○   **What is the ciliary defect in patients with Kartagener's syndrome?**
Absence of dynein side arms on A-tubules.

○   **What is the most common site of CSF leakage from the inner ear into the middle ear in children?**
Oval window (especially in patients with Mondini malformation).

○   **What are the two types of congenital defects that lead to spontaneous CSF otorrhea?**
Preformed bony pathway around the bony labyrinth, often associated with a meningocele and aberrant arachnoid granulations located over a pneumatized area of the skull.

○   **Which of these is associated with meningitis?**
Preformed bony pathway around the bony labyrinth.

○ **How does the defect caused by arachnoid granulations usually present?**

Presents after age 50 as unilateral serous otitis which is at first recurrent and then persistent.

○ **Why does spontaneous CSF otorrhea present late when caused by arachnoid granulations?**

Arachnoid granulations become larger with time; the normal pulsation of CSF pressure can cause bony erosion.

○ **What syndrome is characterized by recurrent episodes of vertigo and ataxia in several members of a family?**

Familial ataxia syndrome.

○ **Of the four variants of this syndrome (EA1, EA2, EA3, EA4), which one does not respond to acetazolamide?**

EA3 or periodic vestibulocerebellar ataxia.

○ **Which of these 4 variants is caused by mutations in a potassium channel gene (KCNA1) on 12p13?**

EA1

○ **What are the two most common variants of this syndrome?**

EA1 and EA2.

○ **Which of these is associated with vertigo and results from mutations of a calcium channel gene on 19p?**

EA2.

○ **What gene mutation is behind EA1?**

Mutation in a potassium channel gene KCNA1 on 12p13.

○ **Which variant is associated with migraine?**

EA2.

CHAPTER 28 Degenerative

○ **What are the two types of esophageal diverticula?**

Pulsion and traction.

○ **Which of these is associated with high intraluminal pressure?**

Pulsion.

○ **Which of these is Zenker's diverticulum?**

Pulsion.

○ **Where do pharyngoesophageal/Zenker's diverticula occur?**

Between the oblique and transverse fibers of the inferior constrictor (Killian's dehiscence), most commonly on the left, and between the cricopharyngeus and the esophagus (Killian-Jamieson area).

○ **What problem results from rupture of the middle meningeal artery?**

Epidural hematoma.

○ **What is a laryngocele?**

Abnormal dilatation of the laryngeal saccule.

○ **What are the three types of laryngoceles?**

Internal, external, and combined.

○ **Where are internal laryngoceles located?**

Beneath the mucosa of the false vocal cord and aryepiglottic folds.

○ **How do laryngoceles become external?**

Penetrate the thyrohyoid membrane at the site of entry of the superior laryngeal artery and nerve.

○ **What are mixed laryngoceles?**

External laryngoceles with a dilated internal component.

○ **When do most laryngoceles present?**

Can present at any time, but most commonly arise in the sixth decade of life.

○ **What are the four etiologies of vocal cord immobility?**

Paralysis, synkinesis, cricoarytenoid joint fixation, and interarytenoid scar.

○ **What condition is characterized by generalized tension in all laryngeal muscles?**

Muscular tension dysphonia.

○ **In which patients is this most commonly seen?**

Untrained occupational and professional voice users.

○ **What are the two main theories of the pathophysiology of BPPV?**

Cupulolithiasis theory: deposits gravitate, attach to, and stimulate the cupula.

Canalolithiasis theory: deposits float freely within the SCCs under the influence of gravity.

○ **What percent of cases occur in the posterior SCC? Horizontal SCC?**

Posterior 80–95%; horizontal 5–20%.

○ **Which theory is currently more favored?**

Canalolithiasis.

○ **How does this theory account for the latency of onset of nystagmus?**

Delay is due to the adherence of deposits to the membranous wall of the labyrinth.

○ **What are the deposits thought to consist of?**

Calcium carbonate crystals, possibly resulting from microfractures of the temporal bone near the round window niche (also near the ampulla of the posterior SCC).

○ **What therapeutic maneuver is based on the cupulolithiasis theory?**

Semont.

○ **What therapeutic maneuver is based on the canalolithiasis theory?**

Epley.

○ **What is the success rate of the Epley maneuver after only one manipulation?**

50–77%.

○ **What is the success rate after two manipulations?**

95–97%.

○ **What toxin is the most common cause of cerebellar degeneration?**

Ethanol.

○ **What is the rate of recurrence?**

30–50% eventually have a recurrence; 10–20% within 1–2 weeks of the maneuver.

○ **What are the two types of tympanic membrane perforations?**

Central and marginal.

○ **Which of these is associated with cholesteatoma?**

Marginal.

○ **What are the two parts of a cholesteatoma?**

Amorphous center surrounded by keratinized squamous epithelium.

○ **What are the two types of cholesteatomas?**

Congenital and acquired.

○ **What are the two types of acquired cholesteatomas?**

Primary and secondary.

○ **What is the difference between a primary and a secondary cholesteatoma?**

Primary usually occurs in the attic at Shrapnell's membrane and starts as a retraction pocket; secondary is associated with chronic middle ear infection and TM perforations.

○ **Which ossicle is most commonly involved in patients with cholesteatoma?**

Incus.

○ **What percent of patients have erosion of the scutum with cholesteatoma?**

42%.

○ **What are the most common sites of origin of primary acquired cholesteatomas?**

Posterior epitympanum, posterior mesotympanum, and anterior epitympanum (in descending order of frequency).

○ **What is the typical route of spread of cholesteatomas originating in the posterior epitympanum?**

Starting from Prussak's space, penetrate posteriorly to the superior incudal space lateral to the body of the incus, and progress to the aditus and the antrum.

○ **What is the typical route of spread of cholesteatomas originating in anterior mesotympanum?**

Descend to the pouch of von Troeltch, and may involve the stapes, sinus tympani, or facial recess.

○ **What percent of cholesteatomas are complicated by a labyrinthine fistula?**

5–10%.

○ **Where does this most often occur?**

Lateral semicircular canal (75%).

○ **In a patient with a cholesteatoma, what factors make the presence of a fistula highly unlikely?**

Disease <20 years, normal bone conduction, negative fistula test, no history of dizziness, and normal facial nerve function.

○ **What is the significance of pain in a patient with cholesteatoma or chronic otitis media?**

Expanding mass or empyema in the antrum.

○ **What are the three layers of the otic capsule?**

Outer periosteal layer, inner periosteal layer (endosteum), and the middle endochondral layer.

○ **Which of these layers does otosclerosis involve?**

Middle endochondral layer.

○ **What are the terms used to describe involvement of the oval window and cochlea?**

Fenestral otosclerosis and retrofenestral otosclerosis, respectively.

○ **What does the "Blue Mantles of Manasse" refer to?**

Basophilic appearance on hematoxylin and eosin staining of bone in the active stage of otosclerosis.

○ **What is the most commonly involved site of otosclerosis in the temporal bone?**

Anterior to the oval window at the fissula ante fenestrum.

○ **What percent of cases of otosclerosis are bilateral?**

85%.

○ **At what age does otosclerosis peak in incidence?**

Third decade.

○ **What conditions accelerate hearing loss in patients with otosclerosis?**

Pregnancy, estrogen replacement.

○ **What genetic mutation has been implicated as a possible cause of otosclerosis?**

Mutation of the COLIA1 gene on chromosome 17q.

○ **What virus is thought to play a role in the etiology of otosclerosis?**

Measles.

○ **What is the inheritance pattern of otosclerosis?**

Autosomal dominant with incomplete penetrance (only 25–40% of carriers express the phenotype).

○ **How is far-advanced otosclerosis (FAO) defined?**

Otosclerosis with an air conduction threshold greater than 85 dB and a bone conduction threshold not measurable.

○ **What are the histopathologic findings of patients with FAO?**

Invasion of otosclerotic foci into the cochlear endosteum and the stapes footplate.

○ **What features on history distinguish FAO from profound SNHL?**

Family history of otosclerosis; progressive hearing loss usually of long duration; history of hearing aid use that is no longer beneficial or present use of a hearing aid with benefit beyond that which would be expected for the severity of the hearing loss; paracusis; and previous audiograms indicating an air–bone gap.

○ **What features on physical exam distinguish FAO from profound SNHL?**

Patients with FAO more likely will have a soft voice with better quality than expected for the degree of hearing loss and the ability to hear a 512 Hz tuning fork placed on the teeth, dentures, or gums.

○ **What is Eagle's syndrome?**

Elongation of the styloid process or ossification of the stylohyoid ligament resulting in nonspecific throat pain, foreign body sensation, and increased salivation.

○ **What is the most common cause of pulsatile tinnitus in patients older than 50?**

Atherosclerotic carotid artery disease.

○ **What are the most common manifestations of vertebrobasilar insufficiency (VBI)?**

Abrupt, transient attacks of vertigo associated with bilaterally reduced caloric responses.

○ **What is the treatment for vertigo secondary to VBI?**

Aspirin or ticlid if aspirin sensitive.

CHAPTER 29 Infectious

○ **What is Gradenigo's syndrome?**

Petrositis involving VI in Dorello's canal causing retro-orbital pain, diplopia, and otorrhea.

○ **What is the most commonly proposed theory of the etiology of Bell's palsy?**

Activation of a latent virus present within the geniculate ganglion leading to entrapment, ischemia, and degeneration of the labyrinthine segment of VII.

○ **What viruses are most commonly implicated in the etiology of Bell's palsy?**

Herpes simplex and herpes zoster viruses.

○ **True/False: Enhancement of the facial nerve is commonly seen on MRI of patients with Bell's palsy and is likely to resolve in 2–4 months.**

True.

○ **What is the outcome of Bell's palsy left untreated?**

Complete recovery in 71%; permanent diminished function in 16%; poorer prognosis if >60 years of age, and if onset of recovery is >3 months after initial onset of paralysis.

○ **True/False: Addition of acyclovir to prednisone for treatment of Bell's palsy has not been shown to result in significant improvement of facial nerve function.**

False.

○ **What is the outcome of patients with Bell's palsy who have 90% or more degeneration on ENoG within the first 14 days of onset and undergo decompression?**

91% have a good outcome (House I or II) 7 months after paralysis.

○ **What is the outcome of these patients who are treated with steroids alone?**

42% have a good outcome.

○ **What is the outcome of these patients who undergo surgical decompression >14 days after injury?**

Similar outcome as patients treated with steroids.

○ **What is the incidence of recurrent facial palsy in otherwise healthy patients with Bell's palsy?**
5–7%.

○ **What is the mean interval to the 1st recurrence?**
10 years.

○ **What factors increase the risk of recurrent Bell's palsy?**
Diabetes mellitus and family history.

○ **What differentiates herpes zoster oticus from Ramsay Hunt syndrome?**
Ramsay Hunt syndrome is herpes zoster oticus + facial nerve paralysis.

○ **What is the incidence of VIIIth nerve involvement in patients with Ramsay Hunt syndrome?**
20%.

○ **Which etiology of facial nerve palsy has a worse prognosis: Bell's palsy or Ramsay Hunt syndrome?**
Ramsay Hunt syndrome.

○ **What are negative prognostic factors for Ramsay Hunt syndrome?**
Increased age and a simultaneous onset of paralysis with vesicular eruption.

○ **Why must the dose of acyclovir be larger for patients with varicella zoster virus (VZV)?**
The thymidine kinase of VZV is much less sensitive to acyclovir than the herpes simplex virus.

○ **What is the recommended treatment for Ramsay Hunt syndrome?**
Acyclovir 800 mg five times a day × 10 days and prednisone taper × 14 days.

○ **What is the treatment for otogenic facial palsy in association with acute suppurative OM?**
Wide myringotomy, cultures, and IV antibiotics.

○ **What organisms are most often associated with facial palsy due to chronic OM?**
Gram-negative organisms and *Staphylococcus aureus*.

○ **What is the incidence of facial palsy as the presenting symptom of tuberculous mastoiditis?**
39%.

○ **What percent of patients with Lyme disease have facial nerve paralysis as the sole manifestation?**
20%.

○ **What is the most common cause of cough in children?**

URI.

○ **Other than URI, what are the most common causes of persistent cough in infants up to 18 months?**

Aberrant innominate artery, cough-variant asthma, and gastroesophageal reflux disease.

○ **In children 18 months to 6 years?**

Sinusitis (50%), cough-variant asthma (27%).

○ **In children 6–16 years?**

Cough-variant asthma (45%), psychogenic (32%), and sinusitis (27%).

○ **What organism is the most common cause of bacterial tracheitis in children?**

S. aureus.

○ **What is the most common cause of laryngotracheobronchitis (croup) in children?**

Parainfluenza virus.

○ **How is croup managed?**

Humidification, dexamethasone, and racemic epinephrine.

○ **What is the most common notifiable and vaccine-preventable disease in children under age 5?**

Pertussis.

○ **How should contacts be treated?**

14 days of erythromycin.

○ **What percent of cultured organisms in patients with recurrent tonsillitis produce β-lactamase?**

Approximately 40%.

○ **In what age group is tonsillitis from group A streptococci most common?**

Ages 6–12.

○ **What is the most common valvular problem resulting from rheumatic fever?**

Mitral valve stenosis.

○ **According to the Paradise study from 1984, what are the criteria for adenotonsillectomy for recurrent tonsillitis?**

At least three episodes in each of 3 years or five episodes in each of 2 years or seven episodes in 1 year—with each episode documented by a physician.

○ **When should an asymptomatic patient with a positive posttreatment culture for group A streptococci be treated?**

If the patient or someone in his family has a history of rheumatic fever.

○ **What proportion of children will have had at least one episode of OM by age 1?**

Two-thirds.

○ **What age group has the highest incidence of OM?**

6–18 months.

○ **What is the mean duration of OM with effusion after acute otitis media (AOM)?**

40 days.

○ **What percent of children with an episode of AOM will still have an effusion present 3 months later?**

10%.

○ **What is the significance of day care on the risk of developing OM?**

Children in group day care are more likely to develop OM after URI compared with those in home care. The rate of tympanostomies and adenoidectomies is 59–67% higher in children <3 who attend day care.

○ **What is the significance of the seasons on the risk of developing OM?**

OM is most common in the winter and lasts longer when it occurs in the winter.

○ **What is the significance of genetics on the risk of developing OM?**

Risk of OM is higher if a sibling has a history of recurrent OM.

○ **What is the significance of breast-feeding on the risk of developing OM?**

The duration of breast-feeding is inversely related to the incidence of OM.

○ **What is the significance of passive smoke exposure on the risk of developing OM?**

A higher incidence of tympanostomy tubes, chronic and recurrent OM, and otorrhea is seen in children whose mothers smoke. High concentrations of serum cotinine (marker for tobacco exposure) are associated with an increased incidence of AOM and persistent middle ear effusion following AOM.

○ **What medical conditions predispose a child to OM?**

Cleft palate, craniofacial anomalies, congenital or acquired immune deficiencies, ciliary dysfunction, enlarged adenoids, sinusitis, and Down syndrome.

○ **Decreased levels of which immunoglobulin are common in children who are prone to OM?**

IgG2.

○ **How do the American Academy of Pediatrics (AAP) and American Academy of Family Physicians (AAFP) define AOM?**

Acute onset (within 48 hours of symptoms), with the presence of middle ear effusion and signs and symptoms of middle ear inflammation.

○ **What is the first-line treatment for AOM in patients 6 months to 2 years of age?**

High-dose amoxicillin (90 mg/kg/day); for patients with severe illness (moderate to severe otalgia or temperature of 39°C or higher) and where there is significant concern for β-lactamase–positive *Haemophilus influenzae* or *Moraxella catarrhalis*, amoxicillin–clavulanate is indicated.

○ **What organisms most frequently cause AOM?**

Streptococcus pneumoniae (30–35%), nontypeable strains of *H. influenzae* (20–25%), and *M. catarrhalis* (10–15%).

○ **Which organisms more frequently cause AOM in infants younger than 6 weeks?**

Escherichia coli, *Klebsiella*, and *Pseudomonas aeruginosa*.

○ **What percent of middle ear fluid cultures are negative for bacteria?**

25–30%.

○ **True/False: The 23-valent pneumococcal vaccine is not effective in children <2.**

True.

○ **How many serotypes of pneumococcus are responsible for 83% of invasive disease in children <4?**

Seven.

○ **What is the reduction in the need for myringotomy tubes in children who receive the heptavalent pneumococcal vaccine?**

Approximately 20%.

○ **Vaccination against what virus had been shown to decrease the incidence of AOM in infants and children?**

Influenza.

○ **What are the three most commonly identified viruses in middle ear fluid?**

Respiratory syncytial virus (RSV) (74%), parainfluenza, and influenza.

○ **What is the mechanism of resistance for *S. pneumoniae*?**

Altered penicillin-binding proteins.

○ **What organisms most frequently cause chronic suppurative OM?**

P. aeruginosa (most common), *S. aureus*, *Corynebacterium*, and *Klebsiella*.

○ **What are the AAO-HNS indications for myringotomy and tympanostomy tubes?**

Three or more episodes of OM in 6 months; four or more episodes in 12 months.

Hearing loss >30 dB from OME.

OME >3 months.

Chronic TM retraction.

Impending mastoiditis or other complication of OM.

Autophony secondary to patulous eustachian tube.

ET dysfunction secondary to craniofacial anomalies or head and neck radiation.

○ **What is the significance of adenoidectomy on OM?**

Data by Gates showed a 47% reduction in recurrent effusion in children who received adenoidectomy and myringotomy tubes compared with a 29% reduction in recurrent effusion in children who received only myringotomy tubes.

○ **What is the incidence of facial nerve paralysis in patients with chronic OM and cholesteatoma?**

1%.

○ **How is this treated?**

Expedient elimination of infection.

○ **What are the intracranial complications of OM?**

Epidural abscess/granulation tissue, sigmoid sinus thrombosis, meningitis, brain abscess, and subdural abscess.

○ **What are the extracranial complications of OM?**

Subperiosteal (Bezold's) abscess, petrositis, labyrinthitis, and facial nerve paralysis.

○ **What factors predispose one to complications from OM?**

Chronic infection, history of mastoid surgery, cholesteatoma, diabetes, and immunocompromise.

○ **What is the most common complication of acute mastoiditis?**

Subperiosteal abscess.

○ **What is the treatment for uncomplicated acute mastoiditis?**

Tympanocentesis for culture and IV antibiotics.

○ **When is a CT scan obtained?**

If signs of progression arise while on IV antibiotics or if the patient presents with possible intracranial complications.

○ **When is mastoidectomy indicated?**

If the CT scan shows coalescent mastoiditis and/or intracranial involvement.

○ **What are the early signs and symptoms of intracranial infection?**

Prolonged suppurative OM, fetid discharge and persistent pain despite adequate treatment, and bony destruction of inner cortex of mastoid on CT scan.

○ **What are the three most common organisms of OM that result in intracranial infections?**

Streptococcus faecalis, Proteus, and *Bacteroides fragilis.*

○ **What is the most common complaint of patients with an epidural abscess/granulation tissue?**

Deep, constant pain in the temporal area that is very steroid responsive.

○ **What are the most common signs and symptoms of sigmoid sinus thrombosis?**

Picket fence fever, cannon ball infiltrates on CXR, torticollis, jugular foramen syndrome, and otitic hydrocephalus.

○ **What are the three most common organisms causing meningitis secondary to OM?**

H. influenzae type b, *S. pneumoniae,* and *Neisseria meningitidis.*

○ **True/False: Since the introduction of the heptavalent pneumococcal vaccine, overall rates of pneumococcal meningitis have decreased in the United States, but rates caused by non-PC7–related serotypes have increased, primarily in children younger than 2.**

True.

○ **What factor strongly correlates with survival and long-term neurologic deficits in patients with a brain abscess?**

Patient's level of consciousness at the time of diagnosis.

○ **What are the most common pathogens cultured from otorrhea after tympanotomy tubes in children younger than 3?**

H. influenzae and *Diplococcus pneumoniae.*

○ **What are the most common pathogens cultured from otorrhea after tympanotomy tubes in children older than 3?**

S. aureus and *P. aeruginosa.*

○ **What is the leading cause of chronic cervical lymphadenopathy in young children?**

Nontuberculous mycobacterium or atypical TB.

○ **What are the most common organisms causing nontuberculous mycobacterium?**

Mycobacterium avium-intracellulare complex and *Mycobacterium scrofulaceum.*

○ **What are the clinical features of cervical nontuberculous mycobacterium?**

Typically affects children ages 1–5 years, unilateral, upper cervicofacial lymph nodes, negative or weakly positive PPD, normal CXR.

○ **What are the clinical features of cervical tuberculosis?**

Affects all ages, bilateral supraclavicular lymph nodes, positive PPD, positive CXR, respond to curettage, and macrolide antibiotics.

○ **What are the two most common inflammatory salivary diseases of childhood?**

Mumps parotitis and recurrent parotitis of childhood.

○ **What are the clinical features of recurrent parotitis of childhood?**

Typically presents at age 5–7, more common in males, unilateral, gets less severe with time, 55% will resolve spontaneously, and frank pus is rarely seen.

○ **What is the most common organism found in patients with atrophic rhinitis?**

Klebsiella ozaenae.

○ **What are the diagnostic criteria for allergic fungal sinusitis (AFS) as described by Bent and Kuhn?**

Allergic mucin.
Nasal polyposis.
CT scan findings consistent with chronic rhinosinusitis.
Positive fungal histology or culture.
Type I hypersensitivity diagnosed by history, positive skin test, or serology.

○ **What is allergic mucin?**

Clusters of eosinophils and their by-products (e.g., Charcot–Leyden crystals and major basic protein).

○ **What are Charcot–Leyden crystals?**

Degraded eosinophils.

○ **What organism is most commonly involved in fungal sinusitis?**

Aspergillus species.

○ **What is the incidence of AFS in cases of chronic rhinosinusitis treated surgically?**

6–7%.

○ **True/False: Fluid collections are rare in all forms of fungal disease.**

True.

○ **What is the difference between acute, chronic, and recurrent acute sinusitis?**

Acute <4 weeks; chronic >12 weeks; and recurrent acute >4 episodes/year with resolution between episodes.

○ **What distinguishes bacterial from viral rhinosinusitis?**

Symptoms that worsen after 5 days, persist longer than 10 days, or are out of proportion to those typical of viral infection are characteristics of bacterial rhinosinusitis.

○ **What percent of patients with viral rhinosinusitis develops bacterial rhinosinusitis?**

0.5–2.0%.

○ **What are host risk factors for chronic rhinosinusitis?**

Hypogammaglobulinemia, selective IgA deficiency, AIDS, cystic fibrosis, granulomatous disorders (especially sarcoidosis), primary ciliary dyskinesia, chronic stress, and asthma.

○ **Patients with perennial allergic rhinitis have a significantly higher rate of nasal carriage of which organism?**

S. aureus.

○ **What local factors predispose to sinusitis?**

Narrow osteomeatal complex, osteomyelitis, polyps, accessory maxillary sinus ostia, nose blowing, and dental disease.

○ **What are the most common organisms causing acute bacterial rhinosinusitis?**

S. pneumoniae, H. influenzae, Branhamella catarrhalis, S. aureus, anaerobes (<10%), and other streptococcal species (7%).

○ **What organisms are commonly cultured from patients with chronic sinusitis but rarely seen in patients with acute sinusitis?**

Gram-negative bacteria.

○ **What organisms are commonly cultured from the middle meatus in healthy patients?**

Coagulase-negative staphylococci (35%), *Corynebacterium* species (23%), and *S. aureus* (8%) in adults. *H. influenzae* (40%), *M. catarrhalis* (34%), and *S. pneumoniae* (50%) in children.

○ **Which organism was found, using PCR techniques, to be present in the sinus tissue of most patients with sarcoidosis?**

Propionibacterium granulosum.

○ **What is the Pretz maneuver?**

Sinus irrigation where saline is flushed into one nostril and aspirated from the other nostril while the patient is supine with the nasopharynx parallel to the floor.

○ **Which adjuvant therapies have proven to hasten recovery from acute sinusitis?**

No adjuvant therapies (e.g., antihistamines, decongestants, and steroids) have proven to hasten recovery from acute sinusitis.

○ **What are the most common intracranial complications of rhinosinusitis?**

Subdural empyema (38%), intracerebral abscess, extradural abscess, meningitis, and cavernous and superior sagittal sinus thrombosis (listed in decreasing order of frequency).

○ **Why are infants more prone to meningitis as a complication of rhinosinusitis?**

The arachnoid mater normally serves as a barrier to infection, but in infants, the arachnoid mater is immature.

○ **What percent of patients who develop an intracranial complication from rhinosinusitis have a prior history of chronic rhinosinusitis?**

10%

○ **What is the most common organism cultured from an intracerebral abscess resulting from rhinosinusitis?**

Streptococcus milleri (commensal found in the mouth, vagina, and feces).

○ **Compared with children with chronic sinusitis, children with recurrent sinusitis are more likely to be what?**

Older.

○ **What is the most common pathogen isolated from opacified maxillary sinuses in children?**

S. pneumoniae.

○ **What is the most common organism cultured from the blood of patients with preseptal orbital cellulitis?**

S. pneumoniae (*H. influenzae* type b if not vaccinated).

○ **What is the significance of age in the etiology and pathogenesis of postseptal orbital cellulitis?**

In children under 9, one organism, usually a streptococcus, is responsible. Older children are more likely to be infected with multiple organisms. The likelihood of resolution with a prolonged course of intravenous antibiotics decreases with age (10% in the 9–15 years old age group to 0% in patients older than 15). At age 12, the maxillary sinus comes in contact with molar tooth roots; infection of the molars can lead to orbital cellulitis.

○ **What are the two types of postseptal cellulitis?**

Extraconal and intraconal.

○ **What is the most common form of extraconal infection?**

Medial subperiosteal phlegmon or abscess caused by extension of bacteria from adjacent ethmoid sinusitis.

○ **What are the indications for emergent surgery in patients with orbital cellulitis?**

CT evidence of an intraconal abscess; massive proptosis with retinal or optic nerve ischemia and loss of vision; and visual acuity of 20/60 or less in an immunocompromised patient with a subperiosteal abscess.

○ **True/False: The risk of intracranial complications from orbital cellulitis is higher in teenagers than in infants.**

True.

○ **What are the most common organisms causing nonfatal bacterial meningitis in children >2.5 years?**
H. influenzae, Neisseria meningitides, and *S. pneumoniae*.

○ **What is the incidence of postmeningitic hearing loss?**
10–20%.

○ **Which organism most commonly causes postmeningitic hearing loss?**
S. pneumoniae.

○ **What sort of hearing loss is typical after meningitis?**
Bilateral, severe to profound, and permanent.

○ **What is the incidence of hearing loss after infection with mumps?**
0.5%.

○ **How does hearing loss caused by mumps usually present?**
Hearing loss develops as the parotitis is resolving.

○ **Of all the viruses associated with hearing loss, which one is most likely to be associated with unilateral hearing loss?**
Mumps.

○ **What signs and symptoms are specific for necrotizing otitis externa (NOE)?**
Persistent otalgia for longer than 1 month.
Persistent, purulent otorrhea with granulation tissue for several weeks.
Diabetes mellitus, another immunocompromised state, or advanced age.
Cranial nerve involvement.

○ **Why are diabetics more prone to NOE?**
The pH of their cerumen is higher and more conducive to bacterial growth.

○ **How does the infection spread from the external canal to the skull base?**
Through the fissures of Santorini.

○ **What is the most common causative organism of NOE?**
P. aeruginosa.

○ **Which cranial nerves are most commonly involved in NOE?**
VII (75%), X (70%), XI (56%).

○ **How is NOE treated?**

6 weeks of two different IV antibiotics directed against the organism cultured; alternatively, ciprofloxacin and rifampin for several months; hyperbaric oxygen is recommended for advanced NOE.

○ **When is surgery indicated in the treatment of NOE?**

Progression of pain despite aggressive medical therapy, persistence of granulation tissue, and development of cranial nerve involvement.

○ **Why is it difficult to treat infections involving the perichondrium or cartilage?**

The metabolic demands of cartilage are low, and its blood supply is hence diminished.

○ **What is the most common cause of epidemic encephalitis in the US?**

West Nile virus

○ **What % of patients infected with West Nile virus will develop symptoms?**

Approximately 20%.

○ **What are the primary symptoms of West Nile fever?**

Fever (lasting about 1 week), headache (lasting about 10 days), fatigue (lasting about 1 month), and a generalized rash.

○ **Which two cranial nerves are most commonly affected in West Nile neuroinvasive disease?**

VII and VIII.

CHAPTER 30 Inflammatory

○ **The triad of recurrent facial palsy, orofacial edema, and lingua plicata is classic for what disease?**

Melkersson–Rosenthal syndrome (orofacial granulomatosis).

○ **What is the most likely cause of bilateral facial palsy in a young adult?**

Sarcoidosis.

○ **Where are intracranial lesions that cause bilateral facial paralysis located?**

Pons.

○ **What is Heerfordt's syndrome?**

Facial nerve palsy with anterior uveitis, parotid gland enlargement, and fever.

○ **What are the two types of aspiration?**

Primary or direct from oral substances and secondary or indirect from gastric substances.

○ **Why are infants more prone to aspiration than adults?**

Compared with adults, infants have a relatively lax epiglottis, large arytenoids, and wide aryepiglottic folds.

○ **What other factors can predispose an infant to aspirate?**

CNS disease, prematurity, mechanical barriers (nasogastric tube, endotracheal tube, tracheostomy), anatomic barriers (esophageal atresia/stricture, vascular rings, tracheoesophageal fistula), scoliosis.

○ **What is intractable aspiration?**

Persistent aspiration despite maximum medical management and minor surgery.

○ **What are the surgical options for treatment of intractable aspiration?**

Narrow-field laryngectomy, endolaryngeal stent, laryngeal closure, and tracheoesophageal diversion (TED) or laryngotracheal separation (LTS).

○ **What is the most common cause of GERD in children?**

Transient lower esophageal sphincter relaxation.

○ **What is the most common sign of GERD in infants?**

Regurgitation.

○ **What is the most common complication of GERD in infants?**

Distal esophagitis.

○ **What are other signs or complications of GERD in infants?**

Failure to thrive, vomiting, recurrent aspiration pneumonia, and acute life-threatening events.

○ **What percent of infants with GERD will spontaneously resolve by 18 months?**

85%.

○ **What is the best initial approach for management of mild GERD with no adverse clinical consequences in an infant?**

Parental reassurance; reverse Trendelenburg; prone positioning after feeding.

○ **True/False: Thickening formula decreases the amount of reflux in children.**

False: No studies have proven any benefit of this. It may decrease the amount of visible regurgitation, but it does not improve reflux.

○ **What is the most common form of immune reaction causing food hypersensitivity?**

Type III reactions.

○ **What are the most common type of antigens causing delayed, immune complex or T-cell–mediated reactions?**

Mold or food antigens.

○ **Why do newborns and infants have an increased incidence of food allergy?**

Their gut mucosa is highly permeable, increasing antigen uptake.

○ **What is a fixed food allergy?**

Type I, IgE-mediated response occurring seconds to hours after contact with the allergen.

○ **What are the different manifestations of fixed food allergies?**

Atopic dermatitis, asthma, allergic rhinitis, urticaria, angioedema, oral allergy syndrome, gastrointestinal distress, or severe anaphylaxis.

○ **What are the most common IgE-mediated food allergens in infants with atopic dermatitis?**

Cow's milk, fish, and eggs.

○ **What are the most common IgE-mediated food allergens causing urticaria and angioedema?**

Shellfish, fish, milk, nuts, beans, potatoes, celery, parsley, spices, peanuts, and soy.

○ **What is oral allergy syndrome?**

IgE-mediated reaction causing immediate swelling of the lips, tingling of the tongue and throat, and blistering of the oral mucosa. Symptoms are commonly associated with the ingestion of various fruits and vegetables that cross-react with their specific allergic rhinitis-inducing pollen.

○ **What is cyclic food allergy?**

Non-IgE-mediated delayed sensitivity to food allergens, primarily the result of type III immune complex disease.

○ **True/False: Cyclic food allergy is not related to dose or frequency of allergen exposure.**

False: Unlike fixed food allergy, cyclic food allergy is dose and frequency dependent.

○ **True/False: Patients with a cyclic food allergy often crave a certain food, feeling better when regularly eating it.**

True: This is known as "masked sensitization."

○ **What congenital disease is associated with a relatively high incidence of latex allergy?**

Spina bifida.

○ **What is the incidence of latex allergy?**

1–6% among the general population; 5–17% among health care workers; 20–60% among those with spina bifida.

○ **A patient develops erythematous, eczematous lesions on her arm 48 hours after having her blood drawn. This reaction is characteristic of which Gell and Coombs reaction?**

Type IV, delayed hypersensitivity.

○ **What is the early-phase allergic response?**

Initial sensitization to an allergen results in cross-linking of IgE antibodies on mast cells upon subsequent exposure. Mast cells then degenerate and release chemical mediators like histamine. Histamine stimulates dilatation of the blood vessels in the nose, mucus glands to produce mucin, and leakage of plasma from capillaries and venules. Resulting symptoms include sneezing, itching, rhinorrhea, and nasal congestion.

○ **What is the late-phase allergic response?**

Approximately 50% of allergic patients will have a late-phase response 3–12 hours after the early-phase response. Mediators released from mast cells cause infiltration of eosinophils and neutrophils to the exposure site. Nasal congestion is the primary symptom. Nasal mucosa becomes more sensitive to subsequent allergen exposure (priming) and to nonspecific environmental stimuli (nonspecific hyperresponsiveness).

○ **What condition is characterized by nasal eosinophils, rhinorrhea, normal IgE levels, and negative skin tests for allergens?**

Nonallergic rhinitis with eosinophilia syndrome (NARES).

○ **What is Sampter's triad?**

Aspirin sensitivity, nasal polyposis, and asthma.

○ **What percent of patients undergoing surgery for chronic rhinosinusitis have Sampter's triad?**

10%.

○ **True/False: The concordance of allergy and chronic rhinosinusitis is higher in the pediatric population.**

True.

○ **What impact does allergic rhinitis have on surgical outcomes in endoscopic sinus surgery?**

The long-term success rate decreases from 90–93% (uncomplicated rhinosinusitis in otherwise healthy patients) to 78–85%.

○ **What is the usual presentation of autoimmune inner ear disease (AIED)?**

Progressive sensorineural hearing loss over weeks to months in middle-aged women, occasionally with a serous middle ear effusion.

○ **What percent of patients with AIED have bilateral hearing loss?**

79%.

○ **What proportion of patients with AIED will not have any vestibular symptoms?**

One-third.

○ **What percent of patients with AIED will also have a systemic autoimmune disease?**

29%.

○ **What is an early sign of relapse following treatment for AIED?**

Loud tinnitus.

○ **According to AAO-HNS, what are the criteria for "definite" Menière's disease?**

1. Two or more episodes of spontaneous rotational vertigo lasting 20 minutes or longer.

2. Audiometrically documented hearing loss on at least one occasion.

3. Tinnitus or aural fullness in the affected ear.

4. Exclusion of other causes.

○ **What are the criteria for "certain" Menière's disease?**

The above criteria plus histopathologic confirmation.

○ **What are the criteria for "probable" Menière's disease?**

Only one episode of vertigo plus the other criteria for "definite" disease.

○ **What are the criteria for "possible" Menière's disease?**

Cochlear or vestibular variants of Menière's disease for which other causes have been excluded.

○ **What percent of patients have bilateral Menière's disease?**

After 2 years, 15% of patients; after 10 years, 25–35%; and after 20 years, 40–60%.

○ **What is the mainstay of treatment for Menière's disease?**

Diuretics and dietary salt restriction.

○ **What percent of patients with Menière's disease do not respond adequately to salt restriction and diuretics?**

10%.

○ **What disease is a necrotizing vasculitis of small- and medium-sized muscular arteries, most commonly involving the renal and visceral vessels, and is a potential cause of hearing loss?**

Polyarteritis nodosa.

○ **What syndrome is characterized by vestibuloauditory symptoms in association with nonsyphilitic interstitial keratitis, mostly in young adults?**

Cogan's syndrome.

○ **What are the typical symptoms of interstitial keratitis?**

Photophobia, lacrimation, and pain.

○ **What syndrome is characterized by vestibuloauditory symptoms in association with uveitis, depigmentation of periorbital hair and skin, loss of eyelashes, and aseptic meningitis?**

Vogt–Koyanagi–Harada syndrome.

○ **What disease is characterized by necrotizing granulomas with vasculitis in one or more organs and focal necrotizing glomerulonephritis?**

Wegener's granulomatosis.

○ **What is the most common otologic manifestation of Wegener's granulomatosis?**

Serous otitis media.

○ **What disease is characterized by recurrent aphthous ulcers, ocular inflammation, cutaneous vasculitis, and SNHL?**

Behçet's disease.

○   **Name the most likely etiology of vertigo.**

Positional vertigo, lasting seconds, associated with rotatory nystagmus	BPPV
Acute, nonprogressive, episodic vertigo lasting for hours to days; no hearing loss	Vestibular neuritis
Acute, episodic vertigo lasting at least 20 minutes, low-frequency SNHL	Menière's disease
Constant, progressive dizziness, Brun's nystagmus, SNHL	Cerebellopontine angle tumor
Transient, orthostatic dizziness with vertical nystagmus	Vertebrobasilar insufficiency
Constant dizziness, high-frequency SNHL, oscillopsia, head-shaking nystagmus	Ototoxicity

○   **What is the term for a keratin plug occluding the external auditory canal?**
Keratosis obturans.

○   **How do patients with keratosis obturans usually present?**
Conductive hearing loss, acute severe otalgia, usually bilaterally; otorrhea is rare.

○   **What are the physical findings in a patient with keratosis obturans?**
Thickened tympanic membrane, widened EAC medially, and hyperemic canal skin with granulation tissue.

○   **How do patients with EAC cholesteatoma present?**
Chronic dull pain, usually unilaterally, with otorrhea and normal hearing.

○   **What are the physical findings in a patient with EAC cholesteatoma?**
Localized erosion and periostitis of the posterior-inferior EAC associated with otorrhea.

○   **Where are vocal nodules most commonly located?**
At the junction of the anterior one-third and posterior two-thirds of the vocal fold.

○   **Why are they commonly located there?**
This is the point of maximum velocity of the vocal cords during forceful adduction.

○   **What are the risk factors for developing a vocal fold granuloma?**
Vocal abuse, GERD, prolonged intubation, trauma, and surgery.

○   **Which type of vocal cord granuloma has the worst prognosis?**
Idiopathic.

○ **What are the most common clinical manifestations of laryngopharyngeal reflux in adults?**

Dysphonia (71%), chronic cough (51%), globus (47%), chronic throat clearing (42%), and dysphagia (35%).

○ **What pathologic changes occur in the larynx as a result of GERD?**

Polypoid corditis (Reinke's edema), posterior glottic edema, and arytenoid edema/erythema.

○ **Which of these is most common?**

Posterior glottic edema.

○ **Where is Reinke's edema located?**

Superficial layer of the lamina propria.

○ **A 40-year-old professional singer comes in for hoarseness. Her vocal quality is notably rough and videostroboscopy shows a linear sulcus along the medial edge of the vocal fold with diminished vocal cord vibratory activity. What is the likely diagnosis?**

Type 2 sulcus/sulcus vergeture.

○ **What are the clinical findings associated with pathologic sulcus vocalis?**

Vocal fold stiffness, fullness, edema, and bowing; capillary ectasia; and vibratory disturbances.

○ **What distinguishes type 1 or physiologic sulcus from pathologic sulcus?**

Preservation of vocal cord vibratory activity on videostroboscopy, signifying intact superficial lamina propria.

○ **What are the operative and pathologic findings of patients with pathologic sulcus vocalis/type 3 sulcus?**

Loss of superficial lamina propria and fixation of a thinned epithelium to underlying vocal ligament.

○ **Breathiness that progressively worsens as the day wears on is classic for which autoimmune disease?**

Myasthenia gravis.

○ **Which area of the larynx is involved in sarcoidosis?**

Supraglottis.

○ **Which area of the larynx is involved in Wegener's granulomatosis?**

Subglottis.

○ **What is the most common inflammatory disease of the thyroid?**

Hashimoto's thyroiditis.

○ **What antibodies are specific for Hashimoto's thyroiditis?**

Antimicrosomal and antithyroglobulin antibodies.

○ **How do patients with Hashimoto's thyroiditis present?**

Firm, diffusely enlarged goiter and hypothyroidism.

○ **What infectious diseases can cause chronic thyroiditis?**

Actinomycosis, tuberculosis, and syphilis.

○ **What thyroid disorder is characterized by replacement of the thyroid gland with fibrous tissue?**

Riedel's struma (invasive fibrous thyroiditis, woody thyroiditis).

○ **What is the preferred treatment for patients with toxic multinodular goiter?**

Thyroid resection (lobectomy to total thyroidectomy) because I^{131} treatment often requires repeated doses, does not reduce goiter size, and may even cause acute enlargement.

○ **What are the indications for surgical treatment of Graves' disease?**

Extremely large glands, the presence of a dominant nodule, failure of I^{131}, massive enlargement with compressive symptoms, pregnant women intolerant to antithyroid drugs, women of childbearing age, and patients who are opposed to radioiodine.

○ **What is the treatment of choice for patients over 40 with Graves' disease?**

Radioactive I^{131}.

○ **What is the pathophysiology behind dysthyroid ophthalmopathy?**

Infiltration of fluid and cells into the extraocular muscles and retrobulbar structures secondary to deposition of abnormal antibody-receptor complexes and glycosaminoglycans.

○ **What is the ATA classification system for eye involvement in Graves' disease?**

Class I—Lid lag and the appearance of a stare.

Class II—Conjunctival chemosis, epiphora, periorbital edema, and photophobia.

Class III—Proptosis.

Class IV—Decreased ocular mobility and diplopia.

Class V—Corneal ulceration.

Class VI—Optic nerve involvement.

○ **What percent of patients with dysthyroid ophthalmopathy suffer from visual disturbances severe enough to warrant surgical intervention?**

5%.

○ **Which muscles are most commonly involved in dysthyroid ophthalmopathy?**

Medial and inferior rectus muscles.

CHAPTER 31 Iatrogenic

○ **What are the two most common causes of vocal cord paralysis in adults?**
Surgical trauma (#1) and lung cancer (#2).

○ **In patients with unilateral vocal cord paralysis, which side is most commonly involved?**
Left.

○ **What position will the vocal cord be in if the nerve is damaged at or above the nodose ganglion?**
Lateral.

○ **What position will the vocal cord be in if the nerve is damaged below the nodose ganglion?**
Paramedian, due to innervation from the superior laryngeal nerve.

○ **If the paralyzed vocal cord is in the paramedian position, why is aspiration less likely?**
Indicates that the superior laryngeal nerve is intact, and hence laryngeal sensation is intact.

○ **What accounts for vocal fold bowing observed with vocal fold paralysis?**
Denervation atrophy of the thyroarytenoid muscle.

○ **What problems are seen more commonly in patients with vocal cord paralysis due to a brainstem disorder?**
Breathiness; pitch changes; chronic aspiration; and velopharyngeal insufficiency.

○ **What is the most common cause of unilateral facial palsy in a newborn infant?**
Forceps delivery.

○ **What effects does radiation therapy have on the skin?**
Dryness secondary to damaged sebaceous and sweat glands, thinning of the epidermis, and telangiectasias.

○ **What is the principle dose-limiting factor of radiation therapy?**
Fibrosis of the subcutaneous tissue and muscle.

○ **What are the ocular complications of radiation therapy?**

Cataracts, radiation retinopathy, optic nerve injury, lacrimal gland damage, and ectropion/entropion.

○ **Cataracts can occur after how much radiation therapy?**

6 Gy.

○ **At what doses can radiation retinopathy or optic neuropathy occurs?**

50–55 Gy.

○ **What effects does radiation therapy have on the brain or spinal cord?**

Transient radiation myelopathy, transverse myelitis.

○ **What is the somnolence syndrome?**

Lethargy, nausea, headache, cranial nerve palsies, and ataxia presenting 2–3 months after radiation therapy and lasting 2–4 weeks.

○ **What clinical factors increase the risk of radiation injury?**

Male gender, extremes of age, higher doses and fractions, and comorbidities.

○ **What is the pathogenesis behind transient radiation myelopathy?**

Demyelination of the posterior columns.

○ **Which cranial nerve is most commonly damaged by radiation therapy to the head and neck?**

XII.

○ **What is the most common hormonal deficiency after radiation therapy for nasopharyngeal carcinoma?**

Growth hormone deficiency.

○ **What are the three most important factors leading to osteoradionecrosis (ORN)?**

Hypovascularity, hypocellularity, and hypoxia (the "3Hs").

○ **What are the three types of ORN?**

Type I occurs soon after radiation therapy; Type II occurs long after radiation therapy and is induced by trauma; and Type III occurs long after radiation therapy and occurs spontaneously.

○ **Which bone in the head and neck is most commonly affected by ORN?**

Mandible, as it has a relatively tenuous blood supply and is stress bearing.

○ **What is the incidence of ORN after radiation to the head and neck?**

10–15%.

○ **What are the risk factors for development of ORN?**

Dose of radiation (>70 Gy), size, and extent of primary, postradiation dental extraction.

○ **How much time must elapse before starting radiation after dental extractions?**

10 days.

○ **What percent of premature infants develop subglottic stenosis (SGS)?**

4%.

○ **What is Cotton's grading system for SGS?**

Grade 1: Less than 50% laryngeal lumen obstruction.
Grade 2: 51–70% laryngeal lumen obstruction.
Grade 3: 71–99% laryngeal lumen obstruction.
Grade 4: Complete obstruction.

○ **What is the biggest risk factor for acquired SGS?**

Prolonged endotracheal intubation.

○ **What are other etiologies of SGS?**

Congenital anomalies, increased infant activity, autoimmune mechanisms (antibodies to type II collagen, antineutrophil cytoplasmic antibodies), infection, GERD, caustic injury, and high tracheostomy.

○ **What are the treatment options for SGS?**

Dilation, steroid injection, lathyrogenic agents, cryotherapy, laser therapy, anterior cricoid split, one-stage laryngotracheoplasty, autogenous cartilage grafts, four-quadrant cartilage division, end-to-end tracheal anastomosis, and flaps.

○ **What are the advantages of serial bouginage for the treatment of SGS?**

Noninvasive growth may take care of the stenosis, avoids concerns regarding the potential for laryngeal growth inhibition with open procedures.

○ **What are the disadvantages of serial bouginage?**

Multiple treatment applications over a prolonged period of time, lack of stabilization if cartilaginous destruction or instability has occurred, generally requires a tracheotomy.

CHAPTER 32 Cosmetic and Reconstructive

○ **What is the primary cause of midface aging?**

Ptosis of the malar fat pads and diminished tone of the zygomatic musculature.

○ **What is the primary cause of jowls in the elderly patient?**

Attenuation of the masseteric cutaneous ligaments.

○ **What is the anatomic basis of "hanging columella"?**

Excessively high arch of the alae, abnormally extreme curvature of the intermediate and medial crura, or overaggressive surgical removal of the lateral crus and adjacent soft tissue with subsequent cephalic contraction of alar margin.

○ **What are the causes of lower lip eversion?**

Skeletal deep bite, lower tooth procumberance, excess lip weight and bulk.

○ **What are the clinical features of photoaged skin?**

Thicker than normal with wrinkling, roughness, sallowness, telangiectasias, mottled hyperpigmentation, and loss of elasticity.

○ **What are the histologic features of photoaged skin?**

Thickened stratum corneum, thinner atrophic epidermis with atypia, irregular dispersion of melanin, decreased glycosaminoglycans, and abnormal elastic fibers in the dermis (solar elastosis).

○ **What causes melasma?**

Genetic predisposition, exposure to UV radiation, pregnancy, oral contraceptives, thyroid dysfunction, cosmetics, phototoxic and antiseizure drugs.

○ **True/False: Complete avoidance of sunlight can reverse some of the histologic signs of photoaging.**

True.

○ **What are the primary theories on the etiology of infraorbital bags?**

1. Congenitally excess fat.
2. Weakening of the orbital septum and attenuation of the orbicularis oculi.
3. Weakening of global support resulting in enophthalmos and lower lid pseudoherniation.
4. Weakening and descent of the Lockwood suspensory ligament.

○ **What is Binder's syndrome?**

Maxillonasal dysplasia with inadequate projection, absent nasal spine, premaxillary hypoplasia, severe columellar–lobular disproportion.

○ **What is the most common cause of hair loss in men and women?**

Androgenetic alopecia or male pattern baldness.

○ **What is the pathophysiology of androgenetic alopecia?**

Affected scalp follicles inhibit androgen, causing terminal hairs to convert to vellus hairs.

○ **Which hair follicles are most likely to be involved in androgenetic alopecia?**

Those in the frontotemporal and crown regions of the scalp.

○ **What landmark is used to determine the correct position of the natural hairline?**

The apex of the frontotemporal triangle should fall on a vertical line intersecting the lateral canthus.

○ **Normally, how many hair follicles are contained within 1 cm³ of scalp?**

200.

○ **Approximately what percent of hair follicles must be lost before hair loss is noticeable?**

30%.

○ **What is the most common form of acquired eyelid ptosis?**

Levator aponeurosis disinsertion or dehiscence.

CHAPTER 33 Metabolic

○ **What is the most common thyroid abnormality in hospitalized patients with nonthyroidal illness?**
Low T3 concentration.

○ **What is the major cause of a decreased T3 concentration in patients with a critical illness?**
Impaired peripheral conversion of T4 to T3 secondary to inhibition of the deiodination process.

○ **What clinical sign is the hallmark of thyroid storm?**
Fever.

○ **What is the most common cause of thyroid storm?**
Untreated Graves' disease.

○ **What are the hemodynamics of thyroid storm?**
Tachycardia, increased cardiac output, and decreased systemic vascular resistance.

○ **What is the initial treatment of thyroid storm?**
Intravenous fluids, hypothermia, acetaminophen, propranolol, propylthiouracil, and iodine.

○ **What are the CNS manifestations of myxedema?**
Depression, memory loss, ataxia, frank psychosis, myxedema, and coma.

○ **What are the most common causes of hypothyroidism?**
Hashimoto's thyroiditis, pituitary tumor, thyroidectomy, and radioactive I^{131} treatment for thyrotoxicosis.

○ **What are the most common causes of hyperthyroidism?**
Graves' disease, toxic multinodular goiter, relapsing thyroiditis, amiodarone-induced thyrotoxicosis, autonomous toxic nodule, subacute thyroiditis, and pituitary tumor.

○ **A 45-year-old woman presents with a 2-year history of diffuse, tender thyroid enlargement, lethargy, and a 20-pound weight gain. What is the most likely diagnosis?**

Hashimoto's thyroiditis.

○ **What is the appropriate treatment for the above patient?**

Thyroid hormone replacement therapy.

○ **A 48-year-old man has a serum calcium of 13 mg/dL and a serum PTH of 400 mEq/mL. What is the most likely diagnosis?**

Primary hyperparathyroidism secondary to a parathyroid adenoma.

○ **A 35-year-old woman has a serum calcium of 8.5 mg/dL, a serum PTH of 400 mEq/mL, and a serum creatinine of 5.6 mg/dL. What is the most likely diagnosis?**

Secondary hyperparathyroidism.

○ **What is the most common cause of hypercalcemia?**

Primary hyperparathyroidism.

○ **What is the most common cause of primary hyperparathyroidism?**

Parathyroid adenoma.

○ **What percent of cases of primary hyperparathyroidism are due to diffuse hyperplasia?**

14–16%.

○ **Which cell is most commonly proliferated in diffuse parathyroid hyperplasia?**

Chief cell.

○ **What percent of cases of primary hyperparathyroidism are due to carcinoma?**

3%.

○ **What is the most common cause of secondary hyperparathyroidism?**

Chronic renal failure.

○ **What is the pathophysiology behind secondary hyperparathyroidism from chronic renal failure?**

Chronic hypocalcemia results from decreased production of $1,25(OH)_2$ vitamin D_3, bone resistance to PTH, and decreased clearance of PTH and phosphate, resulting in parathyroid hyperplasia and increased levels of PTH.

○ **What percent of patients with secondary hyperparathyroidism require parathyroidectomy?**

<5%.

○ **What is tertiary hyperparathyroidism?**

Parathyroid hyperplasia results in autonomous hypersecretion such that hyperparathyroidism continues despite correction of the underlying renal disease.

○ **Which type of multiple endocrine neoplasia is not associated with hyperparathyroidism?**

MEN IIb.

○ **What is the significance of elevated preoperative levels of alkaline phosphatase in patients with chronic renal failure undergoing parathyroidectomy?**

Correlates with a good chance of amelioration of bone pain after parathyroidectomy.

○ **What is the classic bony change associated with hypercalcemia?**

Osteitis fibrosa cystica; manifested as subperiosteal bone resorption in the phalanges, pelvis, distal clavicles, ribs, femur, mandible, or skull.

○ **What is another cause of bone disease in patients with renal failure that should be ruled out prior to parathyroidectomy?**

Aluminum bone disease.

○ **What is calciphylaxis?**

Severe soft tissue calcification that can result in deep nonhealing ulcers and gangrene.

○ **What is the medical management of secondary hyperparathyroidism?**

Dietary phosphate restriction, phosphate binders, calcium and vitamin D supplementation (calcitriol), sodium bicarbonate (for metabolic acidosis), charcoal hemoperfusion (for pruritus), bisphosphonates.

○ **What are the indications for parathyroid exploration in patients with asymptomatic or minimally symptomatic hyperparathyroidism?**

Age less than 50.

History of a life-threatening hypercalcemic episode.

Kidney stones on abdominal X-rays.

Serum calcium 1 mg/mL above the upper limits of normal for the lab.

Creatinine clearance reduced by 30% or more compared with age-matched normal persons.

24-hour urinary calcium excretion >400 mg.

T-score at lumbar spine, hip, or distal radius less than −2.5.

Poor follow-up expected.

Coexistent illness complicating conservative management.

○ **What disease should be ruled out on all patients with hypercalcemia?**

Familial benign hypocalciuric hypercalcemia (FHH).

○ **What are the indications for parathyroidectomy in patients with secondary hyperparathyroidism?**

Bone pain (most common indication), intractable pruritus, calcium–phosphate product over 70 despite medical treatment, calciphylaxis, and osteitis fibrosa cystica.

○ **What is the treatment of choice for patients with hyperparathyroidism associated with MEN-I or MEN-IIa?**

Subtotal (3½ gland) parathyroidectomy or total parathyroidectomy with autotransplantation.

○ **What is the treatment of choice for patients with parathyroid carcinoma?**

Radical resection of the involved gland, the ipsilateral thyroid lobe, and the regional lymph nodes.

○ **A 25-year-old pregnant woman, in her 2nd trimester, presents with hyperparathyroidism and a serum calcium of 12 mg/dL. What is the treatment of choice?**

Prompt parathyroid exploration.

○ **What is the first-line therapy for patients with marked hypercalcemia and/or severe symptoms?**

Intravenous hydration followed by furosemide.

○ **What is the most common presentation of severe hypercalcemia?**

Extreme lethargy.

○ **What are the indications for calcium supplementation after thyroid or parathyroid surgery?**

Circumoral paresthesias, anxiety, positive Chvostek's or Trousseau's sign, tetany, ECG changes, or serum calcium less than 7.1 mL/dL.

○ **What is the immediate treatment for patients with acute symptomatic hypocalcemia?**

Intravenous calcium gluconate.

Section IV

PHARMACOLOGY

CHAPTER 34 Anaphylaxis

○ **A 26-year-old woman complains of skin itching and abdominal cramping frequently when she runs, especially in the summer. Her father describes a similar problem. What is the likely diagnosis?**

Exercise-induced anaphylaxis.

○ **What are the most common causes of anaphylaxis?**

Food (33%), unknown (20%), insect sting (14%), drugs (13%), and exercise (7%).

○ **Which patients are at higher risk for anaphylactic reactions?**

Young children, patients with a prior history of anaphylaxis, patients with active or uncontrolled asthma, and patients taking a β-adrenergic blocker.

○ **What precautions should be considered in treating these patients with immunotherapy?**

Multiple short diagnostic skin testing sessions, slow treatment buildup, wait in the office longer than the traditional 20–30 minutes after allergen injections, obtaining a Medic Alert identification bracelet, avoid home immunotherapy, use of antihistamine premedication before treatment injections.

○ **In confusing or fatal cases, what blood tests can confirm that anaphylaxis did occur?**

Serum tryptase, total IgE, and specific IgE values between 45 minutes and 6 hours after the initial symptoms.

○ **What are the three types of allergy-related reactions?**

Vasovagal events, delayed allergic reactions, and immediate allergic reactions.

○ **At the onset of skin endpoint titration testing, a 20-year-old man complains of feeling faint. His skin is pale and cool and he is sweating. His blood pressure, in the recumbent position, is 110/60 and pulse rate is 90. His respiratory rate is 18 and breathing is nonlabored. What is the diagnosis?**

Vasovagal reaction.

○ **During skin endpoint titration, a 20-year-old man complains of feeling ill. His skin is flushed and warm, but he is not sweating. He has several very large wheals on his back, and he complains of severe itching. His blood pressure, in the recumbent position, is 90/45 and pulse rate is 120. His respiratory rate is 23 and breathing is shallow. What is the diagnosis?**

Anaphylaxis.

○ **What are the early signs and symptoms of anaphylaxis?**

Marked exacerbation of allergic symptoms with nasal, throat, and ocular itching, facial flushing, and throat tightness; tachycardia; bronchospasm and cough, urticaria or pruritus, angioedema, and sense of impending doom; less commonly, diarrhea, cramps, vomiting, and urinary urgency.

○ **True/False: The longer the delay from exposure to onset of anaphylaxis, the less severe the reaction.**

True: The exception is food allergies, where symptoms may not occur until several hours after ingestion.

○ **Why should patients be hospitalized after initial treatment of anaphylaxis?**

Up to 20% may subsequently relapse hours later into protracted late-phase reactions (biphasic reaction).

○ **True/False: Biphasic reactions are more likely to occur when the antigen exposure has been by the oral route and often require greater doses of epinephrine in the initial treatment phase.**

True.

○ **How do β-blockers complicate treatment of anaphylaxis?**

β-Blockers are proallergenic, blocking smooth muscle relaxation and increasing production of anaphylactic mediators. They may also cause hypertensive crisis due to unopposed α-adrenergic effects of epinephrine given to treat the anaphylaxis.

○ **How do tricyclic antidepressants (TCAs) and monoamine oxidase (MAO) inhibitors complicate treatment of anaphylaxis?**

TCAs block reuptake of catecholamines, causing both hypertension and sensitizing patients to arrhythmias, and also have α-adrenergic blocking effects. MAO inhibitors prevent degradation of catecholamines, thus allowing their buildup to levels that can cause symptoms ranging from severe headache to hypertensive crisis.

○ **How do medications with α-adrenergic blocking activity (some antihypertensives, phenothiazines, TCAs) complicate treatment of anaphylaxis?**

α-Blockade can cause refractory hypotension that is not improved with epinephrine (a pure α-agonist, such as phenylephrine, should be used instead).

○ **What is the recommended initial dose of epinephrine for anaphylaxis?**

0.3–1.0 mg IM in adults; 0.01 mg/kg IM in children; and 0.2 mg in elders or those on β-blockers.

○ **How often should epinephrine be given in an anaphylactic reaction?**

Every 3–5 minutes until stable in an adult; every 40 minutes until stable in a child.

○ **What are other methods of administering epinephrine?**

Inhalation, IV, subcutaneous, sublingual, intrathecally.

○ **What adjunctive drugs can be used for anaphylaxis refractory to epinephrine?**

Ipratropium, heparin, H_1 and H_2 antihistamines, corticosteroids, and glucagon.

○ **What is the role of H_1 and H_2 antihistamines in anaphylaxis treatment?**

Reversal of myocardial pump failure; combined H_1 and H_2 blockade has shown to be superior to either one alone.

○ **What is the role of corticosteroids in anaphylaxis treatment?**

Mostly for prevention of late-onset reactions.

○ **Why is heparin a useful drug in anaphylaxis treatment?**

Heparin inactivates histamine, improves anaphylactic-induced coagulopathy, and has anti-inflammatory effects.

○ **What is the usual dose of heparin in patients with anaphylaxis?**

10,000 U IV in adults; 50–75 U/kg in children; followed by heparin drip of 1000 U/h (children 25 U/kg/h).

○ **What medications should be given for bronchospasm during anaphylaxis?**

Initially, combined inhaled β-agonists and anticholinergic drugs; once IV access is established, IV glucagon, magnesium, and vitamin C.

CHAPTER 35 Antibiotics

○ **What percent of all adverse drug reactions among hospitalized patients can be attributed to antibiotics?**
25%.

○ **True/False: The rate of colonization of hospitalized patients with *Clostridium difficile* increases in proportion to the patient's length of stay.**
True.

○ **True/False: The incidence of community-acquired *C. difficile* is higher in patients taking H_2 blockers and proton pump inhibitors.**
True.

○ **How long may the onset of pseudomembranous enterocolitis begin after initiation of antibiotics?**
6 weeks.

○ **What is the incidence of *C. difficile* in cases of antibiotic-associated diarrhea?**
10–20%.

○ **Which class of antibiotic is most commonly associated with the development of *C. difficile*?**
Fluoroquinolones.

○ **What is the sensitivity and specificity of testing for *C. difficile* toxins A and B with ELISA?**
Sensitivity 63–99%; specificity 93–100%.

○ **What are the features of the epidemic strain of *C. difficile* (B1/NAP1/027) that set it apart from other strains?**
It produces 16–23× the amount of toxins A and B; produces a third toxin (binary toxin CDT); and has high levels of fluoroquinolone resistance.

○ **What is the initial drug of choice for treating *C. difficile*?**
Metronidazole.

○ **What drug has shown equal efficacy as vancomycin for the treatment of *C. difficile* infections with a lower rate of recurrence (15% vs. 25% for vancomycin)?**

Fidaxomicin.

○ **What other therapy has been shown to decrease the risk of recurrence of *C. difficile*?**

Intravenous infusion of neutralizing monoclonal antibodies to *C. difficile* toxins A and B.

○ **In patients with postoperative pneumonia, empiric monotherapy should cover which organisms?**

Gram-negative organisms.

○ **Vancomycin is effective against which bacteria?**

Gram-positive cocci, including methicillin-resistant *Staphylococcus aureus* (MRSA), *Staphylococcus epidermidis*, enterococci, diphtheroids, and *C. difficile*.

○ **What is Red Man's Syndrome?**

Flushing of the face and neck, pruritus and hypotension associated with rapid infusion of vancomycin, and subsequent release of histamine.

○ **What organisms do penicillin G and V cover?**

Streptococcal pyogenes, *Streptococcal pneumoniae*, *Actinomyces*, oral anaerobes.

○ **Which penicillins are most active against *S. aureus*?**

Methicillin, oxacillin, dicloxacillin, and nafcillin.

○ **Which of these attains the highest blood levels?**

Dicloxacillin.

○ **Which of these is best for patients with renal failure?**

Nafcillin.

○ **Which of these is not active against *Streptococcus pneumoniae*?**

Methicillin.

○ **What organisms are covered by amoxicillin and ampicillin that are not covered by penicillin?**

Proteus, *Escherichia coli*, *Haemophilus influenzae*.

○ **What percent of patients with mononucleosis will develop a rash after taking amoxicillin?**

50%.

○ **Which penicillin derivatives are active against *Pseudomonas*?**

Ticarcillin–clavulanate and piperacillin–tazobactam.

○ **Which first-generation cephalosporin has the longest half-life?**

Cefazolin.

○ **Which penicillin analogue can be given to patients with a history of anaphylaxis after taking penicillin?**

Aztreonam.

○ **Which macrolide does not cover *H. influenzae*?**

Erythromycin.

○ **What is the mechanism of action of quinolones?**

Inhibition of DNA gyrase, which is needed to package DNA into dividing bacteria.

○ **Why is ciprofloxacin contraindicated in children?**

It has been shown to cause arthropathy of the weight-bearing joints in immature animals.

○ **Which quinolone carries the highest risk for QTc prolongation and CNS toxicity?**

Moxifloxacin.

○ **Which medications, when given concurrently with a quinolone, significantly increase the risk of quinolone-associated tendon rupture?**

Corticosteroids.

○ **What can happen if a quinolone is given to a patient dependent on benzodiazepines?**

Acute withdrawal symptoms from the benzodiazepines.

○ **Approximately what percent of *C. difficile* cases occur after taking quinolones?**

55%.

○ **Which medications can be used to treat people exposed to meningococcus?**

Rifampin, ciprofloxacin, or ceftriaxone.

○ **What is the best medication to eradicate nasal colonization with methicillin-resistant *S. aureus*?**

Mupirocin.

○ **Mitochondrial mutations have been found to produce enhanced sensitivity to the ototoxic effects of which medications?**

Aminoglycosides.

○ **Aminoglycosides are effective against what bacteria?**

Aerobic gram-negative bacilli (including *Pseudomonas aeruginosa*), enterococci, staphylococci, and streptococci.

○ **What risks are associated with the use of aminoglycosides?**

Prolonged neuromuscular blockade, ototoxicity, and nephrotoxicity.

○ **Why is the mg/kg dosage of gentamicin given to infants higher than that given to older children?**

Infants have a higher extracellular fluid volume per weight.

○ **How do aminoglycosides exert their toxic effects on the outer hair cells of the inner ear?**

Bind to the plasma membrane and displace calcium and magnesium; once transported into the cell, bind with phosphatidylinositol, causing disruption of the plasma membrane and inhibition of inositol triphosphate, resulting in cell death.

○ **What region of the inner ear is most susceptible to permanent loss of hair cells?**

Basal turn of the cochlea.

○ **What is the most important factor determining risk of ototoxicity with use of aminoglycosides?**

Duration of therapy >10 days.

○ **After aminoglycoside treatments for Meniere's disease, when is the usual onset of disequilibrium?**

4 days after treatment.

○ **What antibiotic is effective for treatment of Wegener's granulomatosis?**

Trimethoprim/sulfamethoxazole (TMP/SMX).

○ **What is the drug of choice for the prophylaxis of *Pneumocystis carinii* infections in patients with HIV?**

TMP–SMX.

○ **What is the alternate therapy and when should it be initiated?**

Dapsone should be used when severe reactions (e.g., skin blistering, mucosal involvement, or anaphylaxis) to TMP–SMX occur.

○ **What is the treatment for otosyphilis?**

2.4 million U of benzathine penicillin IM every week for at least 3 weeks (up to 1 year) or 10 million U of penicillin G IV every day for 10 days followed by 2.4 million U of IM benzathine penicillin every week for 2 weeks plus prednisone 40–60 mg every day for 2–4 weeks followed by a taper.

○ **What is the primary problem of IM penicillin therapy for otosyphilis?**

Fails to achieve treponemicidal levels in the cerebrospinal fluid (CSF).

○ **What medication extends the half-life and facilitates CSF penetration of penicillin?**

Probenecid.

○ **What is the Jarisch–Herxheimer reaction?**

Fever and flulike symptoms beginning within 4 hours of commencing treatment for secondary syphilis.

○ **What are the four processes of bacterial resistance to antibiotics?**

Inability of the antibiotics to penetrate the bacterial cell, β-lactamase production, altered penicillin-binding protein affinity, and methicillin-resistance pattern.

○ **How do organisms inactivate penicillin?**

Produce β-lactamase.

○ **Which organisms can produce β-lactamase?**

S. aureus, H. influenzae, Moraxella catarrhalis, and oral anaerobes.

○ **What characteristic is common to clavulanate, sulbactam, and tazobactam?**

They are all β-lactamase inhibitors.

○ **Which method is responsible for the resistance of *S. pneumoniae* to penicillins?**

Decreased penicillin-binding protein affinity.

○ **What can be done to overcome this method of resistance?**

Increase the concentration of the drug.

CHAPTER 36 Pain Medications

○ **Which pain medication was removed from the US market in 2010 because of the high risk of cardiac toxicity at standard doses?**

Propoxyphene.

○ **What effect can the maximum daily dose of acetaminophen have on the international normalized ratio (INR) in patients taking warfarin?**

INR may increase.

○ **Which nonsteroidal anti-inflammatory drug (NSAID) has the lowest risk of gastrointestinal side effects?**

Ibuprofen.

○ **When should proton pump inhibitors be used in conjunction with NSAIDs?**

In patients with a previous history of a gastrointestinal event and/or patients taking aspirin, steroids, or warfarin.

○ **Which patients should avoid taking NSAIDs?**

Those with a history of ischemic cardiac disease, stroke, congestive heart failure, and recent coronary artery bypass grafting.

○ **Tramadol is particularly effective for which type of pain?**

Neuropathic.

○ **True/False: Unless contraindicated, all surgery patients should routinely be given acetaminophen and an NSAID in scheduled doses throughout the early postoperative course.**

True.

○ **What is the most reliable method of pain assessment in children 4 years and older?**

Self-report (faces pain scale in children younger than 7 and numerical rating scale in children 7 and older).

○   **Why should codeine and hydrocodone be avoided in neonates and very young children?**

Their metabolism to morphine/hydromorphone depends on the cytochrome P450 2D6 (CYP2D6) enzyme, which is inactive at birth and only 25% active by age 5.

○   **True/False: CYP2D6 has the largest phenotypic variability among the CYPs.**

True.

○   **What is the prevalence of CYP2D6 poor metabolizers?**

7–10% Caucasians; less commonly found in African Americans (3%) and Asians (1%).

○   **Ultra-rapid CYP2D6 metabolizers are more commonly found in which areas of the world?**

Middle East and North Africa.

○   **What drugs are the strongest inhibitors to the CYP2D6 enzyme, rendering opioids less effective?**

Selective serotonin reuptake inhibitors (SSRIs), bupropion, quinidine, cinacalcet, and ritonavir.

CHAPTER 37 Antineoplastic Agents

○ **Other than corticosteroids, what medications can be used to treat hemangiomas?**

Interferon α-2a or -2b.

○ **What are the mechanisms of action of interferon α-2b?**

Inhibit epithelial cell migration and proliferation and inhibit growth factor.

○ **What are the potential side effects of interferon α-2b?**

Fever, weight loss, liver enzyme elevation, and DIC.

○ **What are the potential side effects of cyclophosphamide?**

Hemorrhagic cystitis, leukopenia, sterility, and malignancies of the urinary tract.

○ **What is the mechanism of action of methotrexate?**

Inhibits dihydrofolate reductase, interfering with DNA synthesis, repair, and replication.

○ **What is the most common toxicity of methotrexate?**

Abnormal liver function.

○ **What are the five major approaches of gene transfer, and which is most common?**

Replacement of mutated tumor suppressor genes, introduction of toxic/suicide genes, immunomodulation (most common), delivery of antisense nucleotides, and cytolytic viral therapy.

○ **What are the two main categories of gene delivery agents?**

Viral and nonviral/physical.

○ **What are some physical methods of gene transfer?**

Cationic liposomes, plasmid DNA, ballistic particle, calcium-phosphate–induced uptake, and electroporation.

○ **What are the problems with physical methods of gene transfer?**

Lack of specificity and extremely low efficiency.

○ **What viruses are employed in head and neck gene therapy?**

Adenovirus, adeno-associated virus, herpes virus, retroviruses, and vaccinia virus.

○ **What are the advantages of using adenovirus?**

Adenovirus is highly infective of both quiescent and actively dividing cells, has a known tropism for cells of the upper aerodigestive tract, and can carry large genes.

○ **What are the problems with using retroviruses?**

Can only infect actively dividing cells, are permanently integrated into the host cell's genome, and randomly insert into the host genome.

○ **What does the adenovirus vector do once it enters the host cell?**

Forms a nonreplicating, extrachromosomal entity called an episome that persists for 7–42 days.

○ **Where does the adeno-associated virus vector insert its DNA in the host cell?**

At the 19q13.4 location.

○ **What problems may result from insertion at this location?**

This location is associated with chronic B-cell leukemias and integration into both copies of chromosome 19 may lead to cell death.

○ **What are the characteristics of an ideal oncolytic virus?**

Selective for infection and lysis of cancer cells; stimulates a potent antitumor response with limited local/systemic toxicity.

○ **How does the herpes simplex virus-thymidine kinase gene (HSV-tk) work?**

Expresses a viral thymidine kinase that is foreign to mammalian cells but phosphorylates the drug ganciclovir into a compound that terminates DNA synthesis in tumor cells.

○ **What is a proto-oncogene and what is an oncogene?**

A proto-oncogene participates in normal cellular signaling, transduction, and transcription; an oncogene is a mutant allele of a proto-oncogene.

○ **What are the two most common tumor suppressor genes under investigation for treatment of head and neck cancers?**

p53 and p16.

○ **What is an antisense drug?**

A small, single-stranded nucleotide complementary to a target mRNA molecule that binds to mRNA and halts transcription.

○   **What is immunologic gene therapy?**

Enhancement of an immune response specifically against tumor-associated antigens using viral vectors.

○   **What is adoptive T-cell immunotherapy?**

Ex vivo enhancement of tumor immunogenicity; lymphocytes are removed from the patient then reinfused after in vitro activation against the patient's own tumor cells.

○   **What is an alloantigen?**

A human antigen from a different individual.

○   **What is allovectin-7?**

An alloantigen that encodes for class I MHC HLA-B7. It is plasmid DNA with a liposome vector that is injected directly into the tumor. Partial response without toxicity has been demonstrated in Phase III trials for stages 3 and 4 melanoma.

○   **How is isotretinoin effective in the treatment of SCCA of the head and neck?**

Reduces the incidence of second primary tumors.

○   **What is the most effective chemotherapeutic therapy for anaplastic thyroid cancer?**

Doxorubicin with valproic acid.

○   **What drug targets the BRAF V600E mutation in melanoma and has shown significantly improved survival compared with dacarbazine?**

Vemurafenib.

CHAPTER 38 Skin Modifying Agents

○ **What are lathyrogenic agents?**

Compounds that inhibit collagen cross-linking, such as penicillamine and *N*-acetyl-L-cysteine.

○ **What is mitomycin C?**

Substance produced by *Streptomyces caespitosus* that inhibits DNA synthesis and fibroblast proliferation.

○ **True/False: Large doses of vitamin E enhance wound healing.**

False.

○ **True/False: Exogenous use of TGF-β appears to improve healing in tissues injured by radiation therapy.**

True.

○ **What effects do α-hydroxy acids have on the dermis?**

Increase collagen and glycosaminoglycan production.

○ **What skin preparations have been shown to significantly improve the overall severity of photodamaging but have not been shown to affect wrinkles?**

8–10% α-hydroxy acids.

○ **Which patients are better served by 15–20% α-hydroxy acids?**

Patients with sebaceous, Fitzpatrick type III and IV skin.

○ **What are the clinical effects of tretinoin?**

Decrease in fine wrinkling, roughness, and mottled hyperpigmentation after 6 months of use.

○ **What are the histologic effects of tretinoin?**

Thinner stratum corneum, thickened epidermis, increased collagen, angiogenesis, and more uniform dispersion of melanin granules.

○ **What is the mechanism of action of retinoids?**

Cause a 70% inhibition of AP-1 transcription factor binding to DNA, which decreases the activation of metalloproteases such as collagenase, gelatinase, and stromatolysis.

○ **What is the mechanism of action of hydroquinone?**

Blocks the conversion of dopa to melanin.

○ **What is ochronosis?**

A potential adverse reaction to hydroquinone characterized by a reticulated, sooty pigmentation of the cheeks, forehead, and periorbital regions.

○ **Which bleaching agent is also an effective treatment for acne?**

Azelaic acid.

○ **Which bleaching agent is produced by *Aspergillus* and *Penicillium*?**

Kojic acid.

○ **What are the components of Jessner's solution?**

Resorcinol, salicylic acid, lactic acid, and ethanol.

○ **How deep does Jessner's solution penetrate?**

Remains intraepidermal.

○ **How deep can a 20% trichloroacetic acid (TCA) solution penetrate?**

Down to the papillary dermis.

○ **What are the four levels of TCA peels?**

Level 0—No frost, skin appears slick and shiny representing removal of the stratum corneum.
Level 1—Irregular light frost with some erythema; 2–4 days of light peeling.
Level 2—Pink white frost, full-thickness epidermal peel, 5 days of peeling.
Level 3—Solid white frost, papillary dermis.

○ **What are the initial manifestations of systemic phenol toxicity from a chemical facial peel?**

Hyperreflexia and hypertension.

○ **When are cardiac arrhythmias that develop during a phenol peel most likely to occur?**

Within 30 minutes of the start of the procedure.

○ **What is the purpose of application of topical vitamin C after skin resurfacing?**

To decrease the inflammation associated with prolonged erythema (must wait until reepithelization is complete before applying).

○ **What medication used to treat androgenetic alopecia can reduce libido?**

Finasteride.

○ **What medication used to treat androgenetic alopecia is also used to treat hypertension?**

Minoxidil.

○ **How many serotypes of botulinum toxin exist? Which is the most useful clinically?**

Eight serotypes (A through G) with type A being the most useful.

○ **What is the mechanism of action of botulinum toxin?**

Inhibition of acetylcholine release from cholinergic nerve endings.

○ **How is recovery of function accomplished?**

Via sprouting of new nerve terminals and an increase in the number of postjunctional receptors.

○ **What would be the histologic findings on muscle biopsies at the site of botulinum toxin injections?**

Increased unmyelinated axonal sprouts; no change in muscle fibers histologically.

○ **What factors are thought to account for diminished responses to botulinum toxin?**

Formation of antibodies, high cumulative dose, and drug interactions.

○ **Which drugs potentiate the effect of botulinum toxin?**

Aminoglycoside antibiotics.

○ **Which drugs limit the effect of botulinum toxin?**

Guanidine and aminopyridines.

○ **What are the onset, peak, and duration of effects of botulinum toxin?**

Onset 24–72 hours, peak effect at 10–14 days, duration 3–6 months.

CHAPTER 39 Miscellaneous Drugs

○ **What effect does zinc have on viral upper respiratory tract infections?**

Decreases the duration of symptoms.

○ **Tricyclic antidepressants are most likely to benefit patients with tinnitus who have what other problem?**

Insomnia.

○ **What are the most widely used agents for treatment of acute migraine?**

Ergotamine tartrate and sumatriptan.

○ **Which comorbid conditions are contraindications to use of sumatriptan?**

Hypertension and coronary artery disease.

○ **What are the indications for migraine prophylaxis?**

Two or more migraines a week and/or abortive treatment inadequate.

○ **What are the most widely used agents for prophylaxis of migraine?**

Tricyclic antidepressants, β-blockers, anticonvulsants, and calcium antagonists.

○ **What is the medical treatment for otosclerosis?**

Sodium fluoride, vitamin D.

○ **What is the proper tetanus prophylaxis for a patient with a tetanus-prone wound, who last received a booster 7 years ago?**

0.5 mL absorbed toxoid.

○ **What is the appropriate tetanus prophylaxis for a patient with a tetanus-prone wound, who has not been previously immunized?**

0.5 mL absorbed toxoid and 250 units of human tetanus immune globulin.

○ **What medication is most commonly used to treat hyperthyroidism during pregnancy?**

Propylthiouracil (PTU).

○ **What is the best agent for rapid surgical preparation of thyrotoxic patients?**
Long-acting β-blocker.

○ **When is exogenous T4 used in patients with thyroid carcinoma?**
Postoperatively in patients with TSH-dependent carcinomas (follicular, papillary, and Hürthle cell).

○ **Prior to radioiodine therapy, which medications should be discontinued and at what time?**
T3, 1 week before; T4, 4–6 weeks before; PTU, 2 weeks before.

○ **What medication can be given as an alternate to thyroid hormone withdrawal prior to radioiodine therapy?**
Recombinant human TSH.

○ **In a nonacute setting, what is the maximum useful amount of calcium supplementation?**
2 g of calcium per day.

○ **What is the appropriate calcium supplementation if the maximum amount of calcium has already been given and the patient is still hypocalcemic?**
Calcitriol or other vitamin D preparations should be added.

○ **What is an absolute contraindication to treatment of lymphatic malformations with OK-432?**
Penicillin allergy.

○ **What is the effect of β-adrenergic blockers on the lower esophageal sphincter pressure?**
Increases it.

○ **A 26-year-old man with frequent migraines is requesting medication for migraine prevention. He is otherwise healthy but reports difficulty exercising secondary to cough. He has had an allergic reaction to a tricyclic antidepressant in the past. What test should be ordered prior to starting him on migraine prophylaxis?**
Pulmonary function test.

○ **In a patient with chronic obstructive pulmonary disease (COPD), which β-blocker would be preferred: propranolol or metoprolol?**
Metoprolol.

○ **What are the Beers criteria?**
A list of medications that tend to cause increased side effects in the elderly.

○ **Dr. Mark Beers found that hospitals made mistakes when recording the medications of elderly patients being admitted to the hospital what percent of the time?**
60%.

• • • ANTIVERTIGINOUS MEDICATIONS/ANTIEMETICS • • •

○ **What is the treatment for familial ataxia syndrome?**

Acetazolamide.

○ **What is the mechanism of action of meclizine?**

H_1-receptor antagonist.

○ **Which causes less dry mouth: meclizine or scopolamine?**

Meclizine.

○ **What are the metabolic effects of prolonged thiazide diuretic therapy?**

Metabolic alkalosis with hypokalemia and hypochloremia, hyperglycemia.

○ **What is the mechanism of action of ondansetron and dolasetron?**

Selective antagonists of serotonin 5-HT_3 receptors with no effect on dopamine receptors.

• • • ANTIREFLUX AGENTS • • •

○ **What is the drug class of choice for mild esophagitis?**

H_2-receptor antagonists.

○ **What drug used for gastroesophageal reflux disease (GERD) may cause irreversible tardive dyskinesia and is associated with dystonic reactions in 25% of young adults (18–30 years) who take it?**

Metoclopramide.

○ **Which drug class used for the treatment of GERD is associated with an increased risk of hip fracture in postmenopausal women?**

Proton pump inhibitors (PPIs).

○ **Why should patients on long-term PPI therapy be tested for *Helicobacter pylori*?**

Hagiwara et al. found that long-term PPI administration promotes gastric adenocarcinoma in gerbils infected with *H. pylori*.

• • • TOPICAL AND SYSTEMIC ANTI-INFLAMMATORY AGENTS • • •

○ **In the United States, how are topical corticosteroids classified?**

By their ability to constrict capillaries: Class I agents are the strongest and Class VII agents are the weakest.

○ **What is the primary reason periodic breaks should be taken when using topical corticosteroids for chronic conditions?**

To prevent tachyphylaxis.

○ **What are the criteria for bone densitometry in patients on long-term corticosteroids?**

>5 mg/day for 3 or more months.

○ **What is the mechanism of action of steroids in the treatment of hemangiomas?**

Block the estradiol-17 receptor.

○ **What is the recommended treatment for autoimmune inner ear disease?**

First-line treatment is high-dose prednisone, then methotrexate, then cyclophosphamide.

○ **Why is ticlid only warranted in patients unable to tolerate aspirin?**

Risk of life-threatening neutropenia.

● ● ● NASAL DECONGESTANTS AND ANTIHISTAMINES ● ● ●

○ **What is the most effective monotherapy for allergic rhinitis?**

Intranasal corticosteroids.

○ **True/False: Prolonged use of high-dose nasal steroids has been found to cause ocular hypertension.**

False: This association was found with high-dose *orally inhaled* steroids only.

○ **What effect does daily use of fluticasone have on nasal mucous?**

Decreases the number of eosinophils in the mucous.

○ **How do corticosteroids diminish IgE hypersensitivity reactions?**

Diminish capillary permeability, block migratory inhibiting factor, stabilize lysosomal membranes, and inhibit edema formation.

○ **What is the mechanism of action of nasal cromolyn sodium?**

Inhibits degranulation of mast cells.

○ **What symptom do intranasal anticholinergics treat?**

Rhinorrhea.

○ **What is the only nonsedating antihistamine that is eliminated primarily through the kidneys?**

Cetirizine.

○ **What is montelukast?**

An antileukotriene, believed to stabilize rhinosinusitis in patients with Samter's triad.

○ **What effect does oxymetazoline have on the nasal cilia?**

Paralyzes them.

Section V

BASIC SURGICAL CONCEPTS

CHAPTER 40 Preoperative and Postoperative Care

○ **What is the most effective duration for perioperative antibiotic administration?**

24 hours.

○ **Which hypertensive medications classically cause withdrawal hypertension and, therefore, should not be stopped prior to surgery?**

β-Blockers and clonidine.

○ **Of Goldman's risk factors, which has been shown to be the most significant?**

Congestive heart failure (CHF).

○ **What is the appropriate preoperative workup for a young patient with frequent premature ventricular contractions (PVCs)?**

An electrocardiogram (ECG), holter monitor, and a cardiac stress test.

○ **What are the advantages of a thallium stress test over an exercise stress test?**

The thallium stress test can better identify the location and extent of myocardial ischemia.

○ **When should a patient quit smoking to have the greatest decrease in perioperative pulmonary complications?**

At least 8 weeks before the planned procedure.

○ **A patient with advanced laryngeal cancer comes in for preoperative evaluation. He currently weighs 130 lbs and reports weighing 149 lbs 3 months ago. His serum albumin level is 2.4 g/dL. What should be done prior to his operation?**

He should be hospitalized for 7–10 days prior to surgery for nutritional repletion.

○ **The above patient is hospitalized and started on high-calorie tube feeds at 50 cc/h. The next day he becomes confused and goes into cardiac arrest. What has happened?**

Refeeding syndrome.

○ **What is the accepted stress dose of corticosteroids for patients undergoing major procedures?**

Hydrocortisone, 100 mg, the night before the procedure with repeat administration every 8 hours until the stress has passed.

○ **What is the standard endocarditis prophylaxis for dental, oral, or upper airway procedures in adult patients at risk?**

Amoxicillin 2 g orally, 1 hour before the procedure.

○ **When should oral hypoglycemics be discontinued prior to surgery?**

24 hours.

○ **When should warfarin therapy be discontinued prior to surgery?**

96–115 hours (4 doses).

○ **What factors increase the risk of postoperative pulmonary embolism?**

Age >40 years, history of lower extremity venous disease, malignancy, CHF, trauma, and paraplegia.

○ **Children may have unlimited clear liquids up to how many hours prior to scheduled anesthetic induction?**

2–3 hours.

○ **What role might oral clonidine play in the preoperative period?**

As an α_2-adrenergic agonist, it can reduce anesthetic requirements and has been used to provide sedation and anxiolysis while maintaining hemodynamic stability.

○ **What factors predispose children with viral URIs to airway hyperactivity during surgery?**

Age <5 years; family history of allergic disease; infections secondary to respiratory syncytial virus; parainfluenza rhinovirus, influenza or *Mycoplasma pneumoniae*, coexisting malaise; rhinorrhea and excess mucus production; male sex; and preexisting airway reactivity.

○ **What is the single most important factor that determines the length of stay after general anesthesia in ambulatory patients?**

Postanesthesia nausea.

○ **How are children with von Willebrand disease undergoing tonsillectomy managed perioperatively?**

IV administration of desmopressin (0.3 μg/kg) preoperatively, 12 hours postoperatively, and every morning until the fossae are completely healed; aminocaproic acid pre- and postoperatively. Alternatively, Factor VIII concentrate can be given perioperatively.

○ **How are children with idiopathic thrombocytopenia managed perioperatively?**

CBC is drawn 1 week prior to the procedure, and if thrombocytopenia is present, IVIG is administered preoperatively (400 mg/kg for 4 days).

○ **What anesthetic considerations must be taken into account in a patient with sickle cell disease?**

Adequate hydration and oxygenation. Spinal or local anesthesia should be used whenever possible.

○ **How are children with sickle cell disease managed perioperatively?**

Preoperative transfusion to decrease the hemoglobin S ratio to <40% and preoperative intravenous hydration are recommended.

○ **What are the guidelines set by the AAO-HNS for 23-hour admission after adenotonsillectomy?**

Poor oral intake, vomiting, hemorrhage, age younger than 3, home more than 45 minutes from the nearest hospital, poor socioeconomic situation with possible neglect, and other medical problems.

○ **Which patients are at greatest risk for respiratory problems after adenotonsillectomy?**

Those with polysomnogram-proven obstructive sleep apnea, Down syndrome, cerebral palsy, or congenital defects.

○ **Why are children under 3 routinely admitted after adenotonsillectomy?**

Less likely to cooperate with oral intake and more likely to have surgery for airway obstruction.

○ **A patient who is to undergo surgery reports a positive result on a latex-specific RAST test as part of a job screening process but denies any symptoms of latex allergies. Should any precautions be taken during surgery?**

Yes, the procedure should be performed under latex-free conditions.

○ **What is the incidence of postoperative hypertension in patients with obstructive sleep apnea syndrome (OSAS) without history of hypertension?**

63%.

○ **What is the ideal MAP after surgery for OSAS?**

Below 100 mm Hg.

○ **What are the primary disadvantages of ketorolac?**

Impairs platelet function and can lead to mucosal breakdown in the GI tract.

CHAPTER 41 Anesthesia and Intraoperative Fluids and Medications

○ **What surgical prep solution is contraindicated for use on the face?**
Hibiclens, as it is caustic to the eyes.

○ **Why are iodine solutions superior to chlorhexidine as a surgical antiseptic?**
Chlorhexidine is not effective against viruses and fungi.

○ **Which nasal spray has less cardiac toxicity: oxymetazoline or neosynephrine?**
Oxymetazoline.

○ **Which medication has been shown to decrease the catecholamine response during suspension laryngoscopy?**
Fentanyl.

○ **What factors are responsible for transfusion-induced immunosuppression?**
Serum factors and fragmented debris from white blood cells and platelets.

○ **What should be given to cancer patients who need a blood transfusion to minimize the immunosuppression?**
Washed RBCs.

○ **What is the best time to begin prophylactic antibiotic therapy for elective surgery?**
1 hour prior to the operation.

○ **What are the daily maintenance fluid requirements of a healthy 60-kg woman?**
2100 cc.

○ **What is a reliable alternative induction technique in a 5-year-old struggling child who refuses the mask and cannot be managed by intravenous induction because of lack of accessible veins?**
A sedating intramuscular injection of ketamine (3 mg/kg).

O   **What are the negative side effects of ketamine?**

Increased airway secretions, transient increase in intracranial pressure, and auditory/visual hallucinations.

O   **What is the preferred anesthetic technique for bronchoscopy in adults?**

A modified endotracheal tube or a jetting system used with a relaxant and controlled ventilation.

O   **What is the preferred anesthetic technique for bronchoscopy in infants and children?**

Spontaneous respiration with inhalation anesthesia.

O   **All of the inhaled anesthetics are bronchodilators except for which one?**

Nitrous oxide.

O   **Which neuromuscular blocker's metabolism is independent of renal or liver failure?**

Cisatracurium.

O   **Shortly after induction of general anesthesia, the patient's body temperature significantly rises, PVCs are noted on the electrocardiogram and his skin becomes flushed. What is the likely diagnosis?**

Malignant hyperthermia; other symptoms include masseter spasm, sustained muscle rigidity, and myoglobinuria.

O   **What is the mechanism of action behind malignant hyperthermia?**

Inhibition of calcium reuptake into the sarcoplasmic reticulum of skeletal muscle.

O   **What is the treatment for malignant hyperthermia?**

Total body cooling, vigorous hydration, dantrolene.

O   **A 90-year-old woman is given morphine shortly before beside laryngoscopy. Her respiratory rate drops to 6 and her lips turn blue. She responds only to pain. What medication should be given?**

Naloxone, in 20–40 μg increments.

O   **What is a complication of rapid administration of naloxone?**

Flash pulmonary edema.

O   **What medication is used to reverse benzodiazepines?**

Flumazenil, 200 μg IV over 15 seconds, repeated every 15 seconds up to 1 mg.

O   **Which anesthetic should be discontinued 15 minutes prior to placing a tympanic membrane graft?**

Nitrous oxide.

O   **What is the mechanism of action of local anesthetics?**

Prevent increases in the permeability of nerve membranes to sodium ions.

○ **What are the two main classes of local anesthetics?**

Those with an ester linkage and those with an amide linkage.

○ **How do these classes differ in metabolism?**

Those with an ester linkage are metabolized in the plasma by cholinesterase; those with an amide linkage are metabolized in the liver by the p-450 system.

○ **Which local anesthetics are amide compounds?**

Lidocaine, ropivacaine, and bupivacaine.

○ **Which antihypertensive medication prolongs the effect of regional anesthesia with amide anesthetics?**

Clonidine.

○ **What are the toxic side effects of local anesthetics?**

CNS excitability or depression, myocardial depression, peripheral vasodilation, methemoglobinemia, and allergic reactions.

○ **Which local anesthetic produces toxicity at the lowest dose?**

Tetracaine.

○ **True/False: All local anesthetics are weak bases and produce vasodilation.**

False: Cocaine and ropivacaine are the exceptions.

○ **Which local anesthetics have been shown to induce methemoglobinemia?**

Prilocaine, benzocaine, lidocaine, and procaine.

○ **What is the treatment for methemoglobinemia?**

Slow intravenous infusion of 1% methylene blue solution (total dose, 1–2 mg/kg).

○ **What is the maximum recommended dose of bupivacaine?**

2–3 mg/kg.

○ **What is the duration of action of bupivacaine?**

3–10 hours.

○ **True/False: Bupivacaine has a depressant effect on cardiac contractility four times that of lidocaine.**

True.

○ **How does ropivacaine differ from bupivacaine?**

Ropivacaine is also a long-acting amide with equivalent anesthetic properties to bupivacaine but has less potential to cause serious cardiotoxic reactions and has intrinsic vasoconstrictive properties.

○ **What is the maximum recommended dose of lidocaine in a 60-kg woman?**

300 mg without epinephrine; 420 mg with epinephrine.

○ **How much epinephrine is contained in 1 cc of 1:100,000 epinephrine?**

10 μg.

○ **Where should local anesthetic be injected to block the superior laryngeal nerve?**

Halfway between the hyoid and thyroid cartilages.

○ **Where should local anesthetic be injected to anesthetize the subglottis and preepiglottic space?**

Cricothyroid membrane and thyroid notch, respectively.

○ **What makes midazolam particularly useful in the outpatient setting?**

It has a relatively short onset of action and an elimination half-life of 2–4 hours.

○ **Which benzodiazepine is preferred in patients with liver disease?**

Lorazepam.

○ **Which α-agonist is five to ten times more potent than clonidine and is approved for use as a sedative and analgesic in the operating room and ICU?**

Dexmedetomidine.

○ **True/False: All opioids cause bradycardia.**

False: Meperidine is the exception.

○ **What is the primary advantage of using remifentanil over fentanyl?**

Shorter onset of action (within 30–60 seconds of administration) and offset (within 5–10 minutes after discontinuance).

○ **Allergy to what substance is a contraindication to the use of propofol?**

Soy.

○ **What are the adverse side effects of succinylcholine?**

Cardiac dysrhythmias, fasciculations, hyperkalemia, myalgia, myoglobinuria, increased pressures (ocular, gastric, and cranial), trismus, and allergic reactions; it can also trigger malignant hyperthermia and cause prolonged paralysis in patients with pseudocholinesterase deficiency.

○ **Which patients are more likely to have adverse reactions to succinylcholine?**

Those with closed-angle glaucoma, space-occupying intracranial lesions, or severe crush injuries of the lower extremity.

○ **What is the inheritance pattern and incidence of pseudocholinesterase deficiency?**

Autosomal recessive with an incidence of about 1 in 3000.

○ **What patient population might have a decreased amount of pseudocholinesterase?**

Patients taking anticholinesterase medications for glaucoma or myasthenia gravis, chemotherapeutic drugs, and patients with a genetically atypical enzyme.

CHAPTER 42 Airway Management

○ **What are the two primary disadvantages of the laryngeal mask airway (LMA) compared with endotracheal intubation?**

Easier to displace than a secured endotracheal tube (ETT) and does not protect from aspiration.

○ **What are contraindications to LMA?**

Upper airway obstruction, preexisting pulmonary aspiration, and conditions that restrict pulmonary compliance.

○ **What is the primary advantage of the fast-track LMA?**

It allows placement of an ETT without direct laryngoscopy.

○ **What is the primary advantage of the ProSeal LMA?**

It has an extra lumen to allow suctioning of the stomach.

○ **How is the gum bougie introducer for endotracheal intubation used in a patient with difficult airway?**

Any part of the laryngeal airway, usually the posterior glottis, is visualized with the anterior commissure laryngoscope; the bougie is passed through the scope into the larynx; and the ETT is passed over the bougie.

○ **What are the best options for the "can't intubate, can't ventilate" situations after induction of general anesthesia?**

LMA, transtracheal needle jet ventilation, Combitube, or surgical airway.

○ **What situations are best for the use of the lightwand during endotracheal intubation?**

For patients with cervical spine injury, for children with mandibular hypoplasia, or when copious secretions are present.

○ **What is the esophagotracheal Combitube?**

A twin-lumen device with upper and lower balloons that is inserted blindly into the hypopharynx.

○ **What is the primary advantage of the Combitube over an LMA?**

Prevents aspiration if the patient vomits.

○ **What is the Sanders ventilator?**

Jet ventilator that delivers O_2 at <50 psi directly through a port in the laryngoscope.

○ **Why is jet ventilation contraindicated in patients with tracheal stenosis?**

Expiration of air is more difficult than inspiration during jet ventilation in patients with tracheal stenosis and can result in air trapping and pneumothoraces.

○ **Which laryngoscope blade is especially useful for patients with edematous or redundant tissue obstructing the view of the vocal cords?**

Bainton blade.

○ **Which laryngoscope blade has a high-resolution digital camera incorporated into it?**

GlideScope.

○ **What physical features are predictors of difficult intubation in patients with OSAS?**

Low hyoid (mental protuberance to hyoid distance >30 cm), mandibular deficiency, and large neck circumference (>45 cm).

CHAPTER 43 Wound Care

○ **What are the most commonly isolated bacteria from wound infections following major contaminated head and neck surgery?**

Staphylococcus aureus and beta-hemolytic streptococci.

○ **What are the second most commonly isolated bacteria?**

Gram-negative aerobic bacteria.

○ **Why do hematomas increase the risk of infection?**

They prevent fibroblast migration and capillary formation.

○ **What perioperative factors are associated with an increased risk of postoperative wound infection?**

Long preoperative hospitalization; no preoperative shower; early shaving of the operative site; hair removal; and prior antibiotic therapy.

○ **How much time does it take for a surgical wound to fully heal?**

2 years.

○ **Under what conditions is epithelial migration and replication most facilitated?**

Moist wound surfaces under gas-permeable dressings.

○ **How long does epithelialization take to produce a watertight seal?**

48 hours.

○ **Deficiency of which white blood cell is most likely to compromise wound healing?**

Macrophages.

○ **What is the maximum tensile strength of a surgical scar?**

80% of normal uninjured tissue.

○ **What are the three stages of normal surgical wound healing?**

Inflammation (d1–3), proliferation (d3–week 4), maturation (week 4–2 years).

○ **Which stage is most sensitive to the effects of chemoradiation?**

Inflammatory stage.

○ **What are the first inflammatory cells to enter the wound space?**

Neutrophils.

○ **What is the tensile strength of a wound during the inflammatory stage?**

Less than 5% of normal.

○ **What is the major event during the proliferative phase?**

Accelerated production of collagen.

○ **When does the production of collagen peak during wound healing?**

Day 7 after wound closure (continues at this pace for 2–3 weeks).

○ **What is the tensile strength of a wound after 4 weeks?**

30% of normal.

○ **What are the main events of the maturation stage?**

Reduction in the number of fibroblasts and macrophages, increase in collagen content, and gradual increase in tensile wound strength.

○ **What is the function of epidermal growth factor (EGF)?**

It stimulates DNA synthesis and cell division in a variety of cells, including fibroblasts, keratinocytes, and endothelial cells.

○ **What is the wound bursting strength?**

A direct measure of the force required to separate a healing, linear incision.

○ **What effect does radiation therapy (RT) have on the wound bursting strength?**

Significantly decreases it—after 18 Gy, it is 52% of normal.

○ **Poor wound healing after RT is primarily due to injury to which cell?**

Fibroblasts.

○ **Which suture material loses its strength within 7 days?**

Plain catgut.

○ **Which suture materials incite the greatest inflammatory response?**

Plain catgut and chromic catgut.

○ **What is the absorption rate of chromic catgut sutures?**

20 days.

○ **When should scar revision take place?**

Not for at least 1 year after injury/surgery.

CHAPTER 44

Grafts (Autografts, Homografts, and Alloplasts)

○ **When is return of sensation after skin grafting considered maximal?**

After 2 years.

○ **What are the differences between thin and thick split-thickness skin grafts (STSGs)?**

Thin grafts take better, but thick grafts have better color match, less contraction, and are more resistant to trauma.

○ **What is the most important factor in minimizing hyperpigmentation of skin grafts?**

Protection from UV light for a full year postoperatively.

○ **What are the three phases of healing for skin grafts?**

Imbibition, inosculation, and neovascularization.

○ **What process allows survival of skin grafts in the first 48 hours?**

Plasmatic imbibition.

○ **What is meant by inosculation with regard to skin grafts?**

The process by which vascular buds from the recipient bed make contact with capillaries within the graft.

○ **Why do cranial bone grafts have superior resistance to resorption when compared with other bone graft donor sites (e.g., rib or iliac bone)?**

Cranial bone originates from membranous bone, whereas the other donor sites originate from endochondral bone; cranial bone revascularizes more quickly.

○ **What complications are specific to the iliac crest donor site?**

Injury to abdominal contents or the iliofemoral joint, detachment of the inguinal ligament, interference with tensor fascia lata function, or damage to nearby peripheral nerves.

○ **What complications are specific to the rib donor site?**

Pneumothorax, hemothorax, and intercostal nerve injury.

○ **What complications are specific to the cranial bone harvest?**

Dural exposure, meningitis, CSF leak, sagittal sinus injury, and brain injury.

○ **What are the different types of cranial bone grafts?**

Full-thickness calvarium, split-thickness calvarium, bone chips, and bone dust.

○ **What is the minimum age at which the calvarium can be split?**

Age 4 or 5 (layers of the skull are not defined until then).

○ **What is the thickest part of the skull?**

Parietal bone.

○ **What is the thinnest part of the skull?**

Squamous portion of the temporal bone.

○ **True/False: Sagittally oriented scalp incisions tend to cause less scalp sensory disturbance than do coronally oriented incisions.**

True.

○ **What can be done to minimize the visibility of the bicoronal incision?**

Perform a wavy line incision.

○ **What is the preferred site for harvesting calvarial bone?**

Parietal bone (anterior for a flat graft; posterior for a curved graft).

○ **How is the diploic layer of the skull recognized during in situ harvesting?**

Color changes from yellow-white to red and increased bleeding occurs.

○ **What is the best way to avoid injury to the superior sagittal sinus during harvesting of calvarial bone?**

Maintain at least a 2-cm distance from the sagittal suture.

○ **What factor is most essential to the success of a vascularized bone graft to the mandible?**

Good immobilization.

○ **Which alloplastic implant material forms a surrounding capsule?**

Solid silicone.

○ **Which alloplastic implant material has been reported to cause the least amount of bony resorption deep to the implant?**

Porous polyethylene.

○   **What is the major problem of using Mersilene mesh for genioplasty?**

High potential for resorption.

○   **What are the advantages of using mesh implants for repair of orbital floor fractures?**

No need for a bone or fascial barrier between the orbital contents and the mesh; posterior orbital shape can be simulated more easily than with bone grafts; well tolerated when exposed to open paranasal sinuses; and may facilitate survival of bone grafts in the anterior orbit.

○   **What are the advantages of using cranial bone as an autogenous graft compared with other bone grafts for orbital reconstruction?**

Harvested from the same surgical field; little postoperative pain; donor site complications are rare; large amounts can be harvested; and less likely to resorb than endochondral grafts.

○   **What are the advantages of using porous polyethylene over other alloplastic materials for orbital reconstruction?**

Semirigid; porous allowing fibrous, vascular, and bony ingrowth; minimal inflammatory reaction; and infection and extrusion are rare.

CHAPTER 45 Flaps and Prosthetics

○ **What is the best level for undermining skin flaps?**

In the subdermal layer.

○ **What is the maximum length-to-width ratio for local flaps?**

3:1.

○ **True/False: Axial flaps are more reliable than random flaps.**

True.

○ **What is the blood supply of a random flap?**

The dermal and subdermal plexuses.

○ **What is the term for a flap that is raised and pivoted into a defect, leaving a secondary defect that must be repaired?**

Transposition flap.

○ **What is the term for a flap that is raised from a nearby region and moved to a defect across intact skin?**

Interpolation flap.

○ **Considering rotation flaps, myocutaneous flaps, and random flaps, which of these has the strongest blood supply?**

Rotation flap.

○ **True/False: The surviving length of an axial pattern flap remains constant regardless of flap width.**

True.

○ **How does delaying (elevating the flap in two stages 2–3 weeks apart) improve flap survival?**

Conditions tissue to ischemia, closes A-V shunts, and increases blood flow by sympathectomy.

○ **How long does it take for complete regeneration of the endothelium across a microvascular anastomosis?**

2 weeks.

○ **What is the most common complication from microsurgical reconstruction?**

35% suffer medical complications (pulmonary problems, prolonged ventilatory support, and acute ethanol withdrawal).

○ **When is the risk of thrombosis highest after microsurgical reconstruction?**

15–20 minutes after closure.

○ **What is the most common cause of flap failure?**

Venous thrombosis.

○ **When is arterial thrombosis most likely to occur?**

First 72 hours.

○ **What is the initial treatment for any free flap that appears to be failing?**

Immediate reexploration.

○ **What is the significance of time to reexploration and flap survival?**

If flaps are reperfused in 1–4 hours, 100% survival is likely. If reperfusion is established by 8 hours, 80% survival is likely. If reperfusion is not reestablished by 12 hours, flap survival is unlikely.

○ **If a free flap fails, what is the best option for reconstruction?**

If medical condition allows, a second free flap should be performed instead of a locoregional flap.

○ **What is the most potent natural inhibitor of thrombin?**

Hirudin.

○ **Where is this substance found in nature?**

Salivary glands of leeches.

○ **What are the contraindications to leech use?**

Arterial insufficiency, severely immunocompromised, and allergic reaction to previous leech application.

○ **What organism lives in the gut of leeches and is the most common organism associated with wound infections when leeches are applied?**

Aeromonas hydrophila.

○ **What antibiotics is this organism sensitive to?**

Third-generation cephalosporins, ciprofloxacin, aminoglycosides, sulfa drugs, and tetracycline.

○ **What is the typical order of return of sensation in noninnervated flaps?**

Pinprick, touch, then temperature.

○ **True/False: Significant return of sensation to a free flap occurs even in the absence of neural anastomosis.**

True.

○ **Most medical prosthetics for the head and neck are made of what material and last how long?**

Silicone; 2 years.

○ **What is the most secure way to hold a prosthetic in place in the head and neck region?**

Osseointegration.

○ **What sort of intraoral prosthetic can be used to help with swallowing in a patient who has lost a significant amount of tongue tissue?**

Palatal augmentation device.

○ **When is using a prosthetic preferable to soft-tissue reconstruction in the head and neck?**

In cancer patients who need ongoing monitoring in the area of the face at risk for recurrence and when surgical reconstruction is too complicated.

CHAPTER 46 Endoscopic and Laser Surgery

○ **What is the minimum effective concentration of helium in heliox administration in children with airway obstruction?**

60%.

○ **What are the advantages of using heliox during laser surgery on the airway?**

It reduces the amount of inspired oxygen concentration and thus the chance of tube ignition, and it facilitates rapid dissipation of heat.

○ **What is the major complication of laser resurfacing of darker skinned individuals?**

Depigmentation (hyper- or hypopigmentation).

○ **What factors affect the risk of complications after laser skin resurfacing?**

Number of laser passes, energy densities, degree of pulse or scan overlap, preoperative skin condition, anatomic areas.

○ **What are the normal side effects of laser skin resurfacing?**

Erythema, edema, serous discharge, and crusting.

○ **Which laser is primarily used for coagulation of hemangiomas?**

Argon laser.

○ **Which laser is used for tracheobronchial lesions, hair removal in ethnic patient populations, and nonablative skin resurfacing?**

Nd:YAG laser.

○ **Which laser works by passing an Nd:YAG laser through a crystal and is mainly used for vascular lesions and turbinate reduction?**

KTP-532 laser.

○ **Which laser is highly absorbed by water and is used mainly for superficial skin resurfacing?**

Erbium:YAG

○ **What are the three types of infrared lasers with clinical uses?**

CO_2 laser; Erbium:YAG; and Ho:YAG

○ **Lasers with wavelengths in the UV range and visible range are minimally absorbed by water but significantly absorbed by what?**

Hemoglobin and melanin.

○ **Which laser in clinical use has the deepest penetration?**

Nd:YAG (4 mm).

○ **Collateral thermal damage is less with infrared or visible lasers?**

Infrared.

○ **What is plume radiation?**

When the laser beam hits the smoke plume, its wavelength may change, often in the visible portion of the spectrum, and cause temporary blindness.

○ **During surgery to debulk respiratory papillomas using a CO_2 laser, the endotracheal tube cuff is accidentally punctured and a fire starts. What should be done?**

Discontinue ventilation and oxygen, remove the endotracheal tube, and if a visible flame is still present, douse the field with normal saline. Once the fire has been extinguished, reintubate the patient with a regular endotracheal tube.

○ **How does the orbital anatomy viewed through the endoscope differ on the right and left sides to the surgeon?**

Right nasal meatal anatomy lies visually straight back, whereas on the left, the ethmoids appear to be more medial, especially anteriorly and superiorly.

○ **What is the significance of this difference?**

If the surgeon operating on the left takes the same straight back approach as the right, he or she will contact the lamina papyracea and enter the orbit.

CHAPTER 47   Common Surgical Complications

○ **What is the drug of choice of treatment of catecholamine-excess hypertensive crisis?**

Phentolamine in 5- to 10-mg IV increments every 5–15 minutes.

○ **What is the drug of choice for ventricular ectopy?**

Lidocaine, 1.0–1.5 mg/kg IV bolus; repeat every 3–5 minutes to a maximum of 3 mg/kg; then start IV drip at 2–4 mg/min.

○ **What is the drug of choice for bradyarrhythmias and heart block?**

Atropine, 0.5–1.0 mg IV every 5 minutes to a maximum of 2–3 mg.

○ **What is the treatment for patients on β-blockers who are not responding to initial epinephrine treatment?**

Inhalation or IV infusion of a pure β-agonist, isoproterenol or low-dose IV dopamine.

○ **In which patients is isoproterenol contraindicated?**

In those with coronary artery disease.

○ **Patients requiring an emergency tracheostomy for an obstructed airway are more likely to develop what postoperative pulmonary complication?**

Pulmonary edema.

○ **What are the most common anesthetic complications seen in the PACU?**

Nausea, vomiting, and airway compromise.

○ **In emergency surgery following trauma, which organisms are most likely to cause serious sepsis?**

Gram-negative bacteria.

○ **In patients with postoperative pneumonia, empiric monotherapy should cover which organisms?**

Gram-negative organisms.

○   **What is the most common organism identified in patients with pneumonia after major surgical resection of the upper aerodigestive tract?**

Staphylococcus aureus.

○   **After 2 weeks of intubation for ventilatory support, a 32-week premature infant is extubated and severe upper airway obstruction results. What is the most likely cause?**

Subglottic edema.

○   **What is Grillo's rule?**

Any patient who develops symptoms of airway obstruction, who has been intubated and ventilated in the recent past, must be considered to have an airway lesion until proven otherwise.

○   **What factors increase the risk of postintubation tracheal stenosis?**

Difficult intubation, an over inflated cuff, repeated reintubations, and poorly performed tracheostomy.

○   **What is the treatment for acute airway obstruction secondary to postintubation tracheal stenosis?**

Dilatation with rigid ventilating bronchoscopes; tracheostomy is only performed if a prolonged period is needed prior to definitive treatment of the stenosis.

○   **What can cause postoperative pneumocephalus after anterior craniofacial surgery?**

Overly aggressive drainage of CSF via a lumbar drain or ball-valve action of the flaps used to reconstruct the skull base.

○   **What is the treatment of pneumocephalus?**

Emergent drainage with needle aspiration, airway diversion (i.e., tracheostomy), and nasal repacking.

○   **Where are postintubation granulomas typically located?**

On the vocal process of the arytenoid.

○   **During a neck dissection, large bubbles are noted in the internal jugular vein and the anesthesiologist notes a sudden drop in the patient's blood pressure. What is likely to happen to the end-tidal CO_2?**

Will decrease (the patient likely has a central venous air embolism).

○   **What is the treatment for air embolism?**

Pack wound, compress jugular veins, immediately place the patient in the left lateral decubitus and Trendelenburg position, insert needle into right ventricle from under the xiphoid, switch to 100% O_2, and stop nitrous.

○   **During neck dissection, the patient develops sudden, severe bradycardia while the surgeon is dissecting around the carotid bulb. What should be done?**

Surgeon should inject local anesthetic into the carotid bulb or anesthesiologist should give atropine or glycopyrrolate.

○   **What factor best predicts the risk of a major complication following head and neck oncologic surgery?**

10% loss of baseline body weight.

○   **What are the two important techniques to prevent postoperative fistula formation?**

Tension-free closure and perioperative antibiotics.

○   **What precautions should be taken to prevent cardiotoxicity during phenol peel?**

IV fluid hydration and treatment of the face in separate units, 30 minutes apart.

Section VI

SPECIFIC SURGICAL PROCEDURES

CHAPTER 48 Head and Neck

○ **What is the greatest advantage of bronchoscopic visualization during percutaneous dilational tracheostomy?**

Fewer major complications occur.

○ **What are the contraindications to percutaneous dilatational tracheostomy?**

Large thyroid goiter or other neck mass, marked obesity, coagulopathy, previous neck surgery, neck trauma including burns, and inadequate access to the trachea.

○ **What percent of all instances of tracheal bleeding developing 48 hours or longer after surgery are caused by tracheoinnominate fistulae?**

50%.

○ **What percent of patients with tracheoinnominate fistulae survive?**

25%.

○ **What are the risk factors for innominate artery rupture after tracheostomy?**

Placement of tracheostomy below the third ring; aberrant course of the innominate artery; use of a long, curved tube; over hyperextension of the neck during the procedure; prolonged pressure by inflated cuff; and tracheal infection.

○ **Which patients are at a higher risk of pneumothorax after tracheostomy?**

Children.

○ **What is the most common cause of mortality in patients <1 year of age who undergo tracheostomy?**

Plugging or accidental decannulation.

○ **What should be done if the posterior tracheal wall is disrupted during tracheostomy?**

Tracheostomy tube should be replaced with an endotracheal tube.

○ **Subcutaneous emphysema may prelude what condition after tracheostomy?**

Tension pneumomediastinum.

○ **What precaution should be taken for a patient with a tracheostomy undergoing general anesthesia?**

Nitrous oxide should be avoided, as it diffuses into the cuff and can increase the pressure by up to 40 mm Hg. If it is used during induction, the cuff should be deflated temporarily.

○ **What are the signs of a tracheoesophageal fistula after tracheostomy?**

Copious secretions, food aspiration, and air leak around the cuff with abdominal distension.

○ **What percent of patients with long-term tracheostomies are colonized with *Pseudomonas*?**

>60%.

○ **What effect does tracheostomy have on the incidence of pneumonia?**

Patients on a ventilator are at a higher risk of pneumonia after tracheostomy and also tend to develop more serious pneumonias (*Pseudomonas*) secondary to antibiotic resistance.

○ **How soon will deep mucosal ulcerations and exposure of tracheal cartilage occur when cuff-to-tracheal wall tension exceeds mucosal capillary tension?**

Within 1 week.

○ **When performing a thyroid resection, where should the inferior thyroid artery be ligated?**

It should not be ligated. Branches of the inferior thyroid artery should be ligated individually at the capsule.

○ **What is the incidence of permanent recurrent laryngeal nerve injury after total thyroidectomy?**

1–4%.

○ **What are the indications for prophylactic central neck dissection in patients with well-differentiated thyroid cancer?**

No definite indications. The American Thyroid Association advises that it may be performed for advanced, large, or invasive T3 or T4 tumors.

○ **Your patient has a unilateral vocal cord paralysis after thyroidectomy for goiter. What are the indications for surgical intervention?**

If the paralysis is well tolerated (e.g., no aspiration and voice quality acceptable to the patient), 12 months is allowed for spontaneous recovery before proceeding with surgery. If the symptoms are severe, early surgery, typically a reversible procedure, is indicated.

○ **What is the incidence of permanent hypoparathyroidism after total thyroidectomy?**

1–5%.

○ **What is the most common cause of persistent hyperparathyroidism after parathyroidectomy?**

Undiscovered or supernumerary parathyroid gland.

○ **During exploration for primary hyperparathyroidism, three normal parathyroid glands are found but the fourth cannot be identified. What is the next step in management?**

Extend the exploration through the existing incision, to include the central neck compartment between the carotids, posteriorly to the vertebral body, superiorly to the level of the pharynx and carotid bulb, and inferiorly into the mediastinum.

○ **What intraoperative modality may assist in locating an intrathyroidal parathyroid gland?**

Ultrasound.

○ **What is the most reliable method of differentiating a parathyroid adenoma from parathyroid hyperplasia?**

Visual inspection of all four parathyroid glands.

○ **What intraoperative modality confirms adequate removal of parathyroid tissue in patients with hyperparathyroidism?**

Rapid intraoperative PTH assay (expect a decrease of at least 50%).

○ **What is the surgical treatment of choice for patients with secondary hyperparathyroidism?**

Subtotal ($3^1/_2$) parathyroidectomy or total parathyroidectomy with autotransplantation.

○ **What is the difference between hemilaryngectomy and vertical partial laryngectomy (VPL)?**

Thyroid perichondrium is preserved in VPL and excised in hemilaryngectomy.

○ **What are the contraindications to VPL and laryngoplasty?**

Fixed vocal cord, involvement of the posterior commissure, invasion of both arytenoids, bulky transglottic lesions, invasion of the thyroid cartilage, subglottic extension >1 cm anteriorly (5 mm posteriorly), and transglottic lesions extending to the supraglottis.

○ **What are the contraindications to VPL for treatment of postradiation tumor recurrence?**

Involvement of both vocal cords, involvement of body of arytenoid, subglottic extension >5 mm, fixed vocal cord, cartilage invasion, and different tumor type from original primary.

○ **In which circumstance can a hemilaryngectomy be performed in the presence of vocal cord fixation?**

If the tumor does not extend through the cricothyroid membrane or the perichondrium of the thyroid cartilage.

○ **What technique is most effective in preventing postoperative stenosis after VPL?**

Epiglottopexy.

○ **What is an imbrication laryngectomy?**

A through-and-through excision of a horizontal segment of the larynx with anastomosis of the caudal and cephalic laryngeal margins.

○   **What are the treatment options for Tis, microinvasive, and T1 glottic carcinoma?**

Endoscopic surgical excision, laser excision, thyrotomy and cordectomy, or radiation.

○   **What are the contraindications to laser excision of early glottic carcinoma?**

Involvement of the anterior or posterior commissure and subglottic extension.

○   **What is the purpose of vestibulectomy during excision of early glottic cancer?**

Excision of the false vocal cord enhances intraoperative and postoperative visualization of the entire vocal cord.

○   **What is CHP? CHEP?**

Cricohyoidopexy and cricohyoidoepiglottopexy.

Conservation laryngeal procedures performed in concordance with a supracricoid partial laryngectomy. Require preservation of at least one functional cricoarytenoid unit (superior laryngeal nerve, RLN, arytenoid, cricoid, and cricoarytenoid musculature).

○   **What are the indications for a supracricoid partial laryngectomy with CHP or CHEP?**

1. T2 transglottic (TG) or supraglottic (SG) lesions not amenable to SG laryngectomy secondary to ventricular invasion, glottic extension, or impaired TVC motion.
2. T3 TG/SG lesions with TVC fixation or preepiglottic space involvement.
3. T4 TG/SG lesions with limited invasion of thyroid ala without extension through the outer thyroid perichondrium.
4. Selected glottic tumors at the anterior commissure with preepiglottic space or SG involvement.

○   **What are the major complications of these procedures?**

Aspiration pneumonia, rupture of the pexis, laryngocele, and laryngeal stenosis.

○   **What are the contraindications to supraglottic laryngectomy?**

Vocal cord fixation, extension to apex of pyriform sinus, bilateral arytenoid involvement, extensive involvement of base of tongue of the anterior commissure, invasion of the thyroid cartilage, and invasion into the interarytenoid space.

○   **True/False: Extension of a tumor in the pyriform sinus below the plane of the laryngeal ventricle is an absolute contraindication to supraglottic laryngectomy.**

True.

○   **What are the advantages of transoral laser resection of early supraglottic cancer?**

Oncologically sound, no tracheostomy or feeding tube is usually necessary, early discharge, rapid resumption of deglutition, and more cost effective.

○   **What is the absolute contraindication to endoscopic laser resection of supraglottic cancer?**

Base of tongue involvement.

○ **Patients with supraglottic cancer who undergo both surgery and radiation therapy (vs. surgery alone) are at a significantly higher risk for what?**

Long-term gastrostomy feeding.

○ **What is the most common and serious complication following supraglottic laryngectomy?**

Aspiration pneumonia.

○ **In which subsite of the hypopharynx is cancer more common in females?**

Postcricoid area.

○ **During endoscopic evaluation of a tumor of the hypopharynx, what four questions must be answered?**

1. Can the larynx be saved?
2. Is a partial or total pharyngectomy necessary?
3. Is a partial or total esophagectomy necessary?
4. Does the tumor extend into the prevertebral fascia?

○ **What is the most direct approach for resection of most posterior pharyngeal wall tumors?**

Suprahyoid.

○ **What is the most serious complication of this approach and how can it be avoided?**

Damage to the hypoglossal and superior laryngeal nerves; can be avoided if the greater horn of the hyoid is left undissected.

○ **What approach is used for resection of posterolateral tumors?**

Combined suprahyoid and lateral pharyngotomy.

○ **What is the most serious complication of lateral pharyngotomy?**

Excessive retraction on the great vessels leading to thrombosis or embolism.

○ **Which tumors of the pyriform sinus do not necessarily require total laryngectomy?**

2 cm or smaller, located at least 1.5 cm superior to the pyriform fossa apex, with normal vocal cord movement, and no invasion into adjacent sites; patients must also have good pulmonary function.

○ **What procedure is performed for resection of these lesions?**

Partial laryngopharyngectomy.

○ **When is total esophagectomy indicated?**

If the inferior margin during resection of a postcricoid tumor extends below the mediastinal inlet or if a second primary is present in the distal esophagus.

○   **What are the reconstructive options after partial pharyngectomy?**

Primary closure (if 3 or more cm of tissue is available), skin graft, sternocleidomastoid flap, radial forearm free flap, or deltopectoral flap with a deepithelialized pedicle.

○   **What problem arises when regional or transplanted skin flaps are used for reconstruction of the hypopharynx when the larynx is preserved?**

A large amount of immobile pharyngeal wall interferes with the pharyngeal component of swallowing, making aspiration inevitable.

○   **What are the reconstructive options after total laryngectomy and partial pharyngectomy?**

Primary closure if more than 40% of the pharyngeal circumference is left in situ, regional flap (pectoralis major, deltopectoral), radial forearm free flap, gastric patch, free jejunal patch, tongue base rotation flap.

○   **What are the reconstructive options after total laryngectomy and total pharyngectomy?**

Free jejunal interposition graft, U-shaped pectoralis major + split-thickness skin graft (STSG), tubed thin flap (radial forearm or deepithelialized deltopectoral).

○   **During placement of a tubed flap, where should the longitudinal suture line uniting the sides of the flap into a tube be placed?**

Against the prevertebral fascia.

○   **What are the reconstructive options after total laryngopharyngectomy and cervical esophagectomy?**

Gastric pull-up, free jejunal graft.

○   **What is the primary limitation of the gastric pull-up?**

Obtaining enough length to achieve a tension-free closure.

○   **What is the blood supply to the gastric pull-up?**

Right gastroepiploic and right gastric arteries.

○   **What is the blood supply to the jejunum?**

Superior mesenteric arterial arcade.

○   **What electrolyte problem is disproportionately associated with gastric pull-up?**

Hypocalcemia secondary to impaired calcium absorption and inadvertent parathyroid resection during thyroidectomy.

○   **What length of jejunum is normally harvested for reconstruction?**

15–20 cm.

○ **What can be done for a large discrepancy between the circumference of the pharyngeal stoma and the jejunal segment?**

The proximal jejunum can be opened longitudinally along its antimesenteric border or a redundant piece of jejunum can be inserted into the proximal segment to widen the lumen.

○ **Where do fistulas most often occur after free jejunal transfer?**

At the superior anastomosis between the jejunum and pharynx.

○ **Where do strictures most often occur after free jejunal transfer?**

At the inferior anastomosis between the jejunum and esophagus.

○ **What can happen if the free jejunal graft is too long?**

Pooling of secretions and dysphagia.

○ **What can be done to prevent functional dysphagia due to neuromuscular incoordination?**

Myotomy of the jejunal musculature.

○ **True/False: TEP is not effective in patients reconstructed with gastric pull-up.**

False, although the voice quality is poor.

○ **What is the fistula rate in patients who have had prior irradiation requiring total laryngectomy and partial pharyngectomy?**

15–20%.

○ **What is the fistula rate following free jejunal transfer (nonirradiated patients)?**

10–20%.

○ **What is the rate of major complications after gastric pull-up?**

50%.

○ **What are the most common complications of gastric pull-up?**

Regurgitation, cervical dysphagia, stricture, and anastomotic leak.

○ **What percent of patients require dilatation after gastric pull-up?**

50%.

○ **What sort of gastrointestinal complaints do patients have after gastric pull-up?**

Early satiety, emesis, and dumping syndrome.

○ **What can be done to treat or prevent dumping syndrome?**

Eating small dry meals, restricting fluid intake during meals, and using octreotide (somatostatin analogue).

○ **What portion of patients after total laryngectomy will report loss of olfaction?**

Two-thirds.

○ **What maneuvers help facilitate preservation of olfaction after total laryngectomy?**

Rapid facial or buccal movements, "clicking" of the palate, and movement of the olfactory source.

○ **What is the primary advantage of the midline mandibular osteotomy for resection of oropharyngeal tumors compared with the lateral mandibulotomy?**

Preservation of the inferior alveolar and lingual nerves.

○ **If a marginal mandibulectomy is performed and the bony margin is positive, does one irradiate the remaining bone?**

No, as bone is relatively hypoxic and cannot generate many free radicals with radiation therapy; the patient should be taken back to the operating room for mandibulectomy.

○ **True/False: Due to shrinkage, at least 8–10 mm of in situ margin must be taken to achieve a 5 mm pathologically clear margin for tumors of the oral cavity.**

True.

○ **What factors are most strongly related to overall speech function 3 months after surgery for oral or oropharyngeal cancer?**

Closure type, percentage of oral tongue resected, and percentage of soft palate resected.

○ **What is the differential diagnosis for the etiology of stridor in a patient who has undergone total glossectomy and postoperative radiation therapy?**

Edema secondary to altered lymphatics; recurrent tumor; gastroesophageal reflux disease; and superinfection.

○ **What is the purpose of using an STSG to cover a small defect after excision of a tonsil cancer?**

If the pterygoid muscles are exposed during resection, placing an STSG will help prevent muscle fibrosis and trismus.

○ **What is a functional neck dissection?**

Complete cervical lymphadenectomy sparing the sternocleidomastoid muscle, spinal accessory nerve, and internal jugular vein.

○ **What is the primary blood supply to the skin flaps raised in a neck dissection?**

Transverse cervical artery and facial artery.

○ **Which neck dissection incision results in the best cosmetic outcome?**

MacFee incision.

○ **How should this flap be modified if reconstruction with a deltopectoral flap is planned?**

Inferior incision should be as low as possible.

○ **How far apart should the inferior and superior limbs be with the MacFee incision?**

At least four fingerbreadths apart.

○ **Why is the superior limb placed 1 cm inferior to the mandible?**

To hide the scar in the shadow of the mandible.

○ **What are the recommended indications for elective neck dissection by the National Cancer Comprehensive Network?**

When expected incidence of microscopic or subclinical disease surpass 20% (though many use 25% or 30% as the criteria).

○ **True/False: Neck dissections removed in continuity with the tumor specimen are associated with a significantly higher incidence of survival than those removed separate from the tumor.**

True.

○ **What is the initial treatment for a chyle leak diagnosed 3 days after neck dissection?**

Maintain drains and begin medium-chain triglyceride tube feedings.

○ **If the leak does not resolve, what is the next step in management?**

TPN.

○ **Two weeks after undergoing salvage surgery on the neck, a patient loses 800 cc of blood from the operative site. If a bleeding source is not found on carotid arteriogram, what is the next step in management?**

Venous angiography with endovascular occlusion.

○ **What is the incidence of stroke and mortality from carotid blowout?**

10% stroke and 1% mortality rate if intravascular volume is repleted prior to going to the OR. 50% stroke and 25% mortality rate if intravascular volume is not repleted prior to going to the OR.

○ **What is meant by putting a patient on "carotid blowout precautions"?**

Establish IV access with two large bore IVs, type and cross 2 units PRBCs, have an intubation tray at the bedside, and educate nursing staff.

○ **What are the contraindications to percutaneous endoscopic gastrostomy (PEG)?**

Inability to perform upper endoscopy safely; inability to transilluminate the abdominal wall; and the presence of ascites, coagulopathy, or intra-abdominal infection.

○ **When should PEG be performed when done as part of an oncologic resection?**

After the primary resection to avoid inadvertent spread of tumor cells to the gastrostomy site.

○   **What factor is most important regarding the risk of surgical complications in patients undergoing Zenker's diverticulectomy?**

Size of the diverticulum.

○   **What are the primary advantages of endoscopic versus open resection for Zenker's diverticulum?**

Shorter operative time with no significant difference in complication rate; the absence of skin incision; minimal postoperative pain; quicker resumption of oral feeding; and shorter hospital stay.

○   **True/False: Cricopharyngeal myotomy as an adjunctive procedure to diverticulectomy has been shown to significantly decrease the incidence of recurrence.**

False.

○   **What are the primary limitations to endoscopic diverticulectomy?**

Size of the sac; difficult to perform in very small or large sacs (<2 cm or >10 cm); and limitations in access due to anatomic factors (i.e., inability to extend the neck or limited jaw excursion).

○   **Which complication is most likely to be avoided with endoscopic diverticulectomy versus open diverticulectomy?**

Damage to the RLN.

○   **What is felt to be the safest way to address severe esophageal strictures with dilatation?**

Retrograde technique using Tucker dilators over a guide string.

○   **What factors are associated with the highest likelihood of successful esophageal dilatation for treatment of strictures secondary to caustic ingestion?**

Age <8, injuries caused by agents other than lye, and injuries limited to the upper 1/3 of the esophagus and <5 cm long.

○   **What is the premise behind pursuing long-term dilatation therapy?**

The native esophagus is the best esophagus.

○   **What are the indications for esophageal bypass?**

Complete esophageal stenosis and failure to establish a lumen with dilatation.
Irregularity and diverticuli of the esophagus.
Mediastinitis secondary to dilatation.
Fistula formation.
Inability to maintain a lumen of 40 Fr or greater with dilatation.
Patient intolerance of frequent procedures.

○   **What is the most common esophageal bypass procedure?**

Colon interposition.

○ **What is the difference in using the right versus left colon?**

The right colon is interposed in an isoperistaltic fashion, whereas the left colon is interposed in an antiperistaltic fashion.

○ **What is the most significant early complication of this procedure?**

Cervical anastomotic leak (50%).

○ **What is the most significant late complication of this procedure?**

Cervical anastomotic stricture (44%).

○ **What are the contraindications to surgical resection of esophageal tumors?**

Presence of distant metastases; involvement of prevertebral fascia, trachea, or carotid arteries.

○ **What are the available treatments for cricopharyngeal dysphagia?**

Mechanical dilation, pharyngeal plexus neurectomy, cricopharyngeal myotomy, or botulinum toxin.

○ **What is the plane of dissection for raising flaps during parotidectomy and how can one identify this more easily?**

Between the SMAS and the superficial layer of the deep fascia—identify the platysma first and work superiorly.

○ **What are the six ways to identify the facial nerve trunk during parotidectomy?**

Identification of the tympanomastoid suture line, tragal pointer, posterior belly of the digastric, or styloid process; tracing a distal branch retrograde or tracing the proximal portion forward by drilling out the mastoid segment.

○ **What is the most consistent landmark for identification of the facial nerve trunk?**

Tympanomastoid suture line.

○ **When must the facial nerve be sacrificed during parotidectomy?**

Preoperative facial nerve weakness or paralysis; adenoid cystic carcinoma abutting the nerve; malignant tumor infiltrating the nerve.

○ **What does continuous facial nerve monitoring during parotidectomy prevent?**

Short-term paresis.

○ **What factors are associated with the development of temporary facial paresis after parotidectomy?**

Deep lobe tumor; previous parotid surgery; history of sialoadenitis; addition of a neck dissection to the parotid surgery; increased age; diabetes mellitus; increased operative time; history of parotid irradiation; no EMG monitoring.

○ **Which branch of the facial nerve is most commonly paretic after parotidectomy?**

Marginal mandibular.

○ **When the facial nerve is sacrificed during tumor resection, what must be done prior to reconstruction?**
Frozen section confirmation of negative nerve margins.

○ **Branches of the facial nerve anterior to ____ do not require reconstruction for return of function.**
Vertical line from lateral canthus.

○ **Which methods of facial nerve reconstruction have the potential for spontaneous emotional response?**
Direct anastomosis and cable grafting.

○ **After primary anastomosis, what is the typical return of facial nerve function?**
House grade II or III.

○ **What are some possible nerves used for cable grafting?**
Sural, greater auricular, dorsal radial cutaneous, and supraclavicular nerves.

○ **Which of these is used most often?**
Greater auricular nerve.

○ **Which of these can provide the most length?**
Sural nerve (35 cm).

○ **What is the advantage of the dorsal radial cutaneous nerve?**
It branches as it approaches the wrist, making distal separation into bundles for facial nerve branch anastomosis easier.

○ **What is the best functional outcome of cable grafting?**
House grade III or IV.

○ **Which anastomotic technique is preferred by most surgeons?**
Epineural anastomosis using three to eight sutures of 8-0 or 10-0 synthetic monofilament suture.

○ **True/False: No improvement in functional outcome has been demonstrated with the use of tubes or conduits in facial nerve anastomosis or grafting.**
True.

○ **True/False: Postoperative radiation does not significantly affect the outcome after facial nerve grafting.**
True

○ **What is the minimal time for functional return of the facial nerve after anastomosis or grafting?**
4–6 months.

○ **Which reconstructive options restore facial nerve function most quickly?**

Static slings, gold weights, and tarsorrhaphies.

○ **If a tumor-free proximal nerve stump is unavailable for nerve grafting, what method should be used for optimal functional outcome?**

If reconstruction is undertaken within 2 years of division, grafting of the proximal portion of another cranial nerve to the distal stump of the facial nerve is the next best choice.

○ **Which cranial nerve is most often grafted to the distal facial nerve?**

Ipsilateral hypoglossal.

○ **What is a major contraindication to this procedure?**

Paralysis of IX or X.

○ **What is the primary drawback of hypoglossal-facial nerve grafting?**

Ipsilateral tongue paralysis.

○ **What can be done to ameliorate this problem?**

Use of a mid-tongue Z-plasty; use of only part of the hypoglossal nerve (jump graft); and reinnervation of the hypoglossal nerve with the ansa cervicalis.

○ **What is a jump graft?**

The greater auricular nerve is sutured end to side to XII and end to side to the distal facial nerve.

○ **How can dynamic rehabilitation be achieved in a patient with a 10-year history of facial paralysis following radical parotidectomy?**

Cross-facial nerve graft plus microneurovascular muscle transfer.

○ **What are other indications for free muscle transposition surgery for facial reanimation?**

Möbius syndrome or destruction of muscles secondary to trauma.

○ **What is the advantage of the microneurovascular muscle transfer over the temporalis muscle sling in the treatment of facial paralysis?**

Has the potential to restore spontaneous muscle expressions.

○ **After microneurovascular muscle transfer, what is the maximum muscle power attainable compared with normal?**

55%.

○ **What are some other options for improvement of function after facial paralysis?**

Static facial slings, dynamic muscle slings, free muscle transfers, gold weight upper lid implants, lid-tightening procedures, and brow lift.

○ **What is the significance of the Bell's phenomenon prior to gold weight implantation?**

If the patient has a good Bell's reflex, then the surgeon can be more conservative, choosing a lighter implant to avoid ptosis.

○ **Into which plane is a gold weight placed?**

Suborbicularis.

○ **What happens if the implant is placed too deep?**

Can damage the levator muscle, causing ptosis.

○ **Where on the lid is the implant placed?**

2 mm above the lash line.

○ **What are the complications of gold weight implantation?**

Induced astigmatism, ptosis, migration, extrusion, and persistent inflammation.

○ **What is Frey's syndrome?**

Gustatory sweating, secondary to cross-reinnervation of the divided auriculotemporal nerve with cutaneous nerves, after parotidectomy.

○ **What are the treatment options for Frey's syndrome?**

3% scopolamine cream, section Jacobson's nerve, sternocleidomastoid muscle flap, interpose fascia lata between skin and gland, and botulinum toxin.

○ **What is the most common complication of parotidectomy?**

Hematoma.

○ **What is the best surgical approach for removal of parapharyngeal tumors?**

Transcervical.

○ **What should be done preoperatively for retrostyloid malignancies or tumors suspected to be involving the carotid artery?**

Angiography with balloon occlusion.

○ **What is the significance of tumor size on the incidence of complications with resection of carotid body tumors?**

Tumors >5 cm are associated with a significantly higher rate of complications with removal (67% for tumors >5 cm vs. 15% for tumors <5 cm).

○ **What are the advantages of preoperative embolization of carotid body tumors?**

Decreased intraoperative blood loss and operative time.

○ **When a carotid body tumor is embolized preoperatively, communication between the external and internal carotid circulation may occur through which vessel?**

Occipital artery.

○ **During resection of a carotid body tumor, which vessel can be sacrificed in most cases?**

External carotid artery.

○ **When is radiation considered in lieu of surgery for treatment of carotid body tumors?**

Very large tumors, recurrent tumors, or poor surgical candidates.

○ **What is the "first bite syndrome"?**

Complication after removal of a carotid body tumor where the patient experiences intense pain with the first bite of food.

○ **True/False: The relationship between surgical margins and outcome is not clear in the treatment of Merkel cell carcinoma.**

True.

○ **What are the recommended margins for excision of basal cell skin cancers (BCCs)?**

5 mm.

○ **What are the indications for Mohs surgery?**

Morpheaform BCC, recurrent BCC, and BCC in cosmetically sensitive locations.

○ **What is the recommended excisional margin for a 3-cm melanoma?**

2 cm.

○ **A 72-year-old man has a melanoma on his forehead just above the lateral portion of his eyebrow. Should a parotidectomy be performed in addition to resection of the melanoma?**

Yes.

○ **A 43-year-old woman has a melanoma on her nasolabial fold. What surgery should be performed in addition to resection of the melanoma?**

Submandibular gland excision.

○ **What is the primary contraindication to nasopharyngectomy?**

Tumor involvement of the cavernous sinus or cranial nerves.

○ **What is the anterolateral surgical approach to the nasopharynx?**

The maxillary antrum attached to an anterior cheek flap is developed as an osteocutaneous flap and swung laterally.

○ **What are the most common complications of this approach?**

Trismus and palatal fistula.

○ **What are the advantages of this approach?**

Allows wide exposure of the nasopharynx with low morbidity.

○ **What are other surgical approaches to the nasopharynx?**

Lateral rhinotomy with facial disassembly, transpalatal split, lateral cervical approach with mandibular swing, transparotid temporal bone approach, and infratemporal fossa approach.

○ **What factors make a tumor of the nose or paranasal sinuses unresectable?**

Invasion into the frontal lobe, prevertebral fascia, bilateral optic nerves, or cavernous sinus.

○ **What are the four basic surgical procedures used to resect tumors of the midface?**

Medial maxillectomy, suprastructure maxillectomy, infrastructure maxillectomy, and radical maxillectomy.

○ **What are five adjunctive procedures to the above dissections?**

Orbital exenteration, infratemporal fossa dissection, craniotomy, contralateral maxillectomy, and rhinectomy.

○ **What are the three basic transfacial approaches to resection of midface tumors?**

Lateral rhinotomy, total rhinotomy, and midface degloving.

○ **What is the Weber-Ferguson incision?**

Lip-splitting extension of the lateral rhinotomy incision that permits exposure for a radical maxillectomy.

○ **What is the gold standard of treatment for inverting papillomas?**

Medial maxillectomy via lateral rhinotomy.

○ **What area of the sinonasal tract is better visualized via endoscopy as opposed to medial maxillectomy?**

Posterior ethmoid cells, particularly those lateral to the sphenoid sinus and around the optic nerve.

○ **When is a total rhinotomy approach most useful?**

For midline tumors where exposure of the cribriform plate and the bilateral ethmoids is necessary.

○ **What is the primary limitation of the midface degloving approach?**

Limited exposure of the skull base and anterior ethmoid sinuses.

○ **What are the incisions used for the midface degloving approach?**

Sublabial; intercartilaginous; and complete transfixion.

○ **What type of resection would be best for a tumor confined to the floor of the maxillary antrum?**

Infrastructure maxillectomy.

○ **What structures are preserved with an infrastructure maxillectomy that would be resected with a total maxillectomy?**

Orbital floor and sometimes the infraorbital nerve.

○ **What are the contraindications to radical maxillectomy?**

Involvement of the sphenoid, nasopharynx, middle cranial fossa, or extensive infratemporal fossa; presence of bilateral cervical metastases or distant metastases.

○ **What are the contraindications to craniofacial resection?**

Poor surgical candidate, presence of multiple distant metastases, invasion of the prevertebral fascia, cavernous sinus (by a high-grade tumor), carotid artery (in a high-risk patient), or bilateral optic nerves/optic chiasm.

○ **A patient with an advanced sinonasal tumor has significant diplopia secondary to tumor invasion of the periorbital muscles. What procedure should be done in addition to maxillectomy?**

Orbital exenteration.

○ **What happens if the orbital septum is violated during resection of a sinonasal tumor?**

Lid shortening and ectropion.

○ **Why should the inferior turbinate be removed during resection of a sinonasal tumor?**

To prevent interference with a palatal prosthesis.

○ **What should be done during maxillectomy to prevent epiphora postoperatively?**

Dacryocystorhinostomy.

○ **What are the contraindications to surgical resection of juvenile nasopharyngeal angiofibromas (JNAs)?**

Poor surgical risk, recurrent tumor that has proved refractory to previous excisions, and involvement of vital structures.

○ **What is the best surgical approach to resection of JNAs?**

Medial maxillectomy via lateral rhinotomy or midface degloving approach.

○ **What is the success rate of uvulopalatopharyngoplasty (UPPP) for the treatment of obstructive sleep apnea syndrome (OSAS) in adults?**

Overall, 50% experience a 50% reduction in the apnea–hypopnea index (AHI) or in the amount of oxyhemoglobin desaturation.

○ **What preoperative symptom best correlates with improvement in AHI after UPPP?**

Excess daytime sleepiness.

○ **What preoperative factor on the patient's polysomnogram is associated with a positive long-term response to UPPP?**

AHI <40.

○ **What are the advantages of the uvulopalatal flap?**

Reversible; less pain and less incidence of dehiscence than UPPP.

○ **Why should adenoidectomy be avoided when performing UPPP?**

Increases the risk of nasopharyngeal stenosis.

○ **What are some adjunctive procedures for patients who do not improve after UPPP?**

Base of tongue reduction, mandibular advancement with LeFort I osteotomy and maxillary advancement, genioglossus advancement (GA), and tracheostomy.

○ **What is the minimal mandibular height necessary for performing GA?**

25 mm.

○ **What are the normal dimensions of the osteotomy in GA?**

10 × 20 mm.

○ **How far from the inferior border of the mandible should the osteotomy be placed?**

8–10 mm.

○ **What are the possible complications of GA?**

Mandible fracture; dental injury; failure to advance; infection; anesthesia of lower lip, gums, and chin; and bleeding/hematoma.

○ **What are the general indications for performing tracheostomy on patients with OSAS?**

Oxygen saturation <50%, severe arrhythmias, morbid obesity, and unable to tolerate CPAP.

CHAPTER 49 Laryngology

○ **Which laryngoscopes are best for visualizing the anterior commissure or the subglottis?**
Holinger and Benjamin.

○ **Surgical disruption of which layer of the vocal cord is most likely to lead to vocal fold scarring?**
Vocal ligament (highest amount of collagen and fibroblasts).

○ **What are five ways to restore the airway in patients with bilateral vocal fold paralysis?**
Tracheostomy, stitch lateralization of the arytenoid(s), laser arytenoidectomy, unilateral or bilateral laser cordectomy.

○ **Approximately what percent of patients with bilateral vocal cord paralysis never require tracheostomy?**
50%.

○ **In what percent of patients with bilateral vocal cord paralysis is decannulation possible after one of these procedures?**
70%.

○ **What are the four main categories of procedures for unilateral vocal cord paralysis?**
Medialization thyroplasty, arytenoid adduction, intracordal injection, and laryngeal reinnervation.

○ **True/False: Previous Teflon injection is a contraindication to medialization thyroplasty.**
False.

○ **True/False: When injecting Teflon in the vocal fold, it should be placed as far medially as possible.**
False: It should be placed as far laterally as possible.

○ **When is medialization thyroplasty appropriate for the treatment of vocal cord paralysis?**
Any stable, definitive paralysis in a patient without surgical contraindications.

○ **Under what anatomic conditions is medialization laryngoplasty most efficacious in the treatment of vocal fold scarring?**

When arytenoids are mobile, glottic gap is >1.5 mm, and soft tissue deficiency is confined to the anterior 1/3 of the vocal fold.

○ **What symptom, other than hoarseness, is most likely to be improved by medialization thyroplasty and arytenoid adduction?**

Dysphagia.

○ **Into which plane is the implant placed during medialization thyroplasty?**

Subperichondrial.

○ **What are the advantages of performing this procedure under local?**

Desired voice quality can be precisely obtained and airway can be continually evaluated.

○ **What is the aim of arytenoid adduction?**

To pull the muscular process of the arytenoid laterally, resulting in adduction and lowering of the vocal process.

○ **What substances can be used for temporary vocal cord medialization?**

Autologous fat, Gelfoam, collagen, and micronized Alloderm.

○ **A 69-year-old man with terminal lung cancer has severe hoarseness secondary to left vocal cord paralysis. What would be the best treatment option?**

Left vocal cord medialization with Teflon paste.

○ **What is the most likely cause of prolonged dysphonia and vocal fold stiffness after surgery for Reinke's edema?**

Excessive suctioning of the superficial lamina propria.

○ **What is the aim of laryngeal reinnervation?**

To prevent atrophy of the thyroarytenoid muscle.

○ **What are the two primary techniques of laryngeal reinnervation?**

End-to-end anastomosis of the recurrent laryngeal nerve to the ansa hypoglossi or nerve–muscle pedicle flap to the thyroarytenoid muscle (using the ansa and a small piece of strap muscle).

○ **What would be the best treatment for a 60-year-old woman who experiences severe dysphagia and aspiration after removal of a high right vagal schwannoma?**

Right medialization thyroplasty, arytenoid adduction.

○ **What are the indications for endolaryngeal stenting after open repair of laryngeal injuries?**

Disruption of the anterior commissure; multiple displaced cartilage fractures; and multiple, severe lacerations.

○ **What is the most common immediate complication after repair of laryngeal injuries?**

Granulation tissue.

○ **What is the optimal treatment for presbylaryngeus?**

Speech therapy for 1 year; if that fails, then bilateral medialization thyroplasty.

○ **True/False: Arytenoid adduction is contraindicated for the treatment of presbylaryngeus.**

True: Arytenoid adduction is contraindicated in any patient with mobile vocal folds.

○ **What is the most common complication after insertion of a Blom-Singer indwelling voice prosthesis?**

Granulation tissue.

○ **What is the primary disadvantage of the indwelling voice prosthesis compared with the nonindwelling prosthesis?**

Higher rate of fungal colonization.

CHAPTER 50 Paranasal Sinuses

○ **What are the indications for surgical intervention in patients with sinusitis?**
Well-documented history, failure of medical management, significant quality-of-life issues; history confirmed with CT scan and nasal endoscopy.

○ **What percent of patients with rhinogenic headaches secondary to septal impaction experience relief after surgery?**
50%.

○ **What disease should be considered in an adult patient who underwent sinus surgery prior to 18 years of age?**
Cystic fibrosis.

○ **What adjuvant to endoscopic sinus surgery has been shown to decrease the need for subsequent surgery in patients with cystic fibrosis?**
Serial antibiotic lavage.

○ **What is the basic principle of the Messerklinger approach for functional endoscopic sinus surgery (FESS)?**
Identify the skull base first then follow it in a posterior to anterior direction.

○ **For which patients are gravity-dependent inferior antrostomies required?**
Patients with dysfunctional cilia (immotile cilia, cystic fibrosis).

○ **What problem does an accessory maxillary sinus ostium create?**
Enables mucous to recirculate back into the sinus.

○ **What are the three most important surgical landmarks during endoscopic ethmoidectomy?**
Lamina papyracea, fovea ethmoidalis, and anterior ethmoid artery.

○ **What external structure serves as a landmark for the fovea ethmoidalis?**
Medial canthus.

○ **Where does one enter the posterior ethmoids endoscopically?**

At the junction of the oblique and horizontal portions of the basal lamella.

○ **When attempting to remove a suprabullar cell, care should be taken to look for what structure?**

Anterior ethmoid artery.

○ **When performing an external ethmoidectomy, where is the anterior ethmoid artery found?**

2.5 cm posterior to the lacrimal crest in the frontoethmoid suture line.

○ **Where is the posterior ethmoid artery in relation to the optic nerve?**

5 mm anterior.

○ **Which type of frontoethmoid cells are more likely to necessitate both an above (via trephination) and below (endoscopic) approach for adequate resection?**

Type III and IV.

○ **What is the safest direction to follow when resecting cells from the frontal recess?**

From posterior to anterior, avoiding the skull base.

○ **What procedure maximizes visualization of the frontal recess?**

Agger nasi punch out procedure (POP).

○ **What is the name of the procedure where the floor of the frontal sinus is removed but the superior nasal septum is left intact?**

Draf II.

○ **What are the indications for endoscopic frontal sinus drillout?**

Patients with mucoceles or severe frontal sinusitis in whom previous surgery has failed.

○ **What are the indications for osteoplastic flap and frontal sinus obliteration?**

Chronic frontal sinusitis refractory to endoscopic surgery; mucopyocele; severe trauma with fractures involving the drainage pathways; after resection of large frontal tumors near the frontal recess.

○ **Why must all mucosae be removed during frontal sinus obliteration?**

To prevent mucocele formation.

○ **Where do most osteoplastic flaps for frontal sinus obliteration fail?**

Frontal recess and upper anterior ethmoids.

○ **What is the most common intraoperative complication of FESS?**

Bleeding.

○ **What is the most common postoperative complication of FESS?**

Synechiae.

○ **Where does this most commonly occur?**

Between the middle turbinate and lateral nasal wall.

○ **What is bulgarization?**

Technique to incite synechiae formation between the middle turbinate and septum to prevent the middle turbinate from collapsing and obstructing the osteomeatal complex postoperatively.

○ **What factors increase the likelihood of requiring revision sinus surgery?**

Smoking, severe diffuse disease preoperatively.

○ **What are the most common complications of middle meatal antrostomy?**

Epiphora secondary to nasolacrimal duct injury, synechiae.

○ **What are the most common complications of osteoplastic frontal sinus surgery?**

Hypoesthesia in the region of the supraorbital nerve, wound infection.

○ **What factors predispose to complications from ethmoidectomy?**

General anesthesia, multiple previous surgeries, advanced disease, long-term chronic or fungal disease, intraoperative hemorrhage, right-handed right-sided surgery, endoscopic right-handed left-sided surgery, surgeon inexperience.

○ **Is an orbital hematoma a pre- or postseptal injury?**

Postseptal.

○ **Orbital hemorrhage occurs most frequently from trauma to which vessels?**

Orbital veins lining the lamina papyracea and anterior ethmoid artery.

○ **How can one differentiate between pre- and postseptal orbital bleeding?**

Preseptal hematoma is darker, more diffuse with more lid edema; proptosis, chemosis, and mydriasis are characteristic of postseptal hematomas.

○ **How long can the retina tolerate high intraocular pressures?**

60–90 minutes; 15–30 minutes in the presence of an arterial bleed.

○ **If orbital fat is exposed during the operation, why should the nose not be overly packed?**

Packing may press into the periorbita and posterior chamber, increasing pressure and causing proptosis.

○ **If eye changes occur during surgery, what should be done?**

Awaken patient, massage eye, and administer IV mannitol, +/− steroids; if pressure is not reduced, perform lateral canthotomy and cantholysis. Next, perform medial orbital decompression by Lynch external ethmoidectomy. Lastly, periorbital incisions can be made.

○ **What should be done for a severe arterial hemorrhage during FESS that cannot be controlled with packing?**

Compress carotid artery, induce hypotension under general anesthesia, have blood ready for transfusion, call neurosurgery, perform arteriogram with balloon occlusion test; if balloon occlusion is normal, ligate carotid artery. If changes occur, insert Swan-Ganz catheter, administer Hespan, and repeat occlusion test. If still abnormal, carotid bypass or barbiturate coma is indicated.

○ **Which two eye muscles are most prone to damage during FESS?**

Superior oblique and medial rectus muscles.

○ **What is the treatment for subcutaneous emphysema after FESS?**

Observation and reassurance—usually resolves in 7–10 days.

○ **How can a cerebrospinal fluid (CSF) fistula be detected intraoperatively?**

Diluted fluorescein injected intrathecally can be detected intranasally after 20–30 minutes.

○ **What is the treatment for a CSF fistula detected postoperatively?**

Conservative management initially—if still present after 2–3 weeks, surgical closure.

○ **What are the three transpalatal approaches to the sphenoid sinus?**

Midline palatal split, U-shaped incision, S-shaped incision.

○ **What are the relative contraindications to the transsphenoidal approach to the pituitary gland (TSAP)?**

Active sinus infection, limited air cell development, septal perforation, and giant pituitary tumor or vascular tumor that would require wide exposure.

○ **Why is suprasellar tumor extension not a contraindication to TSAP?**

Resection is facilitated by auto decompression of the tumor into the sphenoid cavity.

○ **What is the optimal graft material for sealing the sphenoid cavity?**

Abdominal fat.

○ **Why is this preferred over muscle?**

Improved take rate, less atrophy, increased resistance to infection, better sealing, and less donor site morbidity.

○ **If there is no evidence of a CSF leak intraoperatively, is a fat graft still used?**

Yes, if a thin, bulging diaphragma sella is left, the fat will help prevent secondary empty sella syndrome and the potential for delayed CSF leak.

○ **What are the complications of TSAP?**

Numbness of teeth and gums, nasal septal perforation, short-term crusting/dryness of nasal mucosa, and CSF leak.

○ **What are the indications for orbital decompression?**

Optic neuropathy, severe proptosis (in excess of 24 mm), exposure keratopathy, acute deterioration in orbital status not responsive to short-term corticosteroids.

○ **Which area of the orbital floor should be preserved during endoscopic orbital decompression?**

Portion lateral to the infraorbital nerve canal to prevent vertical subluxation.

○ **What is the primary advantage of the inferior orbital decompression technique?**

Large volume for decompression.

○ **What is the reduction in proptosis after endoscopic medial orbital decompression?**

3.5 mm.

○ **What is the reduction in proptosis after endoscopic medial decompression and external lateral decompression?**

5.4 mm.

○ **What is the landmark for the posterior extent of bone resection during medial orbital decompression?**

Posterior ethmoid artery.

○ **What are the complications from excessive orbital decompression?**

Intractable strabismus and hypoglobus.

○ **What complication after orbital decompression is most threatening to the vision?**

Retinal artery occlusion.

CHAPTER 51 Otology

○ **Where do most facial nerve injuries occur during middle ear surgery?**

Tympanic segment.

○ **What are the surgical landmarks for the tympanic segment of VII?**

Cochleariform process, oval window, pyramidal process, semicanal for the tensor tympani, vertical groove on promontory for the tympanic nerve.

○ **What are the landmarks of the tympanic segment of VII from the mastoid approach?**

Lateral semicircular canal (SCC) and the cog.

○ **How is the facial nerve identified using the tympanic nerve?**

Groove for the tympanic nerve is followed superiorly to the cochleariform process.

○ **What are the surgical landmarks for VII in its mastoid segment?**

Lateral SCC, fossa incudis, and the digastric ridge.

○ **What are some clinical clues to an aberrant facial nerve?**

Congenitally malformed auricle, ossicular abnormalities, craniofacial anomalies, and conductive hearing loss.

○ **Where is the facial nerve most commonly injured during mastoid surgery?**

Near the second genu as it enters the mastoid cavity.

○ **What is the management of intraoperative facial nerve transection?**

Immediate repair with primary anastomosis if possible.

○ **What if primary anastomosis is not possible?**

Use a cable graft with great auricular nerve as the donor.

○   **What if the nerve is only partially transected?**

If greater than 1/2 remains, reapproximate the remaining nerve and perform regional decompression. If less than 1/2 remains, remove the injured segment and repair as with complete transection.

○   **What are the indications for surgical exploration of the facial nerve following temporal bone trauma?**

NET >3.5 mA side-to-side threshold differences or ENoG >90% degeneration.

○   **Which approach is best in patients with normal hearing?**

Supralabyrinthine approach.

○   **What is Donaldson's line?**

Imaginary line in the plane of the horizontal SCC back to the sigmoid sinus marking the top of the endolymphatic sac.

○   **What is the relation of the lateral SCC to the fossa incudis?**

Short crus of the incus is inferolateral to the lateral SCC; the fossa incudis is at the tip of the short crus.

○   **What is the relationship of VII to the lateral SCC and the fossa incudis?**

Medial to the fossa incudis and inferior to the lateral canal.

○   **What is the most important question to answer in the preoperative evaluation of a temporal bone tumor?**

Is the carotid artery or brain involved?

○   **What surgical approach is used for small, localized tumors of the cartilaginous ear canal that have not invaded deep structures?**

Sleeve resection.

○   **What surgical approach is used for tumors that involve both the cartilaginous and bony ear canal without extension into the middle ear?**

Lateral temporal bone resection.

○   **What procedures are often performed in conjunction with a lateral temporal bone resection?**

Neck dissection, parotidectomy, and, occasionally, partial mandibulectomy.

○   **Is the facial nerve sacrificed during lateral temporal bone resection?**

Only if it is involved with tumor.

○   **What surgical approach is used for tumors involving the middle ear that appear confined to the temporal bone?**

Subtotal temporal bone resection.

○ **What structures are resected in a subtotal temporal bone resection?**

External auditory canal, middle ear, petrous bone, TMJ, and parotid gland with facial nerve.

○ **What other procedures are routinely performed with a subtotal temporal bone resection?**

Neck dissection, temporal craniotomy to rule out transdural extension.

○ **True/False: After subtotal temporal bone resection, all patients will have facial nerve paralysis and a dead ear.**

True.

○ **What operation is performed for tumors that involve the medial aspect of the temporal bone in the region of the petrous apex?**

Total temporal bone resection.

○ **What are the three surgical approaches to resection of an acoustic neuroma?**

Translabyrinthine, middle fossa, and retrosigmoid.

○ **What are the two most important landmarks in the middle fossa approach to the internal auditory canal?**

Arcuate eminence and hiatus for the greater superficial petrosal nerve.

○ **Which approach is best in patients with tumors >2.5 cm with good hearing?**

Retrosigmoid.

○ **Which approach is best in patients with tumors <2.5 cm with good hearing?**

Middle fossa.

○ **Which approach offers the best exposure?**

Translabyrinthine.

○ **Which approach results in the best facial nerve outcome?**

Translabyrinthine.

○ **What is the primary disadvantage of the translabyrinthine approach?**

Destroys hearing permanently.

○ **Which approach is best in the high-risk surgical patient, regardless of tumor size?**

Translabyrinthine.

○ **What are the most common complications of acoustic neuroma resection?**

Sensorineural hearing loss, paralysis of VII, cerebrospinal fluid leak (10–35%), meningitis (1–10%), and intracranial hemorrhage (0.5–2%).

○ **What factor is most related to hearing outcome after surgery?**

Size of tumor; significantly more likely to have preservation of hearing if <1.5 cm.

○ **Following acoustic neuroma resection, what problem do patients perceive as most troublesome?**

Hearing loss.

○ **A patient develops a CSF leak after resection of an acoustic neuroma. A pressure dressing and lumbar drain are placed with no improvement. Wound exploration and reclosure are performed, and the leak recurs. What is the next step?**

It the tympanic membrane is intact and hearing is present, plug the eustachian tube via a middle fossa approach. If the tympanic membrane is not intact and hearing is not present, perform a blind sac closure of the external auditory canal and obliterate the middle ear and eustachian tube.

○ **What nerve is involved in paroxysmal lacrimation?**

Nervus intermedius.

○ **Of the disorders of lacrimation, taste, and salivation, which is the first to return after injury to the nervus intermedius?**

Taste.

○ **When is surgical exploration indicated after temporal bone fracture?**

For massively displaced fractures with compromise of the carotid artery or VII; or for VIIth nerve paralysis with >90% degeneration documented on electroneurography (ENoG) within 14 days of the injury.

○ **What approach is most often used for longitudinal fractures?**

Combined transmastoid/middle fossa.

○ **What are the most common injuries encountered on surgical exploration?**

Hematoma and contusion with bony spicules impinging on the nerve sheath.

○ **When is surgical exploration indicated for facial nerve paralysis after gunshot injuries?**

When >90% degeneration is documented on ENoG within 14 days of the injury.

○ **What is the best surgical approach for facial nerve exploration in a patient with a temporal bone fracture distal to the geniculate ganglion with intact hearing?**

Combined transmastoid/middle fossa approach.

○ **What are the indications for surgical treatment of BPPV?**

Incapacitating symptoms >1 year, confirmation of BPPV with Dix-Hallpike on at least three visits, failure of conservative treatment, normal head MRI.

○ **What are the surgical options for treatment of BPPV?**

Singular neurectomy, posterior SCC ablation.

○ **What are the disadvantages of singular neurectomy?**

Technically difficult, 10% risk of SNHL, and nerve may be inaccessible under the basal turn of the cochlea in a small number of patients.

○ **Why is posterior SCC ablation most often the procedure of choice?**

Relatively easier, less risk to hearing, and excellent long-term results (approaches 100%).

○ **How is electrocochleography helpful prior to destructive surgery for Menière's disease?**

In patients with unilateral disease, abnormalities in the asymptomatic ear (SP:AP >35%, distorted CM with after-ringing) predict development of hydrops in that ear.

○ **What is the prognostic significance of a normal AP–SP prior to surgery?**

Outcomes are significantly better.

○ **In terms of functional level, which patients with Menière's disease are candidates for chemical or surgical labyrinthectomy?**

Patients with functional levels of 4, 5, or 6.

○ **What is the most common and most difficult to manage problem after any vestibular destructive surgery?**

Persistent disequilibrium (20%).

○ **What are the surgical options for treatment of Menière's?**

Endolymphatic shunt, destructive labyrinthectomy, and vestibular nerve section.

○ **Which of these is the only surgical procedure considered in an only-hearing ear?**

Endolymphatic shunt.

○ **Which of these is most commonly performed?**

Endolymphatic shunt.

○ **Where is the endolymphatic sac?**

Anterior to Trautmann's triangle within the dura, medial and inferior to the posterior SCC.

○ **What percent of patients will have improved tinnitus and hearing after endolymphatic sac surgery?**

50% experience improvement in tinnitus and 30–40% experience improvement in hearing.

○ **What percent of patients have improvement of vertigo after endolymphatic sac surgery?**

70% experience complete relief, 20% experience decreased vertigo.

○ **What are the four primary approaches to vestibular nerve section?**
Middle fossa, retrosigmoid, transcochlear, and retrolabyrinthine.

○ **Which of these is associated with the greatest risk of damage to VII?**
Middle fossa.

○ **Which of these is most likely to result in postoperative headaches?**
Retrosigmoid.

○ **What increases the likelihood of headaches after the retrosigmoid approach?**
Drilling out of the medial portion of the IAC.

○ **Which way is the sigmoid sinus retracted in the retrosigmoid approach to vestibular nerve section?**
Anteriorly.

○ **Which way is the sigmoid sinus retracted in the retrolabyrinthine approach to vestibular nerve section?**
Posteriorly.

○ **Which of these approaches is at higher risk for a CSF leak?**
Retrolabyrinthine.

○ **What portion of the VIIIth nerve is sectioned in vestibular nerve section?**
Lateral portion (superior and inferior vestibular nerves) in the IAC.

○ **What are the landmarks for identification of the IAC during middle fossa approach to vestibular nerve section?**
Greater superficial petrosal nerve, malleus head, and superior SCC.

○ **What is the success rate of vestibular nerve section?**
For the middle fossa approach, complete elimination of vertigo is achieved in >90%; for the posterior approaches, complete elimination of vertigo is achieved in >80%.

○ **What are the contraindications to vestibular nerve section?**
Only hearing ear, signs of central vestibular dysfunction, and poor medical health.

○ **What are the two approaches to labyrinthectomy?**
Transmastoid and transcanal.

○ **Which of these is superior in complete elimination of vertigo?**
Both are equally effective.

○ **Using the rating system developed by Jahrsdoerfer, what score is associated with the best outcome after surgical treatment of aural atresia?**

8 or greater (80% chance of obtaining an SRT 15–25 dB).

○ **True/False: A patient with a score of 5 or less is considered a very poor operative candidate.**

True.

○ **What is the most important factor in assessing the possibility of surgery in a patient with congenital aural atresia?**

Presence of the stapes.

○ **Why should surgery be delayed until age 5?**

To allow for completion of pneumatization of the temporal bone.

○ **True/False: Surgery is contraindicated in children with unilateral atresia.**

False: Many will operate if the patient is likely to achieve a residual conductive deficit of 30 dB or less.

○ **What factors are considered contraindications to correction of unilateral atresia?**

Poor mastoid pneumatization, anterior displacement of the middle ear, and facial nerve anomalies.

○ **What are the two basic approaches for repair of aural atresia?**

Transmastoid and anterior approaches.

○ **What are the two most important landmarks of the anterior approach?**

The middle cranial fossa dura superiorly and the TMJ anteriorly.

○ **What advantage does hugging the middle fossa dura have on protecting the facial nerve?**

One will enter the middle ear first in the epitympanum; the facial nerve will always lie medial to the ossicular heads in the epitympanum.

○ **What are the reasons for persistent conductive hearing loss after aural atresia repair?**

Inadequate mobilization of the ossicular mass from the atretic bone, an unrecognized incudostapedial joint discontinuity, or a fixed stapes.

○ **What are the reasons for recurrent conductive hearing loss after aural atresia repair?**

Refixation of the ossicular chain or tympanic membrane lateralization.

○ **What is the best method of excising a glomus tympanicum tumor?**

Laser.

○ **Which laser can be used on the tympanic membrane to treat atelectasis?**

CO_2 laser.

O **What are the indications for performing a lateral tympanoplasty?**

Anterior or large perforations, revision tympanoplasty, or if the anterior canal wall is in the way.

O **What are the advantages of lateral tympanoplasty?**

Excellent exposure, high graft take rate (95%), and most versatile approach.

O **What are the disadvantages of lateral tympanoplasty?**

Longer healing time, potential for anterior blunting or lateral healing, and technically more difficult.

O **What are the complications of lateral tympanoplasty?**

Anterior blunting, lateralization, epithelial pearls, and canal stenosis.

O **What vessels can be injured in the middle ear during tympanoplasty?**

Persistent stapedial artery, superficial petrosal branch of the middle meningeal artery, high-riding jugular vein, and anomalous carotid artery.

O **What are the most common reasons for recurrent conductive hearing loss after tympanoplasty?**

Recurrent perforation, blunting of the angle between the tympanic membrane and the external auditory canal, graft lateralization, graft thickening and adhesions, and severe graft atelectasis.

O **What are the indications for simple mastoidectomy?**

Acute coalescent mastoiditis with complications or acute mastoiditis that does not resolve after appropriate antibiotic therapy and myringotomy.

O **What is a modified radical mastoidectomy?**

Conversion of the mastoid, epitympanum, and external auditory canal into a common cavity by removal of the posterior and superior external bony canal walls.

O **True/False: The modified radical mastoidectomy does not involve a tympanoplasty.**

True.

O **What is a radical mastoidectomy?**

Conversion of the mastoid, antrum, and middle ear into a common cavity, with removal of the tympanic membrane, malleus, incus, chorda tympani, and mucoperiosteum.

O **Should a cholesteatoma be removed over a fistula?**

Controversial, in that leaving a piece of matrix to seal the fistula increases the risk of recurrent cholesteatoma, while completely removing the matrix and exposing the fistula increases the risk of hearing loss and vertigo.

○ **What are the indications for second look surgery after removal of a congenital cholesteatoma?**

Obvious recurrent disease, unexplained deterioration in hearing, and concern about the adequacy of the initial surgery or disease found to extend into the antrum or mastoid.

○ **How do the surgical findings differ during removal of a congenital cholesteatoma from removal of a cholesteatoma associated with chronic suppurative otitis media?**

Absence of inflammatory changes/adhesions and easier removal with potential for complete preservation of the middle ear mucosa.

○ **What are the boundaries of the facial recess?**

Chorda tympani laterally, upper mastoid segment of VII medially, and bone of fossa incudis superiorly.

○ **What type of cholesteatoma is most frequently found in the facial recess?**

One associated with a perforation below the posterior malleolar fold.

○ **Which areas of the middle ear are most difficult to see during mastoidectomy?**

Infrapyramidal and tympanic recesses.

○ **What is the management of injury to the sigmoid sinus during mastoidectomy?**

Apply gentle pressure, place a Surgicel or Gelfoam patch, and continue with surgery.

○ **What is the management of injury to the dura with CSF leak during mastoidectomy?**

Repair with temporalis fascia held in place with sutures or packing and continue with surgery; small tears can be managed with a Surgicel or Gelfoam patch.

○ **Unbeknownst to the surgeon, the dura is torn during mastoidectomy, and postoperatively, the patient develops a severe headache, followed by hemiplegia and coma. What has likely happened?**

Pneumocephalus; torn dura can create a ball valve-like effect and trap air from the middle ear. Influx of air may occur during Valsalva or as a result of high intracranial negative pressure due to the rapid escape of CSF through the tear.

○ **According to Sheehy, in which situations is the canal wall down (CWD) approach most appropriate?**

Only-hearing ear, very contracted mastoid, mastoid with a labyrinthine fistula, or presence of canal wall erosion due to disease.

○ **What are the disadvantages of the CWD procedure in the management of cholesteatoma?**

Healing is slower, indefinite periodic cleaning and dry ear precautions are required, and hearing aids are more difficult to fit in the meatus.

○ **What are the two most important principles of CWD procedures?**

Lowering the posterior canal wall to create a round cavity and creating a large meatus.

○ **Why is it important to saucerize the cavity margins?**

The soft tissues and auricle will assume a more medial position during healing, resulting in a smaller cavity.

○ **What is the benefit of amputating the mastoid tip?**

Reduces cavity size and eliminates a dependent cavity area that is not visible.

○ **Which portions of the ossicular chain are always removed in CWD procedures?**

Incus and head of the malleus.

○ **If a CWD procedure is used to treat a posterior-superior retraction cholesteatoma, what would be the most likely site of residual cholesteatoma?**

Sinus tympani.

○ **What are the disadvantages of the canal wall up (CWU) approach?**

Limited exposure of the anterior epitympanum, sinus tympani, and facial recess.

○ **If the CWU procedure is chosen, what are the indications for a second look?**

Missing middle ear mucosa or extensive cholesteatoma.

○ **What is the single most important factor affecting hearing results after CWD tympanomastoid surgery?**

Maintenance of a pneumatized space juxtaposed to the round window.

○ **What techniques can be used to accomplish this?**

Placement of the fascia graft such that it does not obliterate the space between the eustachian tube orifice and the round window; placement of silastic crescent in the hypotympanum.

○ **What other techniques can help improve hearing results?**

Shielding the round window to increase the difference in sound pressure between the oval and round windows; placing the graft directly atop the head of the stapes when the suprastructure is present; using a TORP or placing the graft directly on the stapes footplate when the suprastructure is not present (type IV tympanoplasty).

○ **What are the potential problems with a type IV tympanoplasty?**

Narrowing of the middle ear space and graft lateralization.

○ **What are the indications for using a TORP when the stapes suprastructure is present?**

Stapes tilted toward the promontory, partial arch necrosis, and unusually deep oval window niche where a PORP might contact the fallopian canal and/or promontory.

○ **What are the expected residual hearing levels after PORP and TORP?**

15 dB conductive hearing loss PORP; 25 dB conductive hearing loss TORP.

○ **What are the advantages of using porous polyethylene prostheses over fitted autograft ossicles?**

Hearing is more stable, decreased incidence of residual and recurrent cholesteatoma.

○ **What is the most common cause of failure using a fitted ossicle for middle ear reconstruction?**

Separation of the ossicle from the stapes.

○ **What factors contribute to extrusion of middle ear prostheses?**

Eustachian tube dysfunction (70%), graft failure, and cartilage resorption.

○ **What technique is employed during ossiculoplasty to decrease the risk of prosthesis extrusion?**

Placement of cartilage between the prosthesis and the tympanic membrane.

○ **How should an extruded prosthesis be managed?**

Allow spontaneous extrusion; TM may heal and make a spontaneous connection.

○ **What are the indications for using plastic sheeting in middle ear surgery?**

Absence of mucosa on the promontory, in most of the middle ear, or in the middle ear cleft (except in the eustachian tube).

○ **What is the purpose of the plastic sheeting in these conditions?**

To prevent adhesions from forming and to allow mucosa to grow over denuded areas.

○ **What are the indications for staging a tympanoplasty without mastoidectomy?**

Extensive mucous membrane destruction, stapes fixation.

○ **What can cause persistent cavity discharge after CWD procedures?**

High facial ridge, particularly large cavity, open middle ear space, inadequate meatal opening, poor postoperative care leading to infection.

○ **What are the options for surgical management of the chronically draining mastoid cavity?**

Autologous cultured epithelial graft (from buccal mucosa), large meatoplasty, revision mastoidectomy, reconstruction of canal wall with an aerated cavity, mastoid cavity obliteration, and mastoid/middle ear obliteration.

○ **When is mastoid and middle ear obliteration most appropriate?**

In a dead ear, without cholesteatoma.

○ **What is the Palva flap?**

Technique used for mastoid obliteration where the soft tissue off the back of the ear is swung into the mastoid.

○ **What are the most common reasons for mastoid surgery failure without recurrent cholesteatoma?**

Persistent suppurative disease in unexenterated air cells (most commonly at the sinodural angle and along the tegmen) and technical factors such as high facial ridge or meatal stenosis.

○ **What is the most common postoperative complication of pressure equalizing tube insertion?**

Persistent otorrhea.

○ **What is the most common cause of perilymph fistula?**

Otologic surgery (stapedectomy).

○ **What congenital ear malformation is most commonly associated with perilymph fistula in children?**

Mondini deformity.

○ **What is the most common location for iatrogenic labyrinthine fistula formation during mastoidectomy?**

Lateral SCC.

○ **What is the management of intraoperative violation of the labyrinth?**

Immediate application of a Gelfoam patch or other tissue seal (other than fat).

○ **What is the prognosis after such an injury?**

Good if immediately recognized and treated.

○ **During stapedectomy, the entire stapes footplate falls into the vestibule. What should be done?**

It should be left in the vestibule, as attempts to retrieve it are more likely to cause damage than leaving the footplate where it is.

○ **Where is the safest place to create an opening in the stapes footplate?**

Central area.

○ **What is a "perilymph gusher"?**

Rapid release of perilymph after stapes footplate fenestration due to pressure and fluid from the CSF compartment venting through the inner ear.

○ **Which patients are at greater risk for a "perilymph gusher"?**

Patients with congenital stapes fixation and a patent cochlear aqueduct or a large vestibular aqueduct.

○ **What is the management of a "perilymph gusher"?**

Reduction of CSF pressure with mannitol and/or a lumbar drain; application of a tissue seal over the oval window fistula using fascia, perichondrium, or fat and secured with a stapes prosthesis; and postoperative hospitalization with continued reduction in CSF pressure.

○ **Ten days after stapedectomy, your patient complains of progressive hearing loss and vertigo that does not respond to steroids. What do you do?**

Take the patient back to the operating room to explore for a granuloma. If one is found, remove the granuloma and place a new prosthesis with a tissue seal over the oval window.

○ **What are the signs and symptoms of a poststapedectomy perilymph fistula?**

Episodic vertigo, especially with exertion, SNHL, loss of speech discrimination, and nystagmus with changes of air pressure on the TM.

○ **What is the most common complication of stapedectomy?**

Prosthesis displacement.

○ **What is Tullio's phenomenon?**

Vertigo with loud noise.

○ **What is the significance of Tullio's phenomenon after stapedectomy?**

Suggests that the prosthesis is too long and impinging on the saccule.

○ **What are the five primary causes of conductive hearing loss after stapedectomy?**

Failure to recognize obliterative otosclerosis of the round window; displacement of the prosthesis after head trauma or large changes in middle ear pressure; necrosis of the long process of the incus; migration of the prosthesis in the oval window; and adhesions.

○ **What is the significance of SNHL after stapedectomy?**

If no tissue graft was used, 50% of SNHL will be due to fistulas and should be revised.

○ **During stapedectomy, how is the round window evaluated for normal movement?**

The membrane is not readily visible, so a drop of saline is placed in the niche and movement is seen as a change in light reflection on the meniscus when the prosthesis is palpated.

○ **Revision stapedectomy is performed. What should be done with the original prosthesis?**

If possible, it should be left in place, and a second fenestra and prosthesis should be placed.

○ **In patients with bilateral otosclerosis, which ear should be operated on first?**

Poorer hearing ear.

○ **In patients where one ear has previously been operated on and hearing loss is equal bilaterally, which ear should be operated on?**

The unoperated ear.

○ **In patients with bilateral otosclerosis and equal hearing loss, which ear should be operated on?**

Right-handed surgeon should work on the left ear (or patient preference).

○ **When is stapedectomy contraindicated?**

In young children until it has been demonstrated that they are not prone to otitis media, in the presence of active middle or external ear disease or active URI, tympanic membrane perforation, Menière's disease.

○ **Why is stapedectomy dangerous in patients with Menière's disease?**

A dilated saccule may sit immediately beneath the footplate and be injured upon entry into the vestibule.

○ **What is obliterative otosclerosis?**

Margins of the footplate cannot be seen or removed.

○ **What is the significance of a white versus a blue floating footplate?**

Hearing success is much less in the presence of a white floating footplate (52%) versus a blue floating footplate (97%).

○ **Why should visible lasers not be used for revision stapedectomies?**

These lasers depend on pigment for absorption so when working around white bones and tendons, inner ear damage is more likely.

○ **The STAMP procedure is advantageous for which type of otosclerosis?**

Otosclerosis confined to the fissula ante fenestram.

○ **How is the STAMP procedure different from traditional laser stapedotomy?**

No prosthesis is used; the anterior crus and anterior 1/3 of the footplate are vaporized using a hand-held argon laser.

○ **What is the incidence of malleus ankylosis during primary surgery for otosclerosis?**

1–2%.

○ **What is the incidence of malleus ankylosis during revision surgery for otosclerosis?**

5–14%.

○ **What two inner ear malformations are contraindications to cochlear implantation?**

Michel deformity and small IAC syndrome (<3 mm).

○ **What psychological problems are contraindications to cochlear implantation?**

Organic brain dysfunction, mental retardation, psychosis, and unrealistic expectations.

○ **Into which ear is the implant placed if there is no difference acoustically between ears?**

Into the better surgical ear as determined by CT scan (side with the least amount of ossification or fibrosis within the scala tympani).

○ **Into which ear is the implant placed if the patient has had different durations of hearing impairment in each ear?**

Into the ear that has had the shortest duration of deafness.

○ **A patient with Meniere's disease and profound SNHL is being evaluated for cochlear implantation. She still has infrequent episodes of vertigo. What test should be ordered prior to surgery?**

ENG.

○ **What percent of patients will have new bone growth covering the round window niche and membrane during cochlear implantation?**

50%.

○ **What condition increases the likelihood of this happening?**

History of meningitis.

○ **What is the incidence of ossification after pneumococcal meningitis?**

20–30%.

○ **A 45-year-old man is being evaluated for cochlear implantation. He has a long history of chronic ear disease that is now dormant and has a modified radical mastoid cavity. What other procedures may be considered in conjunction with cochlear implantation?**

Close the external auditory canal and obliterate the mastoid and middle ear.

○ **True/False: Presence of PETs is a contraindication to cochlear implantation.**

False.

○ **True/False: The electrode of the cochlear implant is normally placed into the scala tympani.**

True.

○ **True/False: Results of cochlear implantation in children with congenital inner ear malformations are comparable with those without malformations.**

True (if the cochlea is fully intact).

○ **What are the most common complications of cochlear implantation?**

Flap complications, electrode dislocation or malinsertion, facial nerve injury, and stimulation of facial nerve postoperatively.

○ **Which complication is more likely in patients with a history of otosclerosis who undergo cochlear implantation?**

Unwanted facial nerve stimulation due to demineralization of surrounding bone.

○ **Which complication is more likely in patients with cochlear dysplasia who undergo cochlear implantation?**

CSF leak.

○ **A patient who recently had a cochlear implant placed complains of throat pain every time someone talks to him. What has happened?**

One of the electrodes of the cochlear implant is stimulating Jacobson's nerve on the promontory.

○ **How can this be treated?**

Removal of the electrode(s) stimulating the nerve (probably 17 or 18).

○ **What factors are associated with improved outcome after cochlear implantation?**

Shorter duration of auditory deprivation; postlingual onset of deafness; etiology of deafness (meningitis patients have poorer outcomes); higher IQ; better preoperative word and sentence recognition; lip reading ability; better preoperative residual hearing; optimized implant technology and processing; an intact, nonossified cochlea; and in kids, younger age at the time of implantation, motivated family, oral preoperative education, and oral education rehabilitation.

CHAPTER 52 Pediatric Otolaryngology

○ **What are the indications for antireflux surgery in children?**

Mild to moderate symptoms that fail medical therapy; severe gastroesophageal reflux disease with life-threatening symptoms.

○ **What is the difference between a Nissen and a Thal fundoplication?**

Nissen is a 270-degree wrap and Thal is a 360-degree, or complete, wrap.

○ **What are the three laryngeal closure procedures?**

Epiglottic flap, glottic closure, and vertical laryngoplasty.

○ **What are the primary disadvantages of glottic closure?**

It does not allow speech, is difficult to reverse, and rarely works unless the larynx is bilaterally denervated.

○ **Of tracheoesophageal diversion (TED) and laryngotracheal separation (LTS), which is technically easier?**

LTS.

○ **Which is easier to reverse?**

TED.

○ **Which is preferred if the patient has or has had a tracheostomy?**

LTS.

○ **Can these patients talk?**

Potentially, via esophageal speech.

○ **What approach is used for revisions of failed choanal atresia repairs?**

Transpalatal.

○ **What is the best treatment for nasal pyriform aperture stenosis?**

Sublabial medial maxillectomy.

○ **What surgical procedure is the most common cause of iatrogenic vocal cord paralysis in children?**

Tracheoesophageal fistula repair.

○ **What is the most likely cause of stridor after ligation of a patent ductus arteriosus?**

Iatrogenic injury of the left recurrent laryngeal nerve.

○ **What is the term for the treatment of airway obstruction in children with craniofacial abnormalities where the mandible is gradually elongated?**

Distraction osteogenesis.

○ **What are some predictors of failure for endoscopic CO_2 laser treatment of subglottic stenosis?**

Circumferential scarring, scarring longer than 1 cm, tracheomalacia and loss of cartilage support, history of severe bacterial infection associated with tracheostomy, posterior laryngeal inlet scarring with arytenoid fixation, and multiple stenotic sites.

○ **What effects do multiple laser procedures have on the airway?**

Increased scarring, ossification of the cricoid cartilage.

○ **What criteria should be met before performing single-stage laryngotracheal reconstruction (LTR) in neonates?**

At least two failed attempts at extubation, documentation of stenosis endoscopically, weight >1500 g, spontaneous ventilation with F_{IO2} <35%, no evidence of lower respiratory tract infection or congestive heart failure within 30 days of the operation, and no hypertension.

○ **What must be done prior to single-stage LTR?**

Assess for adequate vocal cord mobility and treat GERD.

○ **What are the advantages of single-stage LTR?**

Avoidance of prolonged indwelling stents with associated danger of displacement or breakage, no need for tracheotomy care, single procedure, long-term antibiotic therapy (such as with stenting) is not required.

○ **How long should the patient remain intubated after single-stage LTR?**

3–7 days with anterior graft only; 12–15 days with anterior and posterior grafts.

○ **What are the contraindications to single-stage LTR?**

Abnormal pulmonary function, coexistent medical problems that require a tracheostomy, and severe grade 4 stenosis.

○ **What is the most important factor associated with successful and permanent decannulation after LTR?**

Age >24 months at the time of LTR.

○ **True/False: Children with congenital laryngotracheal stenosis have a better voice outcome after surgical correction compared with children with acquired stenosis.**

True.

○ **What is the primary advantage of early LTR?**

Better speech acquisition.

○ **What is the best approach for the treatment of the funnel-like morphologic variant of congenital long-segment tracheal stenosis?**

Single-stage anterior LTR with cartilage or pericardium grafting.

○ **What are the indications for four-quadrant cartilage division?**

Congenital elliptical cricoid cartilage, severe congenital or acquired SGS, and calcification of the cricoid cartilage from failed LTRs.

○ **What is the primary disadvantage of this technique?**

Requires long-term stenting (1–12 months).

○ **Why is end-to-end tracheal anastomosis rarely used in children?**

Difficult to perform in the subglottic region without damaging the vocal cords.

○ **True/False: Division of the cricoid cartilage has been shown to inhibit its further growth.**

False.

○ **In placing an autogenous cartilage graft, where does the surface bearing perichondrium face?**

Toward the lumen of the larynx.

○ **How does one identify the anterior commissure during laryngofissure?**

By identifying Montgomery's aperture, a small hole just inferior to the anterior commissure or through direct laryngoscopy.

○ **What is the procedure of choice for reconstruction of the anterior commissure?**

Epiglottopexy laryngoplasty.

○ **What is the microtrapdoor flap used for?**

To correct posterior glottic stenosis.

○ **How does one avoid postoperative hemorrhage from the innominate artery after repair of tracheal stenosis?**

Dissect immediately on the trachea without disrupting the artery or its investments; if the artery has been previously dissected or the lesion is fixed to it, interpose a pedicled strap muscle between the anastomosis and the artery.

○ **How does one avoid injury to the recurrent laryngeal nerves during repair of tracheal stenosis?**

Avoid dissecting out the nerves and carry out dissection immediately on the trachea.

○ **Why is it important to avoid dissection of the trachea for more than 1–1.5 cm proximal or distal to the anastomotic site?**

To protect the blood supply to the trachea.

○ **When is hilar release contraindicated?**

In patients with poor pulmonary reserve.

○ **What is the primary advantage of slide tracheoplasty compared with end-to-end anastomosis for the repair of tracheal stenosis?**

Ability to span longer segments.

○ **Slide tracheoplasty increases the cross-sectional airway area by how much?**

Fourfold.

○ **What is the primary disadvantage of augmentation tracheoplasty for the treatment of tracheal stenosis?**

Need for multiple bronchoscopies due to recurrent granulation tissue formation at cartilage graft sites (thought to be secondary to the need for prolonged intubation postoperatively).

○ **After pericardial patch augmentation tracheoplasty, what factors significantly increase the likelihood of fatal outcome?**

Tracheal involvement within 1 cm of the carina or involvement of either mainstem bronchus.

○ **What are the contraindications to tracheal sleeve resection?**

Involvement of the glottis or subglottis, stenosis longer than 6 cm, temporary or chronic respiratory failure or neurological deficit.

○ **What are the treatment options when sleeve resection is contraindicated?**

Endotracheal prosthesis, tracheostomy with a cannula, or a Montgomery T tube.

○ **What has been shown to decrease the incidence of postoperative granulomas after LTR?**

Use of absorbable suture.

○ **What is the significance of hemoptysis after tracheal sleeve resection?**

May portend rupture of the innominate artery.

○ **How much trachea can be resected without using a release technique?**

3 cm (possibly 4 cm with the patient's head in extreme flexion).

○ **What ten techniques are available to gain additional tracheal length in resection cases?**

Extreme flexion, suprahyoid release, infrahyoid release, inferior constrictor release, peritracheal mobilization, intercartilaginous incisions, dissection and mobilization of the right hilum, release of the inferior pulmonary ligament, dissection of the pulmonary vasculature, and transection and reimplantation of the left main stem bronchus.

○ **Which of these is most likely to result in prolonged postoperative dysphagia?**

Combined infrahyoid and inferior constrictor release.

○ **Which of these allows the greatest amount of mobilization?**

Mobilization of the right hilum with release of the inferior pulmonary ligament, dissection of the pulmonary vasculature, and transection and reimplantation of the left main stem bronchus allow up to 6 cm of superior mobilization.

○ **How much mobilization can be achieved with peritracheal mobilization (dissection of the annular ligaments)?**

Up to 1.5 cm.

○ **How much mobilization can be achieved with the suprahyoid release?**

Up to 5 cm.

○ **What structures are removed or transected with the suprahyoid release?**

Stylohyoid, mylohyoid, geniohyoid, and genioglossus muscles are transected, and the body of the hyoid bone is transected at its attachments to the greater and lesser cornus.

○ **What is a Grillo stitch?**

Nonabsorbable suture extending from the periosteum of the mentum to the sternum used to keep the neck flexed after tracheal resection.

○ **What structure is most at risk during removal of a 1st branchial arch sinus?**

Facial nerve.

○ **Why should general anesthesia be avoided in patients with mononucleosis?**

They are at a heightened risk of suffering hepatotoxicity from the anesthetics.

○ **What are the indications for polysomnography prior to adenotonsillectomy for obstructive sleep apnea?**

If history and physical exam are not in agreement or if the child is at an unusually high risk for perioperative complications.

○ **Which patients are at increased risk for atlantoaxial subluxation during tonsillectomy?**
Patients with Down syndrome, achondroplasia, Arnold–Chiari, and rheumatoid arthritis.

○ **What percent of patients with Down syndrome have an unstable transverse ligament of the atlas?**
10%.

○ **What test should be performed prior to operating on these children?**
Flexion and extension lateral neck films.

○ **When should aspirin, naproxen, and all other NSAIDs be discontinued prior to surgery?**
2 weeks, 4 days, and 3 days, respectively.

○ **What tests confirm the diagnosis of von Willebrand's disease?**
Elevated PTT and bleeding time, decreased or absent von Willebrand factor serum levels.

○ **What is the most cost-effective predictor of posttonsillectomy hemorrhage?**
Personal and family history of bleeding.

○ **What group of patients is at increased risk for hemorrhage?**
Age >20 who have surgery during winter.

○ **Which subtype of von Willebrand's disease responds to treatment with desmopressin?**
Type I, the most common, where qualitatively normal von Willebrand factor is present in subnormal levels.

○ **When do serum levels peak after administration of IV desmopressin?**
45–60 minutes.

○ **What are the adverse effects of desmopressin?**
Hyponatremia, seizures, and tachyphylaxis.

○ **Why is pulmonary edema a potential complication after adenotonsillectomy?**
Long-standing partial airway obstruction from enlarged tonsils serves as a natural PEEP. Sudden relief of the obstruction/PEEP can result in transudation of fluid into the interstitial and alveolar spaces.

○ **What is the initial management of posttonsillectomy pulmonary edema?**
Reintubation and administration of PEEP, gentle diuresis.

○ **What factors affect pain after adenotonsillectomy?**

Old age and use of electrocautery are associated with greater pain; postoperative administration of antibiotics has been shown to decrease pain.

○ **What has been shown to accelerate the return to a normal diet after tonsillectomy?**

A single intraoperative dose of steroids.

○ **What is the incidence of clinically significant VPI after adenoidectomy?**

1:1500–3000.

○ **What is the treatment for postadenoidectomy VPI?**

If it persists beyond 2 months, speech therapy; beyond 6–12 months, palatal pushback, pharyngeal flap surgery, or sphincter pharyngoplasty.

○ **Which of these procedures is best for patients with poor palate movement and good lateral wall movement?**

Superior pharyngeal flap.

○ **Which of these procedures is best for patients with poor lateral wall movement and good palate movement?**

Sphincter pharyngoplasty.

○ **Which of these procedures creates lateral ports through the nasopharynx for breathing?**

Superior pharyngeal flap.

○ **Why is tonsillectomy recommended prior to or in conjunction with these procedures?**

Hypertrophied tonsils may tether the palate and contribute to the VPI; raising the flaps is more difficult in the presence of tonsils; keeping the tonsils increases the risk of obstructive sleep apnea postoperatively.

○ **What are the most common complications of pharyngeal flap surgery?**

Bleeding, airway obstruction, and obstructive sleep apnea.

○ **What disease increases the risk of nasopharyngeal stenosis after adenotonsillectomy?**

Syphilis.

○ **What is Grisel's syndrome?**

Vertebral body decalcification and laxity of the anterior transverse ligament secondary to infection in the nasopharynx.

○ **How is adenoidectomy related to Grisel's syndrome?**

Traumatic adenoidectomy can result in Grisel's syndrome.

○ **What is the standard surgical approach for removal of thyroglossal duct cysts (TGDCs)?**

Sistrunk procedure.

○ **What is the recurrence rate following the Sistrunk procedure?**

1–4%.

○ **What is the recurrence rate following excision of a TGDC without removal of the midportion of the hyoid and the ductal remnant?**

38%.

○ **What is the most common complication after repeated laser treatments for recurrent respiratory papillomatosis (RRP)?**

Anterior glottic webs.

○ **When is open repair of posterior glottic stenosis in a patient with RRP possible?**

When there has been no papilloma regrowth 8 or more weeks after ablation.

○ **What is the surgical treatment of choice for giant congenital melanocytic nevi?**

Tissue expansion followed by total excision.

CHAPTER 53

Plastic and Reconstructive

○ **What is the appropriate ratio of the long and short axes for elliptical incisions?**

4:1.

○ **What complication will occur if the above ratio is not met?**

A dog-ear deformity.

○ **What are the four ways to correct hypertrophic or wide scars?**

Excision/undermining, Z-plasty or W-plasty, geometric broken line closure, and dermabrasion.

○ **What are the two most common complications of dermabrasion?**

Milia and hypopigmentation.

○ **What are the mild complications of laser skin resurfacing?**

Prolonged erythema, acne or milia, contact dermatitis, and pruritus.

○ **What percent of patients develops postinflammatory hyperpigmentation?**

33% (more for darker skin types).

○ **What treatments can be used to help this problem?**

Hydroquinone or retinoic acid plus a topical class I corticosteroid, glycolic acid.

○ **What should be used to prevent this problem?**

Sunscreen (pretreatment regimens have not been proven to help).

○ **What factors increase the risk of prolonged erythema?**

Regular use of tretinoin or glycolic acid, rosacea, multiple passes, inadvertent pulse stacking, aggressive intraoperative rubbing.

○ **When does hypopigmentation after laser skin resurfacing present?**

6–12 months after treatment.

○ **What percent of patients develops contact dermatitis after laser resurfacing?**

65%.

○ **How is it treated?**

Bland emollients (avoid topical antibiotics), topical class I corticosteroids, cool and wet compresses.

○ **What percent of patients develops herpes simplex virus (HSV) despite antiviral prophylaxis?**

2–7%.

○ **How should an outbreak of HSV be treated?**

Switch to a different antiviral and administer the maximum dose.

○ **Which anatomic areas are more prone to scarring after laser treatment?**

Infraorbital area, mandible, and anterior neck.

○ **What other factors increase the risk of scarring?**

Development of wound infection or contact dermatitis, recent use of isotretinoin, history of radiation therapy, and history of keloids.

○ **What can be used to treat scarring after laser skin resurfacing?**

Intralesional or topical corticosteroids, 585 nm pulsed-dye laser (two to three treatments at 6–8 weeks intervals).

○ **Patients who have previously undergone blepharoplasty are at increased risk for which complication after laser skin resurfacing?**

Ectropion.

○ **Which injectable filler is approved by the FDA for treatment of lipoatrophy in HIV patients?**

Poly-L-lactic acid (Sculptra).

○ **How long does Sculptra last?**

Up to 3 years.

○ **Which type of injectable fillers can be diminished with hyaluronidase in the case of over augmentation?**

Hyaluronic acid derivatives (Restylane, Juvederm, Captique).

○ **Which injectable fillers require a skin test prior to use?**

Bovine collagen fillers (Zyplast and Zyderm).

○ **What is the incidence of positive responses to skin tests for injectable collagen?**

3%.

○ **How long does injectable collagen remain in the tissue?**

3–6 months.

○ **What is the primary advantage of AlloDerm?**

Semipermanent (20–50% persistence beyond 1 year).

○ **What is isolagen?**

Injectable autologous soft tissue material derived from cultured human fibroblasts.

○ **How many hairs are contained in a minigraft?**

3–8.

○ **How many hairs are contained in a micrograft?**

1–2.

○ **How long does it take for hair to start growing after transplantation?**

10–16 weeks.

○ **How much time should be allotted between transplantation sessions?**

4 months.

○ **Alopecia in which area of the scalp is not improved by scalp reduction?**

Frontal.

○ **What procedure is normally performed prior to extensive scalp reductions?**

Ligation of the occipital vessels 2–6 weeks before the reduction.

○ **Between which layers of the scalp are tissue expanders placed?**

Between the periosteum and the loose areolar tissue.

○ **What transposition flap restores the frontal hairline?**

Juri flap.

○ **What is the blood supply to this flap?**

Superficial temporal artery.

○ **How many stages are required for completion of the Juri flap?**
Four stages.

○ **When should micro- and minigrafts be placed in relation to flap or reduction procedures?**
After the flap or reduction procedures have healed.

○ **Which patients are good candidates for the pretrichial forehead lift?**
Women with a high hairline and long vertical height to the forehead.

○ **Which patients are good candidates for the midforehead lift?**
Men with deep rhytids in whom a coronal lift is contraindicated.

○ **Which patients are good candidates for direct brow lift?**
Those with brow asymmetries (i.e., from facial nerve paralysis) and marked ptosis of the lateral eyebrow.

○ **What are the relative contraindications to the coronal forehead lift?**
Male-pattern baldness in men and high hairlines in women.

○ **What is the plane of dissection in the coronal forehead lift?**
Subgaleal.

○ **In what region is division of the frontalis muscle prohibited?**
Between the lateral brow and the temporal hairline.

○ **Which patients are not good candidates for endoscopic brow lift?**
Women with high hairlines, patients with male-pattern baldness or tight, thick skin with extensive bony attachments (more common in Asians and native Americans).

○ **Where is the frontal branch of VII most vulnerable during brow lift?**
Just above the lateral brow, 1–2 cm from the orbital rim.

○ **Where should subperiosteal undermining begin during brow lift?**
2.5 cm above the lateral orbital rim to avoid injury to the supraorbital nerve.

○ **When dissecting from the temporal region to the zygomatic arch, where does the deep temporal fascia divide into superficial and deep layers?**
The temporal line of fusion at the level of the superior orbital rim.

○ **What happens to the fascia as dissection continues toward the zygomatic arch?**
The temporoparietal fascia and the superficial layer of the deep temporal fascia fuse 1 cm above the zygomatic arch.

○ **What is the proper plane of dissection in the temporal region to avoid injury to VII?**

Within the subaponeurotic plane (deep to the temporoparietal fascia).

○ **What is the safest plane of dissection in the temporal region when exposure of the zygomatic arch is necessary?**

Within the superficial temporal fat pad deep to the superficial layer of the deep temporal fascia.

○ **In what region of the face can transection of the SMAS directly injure a branch of VII?**

Temporal region.

○ **Where in the midface is the facial nerve most vulnerable during SMAS undermining?**

Anterior to the parotid gland.

○ **What is the safest plane of dissection in the malar region?**

Along the superficial surface of the elevators of the upper lip (zygomaticus major and minor).

○ **How does the facelift incision differ between men and women?**

In women, the incision runs along the posterior margin of the tragus (posttragal); in men, the incision is placed in the preauricular crease (pretragal) so that facial hair does not grow on the tragus postoperatively. Also, a margin of non–hair-bearing skin is preserved around the inferior attachment of the earlobe in men.

○ **What is the difference between SMAS imbrication and SMAS plication?**

Imbrication involves undermining and cutting the SMAS prior to suspension; plication involves folding the SMAS on itself.

○ **What is the difference in outcome between these approaches?**

No significant difference in outcome.

○ **In what direction are the flaps pulled during SMAS suspension?**

Primarily superiorly and partially posterior.

○ **What complication results from pulling too far posteriorly?**

Widening and flattening of the oral commissure.

○ **What is the significance of the position of the hyoid bone in rhytidectomy?**

Dictates the maximum improvement possible in the cervicomental angle; ideal position is high and posterior.

○ **What effect does SMAS suspension have on the nasolabial folds?**

Deepens them.

○ **Which approach to rhytidectomy improves the nasolabial folds?**

Deep plane rhytidectomy.

○ **In which plane is the neck dissected during deep plane rhytidectomy?**

Preplatysmal.

○ **In which plane is the lower face dissected during deep plane rhytidectomy?**

Sub-SMAS plane.

○ **In which plane is the midface dissected during deep plane rhytidectomy?**

Subcutaneous for 2–3 cm anterior to the tragus, then immediately superficial to the orbicularis and zygomaticus muscles.

○ **What is a pixie or satyr earlobe?**

Common complication of rhytidectomy where the earlobe is elongated and directly attached to the facial cheek skin.

○ **What is the most common complication of rhytidectomy?**

Hematoma.

○ **When do most major hematomas occur after rhytidectomy?**

First 12 hours postoperatively.

○ **What is the most commonly injured nerve during rhytidectomy?**

Greater auricular nerve.

○ **What is the consequence of overly aggressive resection of upper eyelid skin?**

Loss of crease definition.

○ **Why should extra caution be taken during lateral dissection of the upper eyelid?**

To avoid prolapsing the lacrimal gland.

○ **What is the most severe, yet rarest, complication of blepharoplasty?**

Retrobulbar hemorrhage—incidence 0.04%.

○ **When should lid malposition after blepharoplasty be corrected?**

No sooner than 6 months after the initial surgery.

○ **What happens to the position of the globe when 2.5 cc of fat is removed?**

Globe moves 1 mm inferiorly and 2 mm posteriorly.

○ **How does release of the arcus marginalis affect eye contour?**

Creates a more convex, youthful eye contour.

○ **What are two major limitations of the transconjunctival approach to lower lid blepharoplasty?**

Redundant skin cannot be removed and orbicularis hypertrophy cannot be treated.

○ **Identification of what structure is essential in safely exposing the medial and central fat pads during a transconjunctival lower eyelid blepharoplasty?**

Inferior oblique muscle.

○ **What are the two types of lower lid malposition after blepharoplasty?**

Retraction and ectropion.

○ **Which is more common?**

Retraction.

○ **What is the difference between retraction and ectropion?**

Retraction is vertical lid shortening due to fibrosis in the middle lamellar plane; ectropion is lid eversion caused by shortening of the anterior lamella, skin, and orbicularis oculi.

○ **What is the most common cause of lower lid retraction after blepharoplasty?**

Accumulation of small amounts of blood in the middle lamellar plane.

○ **What are five lower lid blepharoplasty techniques that help prevent postoperative retraction?**

1. Horizontal alignment of lower lid incisions.
2. Preservation of a strip of orbicularis attached to the tarsal plate.
3. Draping of the flap medially and superiorly.
4. Placement of a suspension suture between the deep surface of the orbicularis and the orbital periosteum.
5. Triamcinolone injection into plane of orbital septum.

○ **What factors predispose to lid malposition after lower lid blepharoplasty?**

Proptosis or unilateral high myopia; preexisting scleral show; malar hypoplasia; lower lid laxity from previous surgery; and females >65 years and all males.

○ **What is the most effective treatment for entropion that fails to resolve with massage?**

Placement of a spreader graft (i.e., palatal mucosal graft) in the posterior lamella.

○ **What is the proper plane of dissection during rhinoplasty?**

Deep to the subcutaneous tissue and SMAS layers.

○ **Reduction of what structure accomplishes the majority of profile changes in patients requesting reduction rhinoplasty?**

Cartilaginous dorsum.

○ **What is the most common reason for rhinoplasty revision?**

"Polly beak" deformity or supratip swelling.

○ **What are the complications of radical septal resections?**

Columellar retraction, dorsal saddling, airway collapse, increased nasal width, loss of tip support, and septal perforation.

○ **How much auricular cartilage can be harvested without affecting the structural integrity of the ear?**

The entire concha can be removed as long as the antihelix is kept intact.

○ **When should a posterior incision be used to harvest auricular cartilage?**

Small grafts and when epithelial and soft tissues are to be incorporated with the graft.

○ **What is the advantage of leaving a small amount of soft tissue on the auricular graft?**

More rapid host bed fixation.

○ **What is the one way to improve the stability of a columellar strut?**

Carve the base into a V or fork or rest a large strut on a cartilage platform (plinth).

○ **What is the most common cause of alar margin elevation?**

Overaggressive resection of the lateral crus.

○ **What is the most important surgical component of the septum?**

Quadrangular cartilage—provides midline support and can significantly influence the external appearance of the nose.

○ **What are the different approaches used in septoplasty?**

Complete, partial, hemi- and high transfixion incisions.

○ **Which major tip support mechanism is violated by the complete transfixion incision?**

Attachment of the medial crura to the caudal septum.

○ **What effect does the complete transfixion incision have on tip projection and rotation?**

Decreases tip projection and increases tip rotation (resulting in nasal shortening).

○ **What is the difference between the hemitransfixion incision and the Killian incision?**

The hemitransfixion incision is made unilaterally at the junction of the caudal septum and the columella, whereas the Killian incision is made unilaterally 2–3 mm cephalic to the mucocutaneous junction.

○ **What are the three primary incisions used in tip surgery?**

Intercartilaginous, transcartilaginous, and marginal incisions.

○ **Which major tip support mechanism is violated by the inter- and transcartilaginous incisions?**

Attachment of the caudal edge of the upper lateral cartilages to the cephalic edge of the alar cartilages.

○ **What are the two major approaches to tip surgery?**

Delivery and nondelivery.

○ **What are the two types of nondelivery approaches?**

Transcartilaginous and retrograde.

○ **What are the advantages of using a nondelivery approach?**

Requires minimal dissection ensuring more symmetric and predictable healing; resists cephalic rotation; single incision; preserves existing tip projection; and resists tip retrodisplacement and postoperative tip ptosis.

○ **What are the disadvantages of using a nondelivery approach?**

Technically more difficult if inexperienced.

○ **What are the advantages to the open approach?**

Wider exposure, allowing the use of binocular vision, bimanual dissection, and microcautery for hemostasis; enables direct vision of the domes and the nasal profile; and can secure tip grafts directly with suture and approach the septum from above-down as well as from below-up.

○ **What are the disadvantages of the open approach?**

Transcolumellar external scar; risk of disturbing normal anatomy in the infratip lobule and caudal aspects of the alar cartilages; prolonged edema in thick-skinned patients; potential for excess trauma to the tip and dorsal skin flap; increased operative time; increased difficulty in judging the exact tip–supratip relationship after skin flap replacement; grafts must be suture fixated.

○ **When can the transcartilaginous incision not be used?**

In patients with widely divergent intermediate crura where the domes need exposure for narrowing.

○ **Which incisions can be used for exposure and delivery of the alar cartilages?**

Intercartilaginous and marginal incisions.

○ **In the delivery approach, what are the indications for using a complete, rather than hemi-, transfixion incision?**

Severely deviated caudal septum; when access to the nasal spine is necessary; when tip rotation and nasal shortening are desired.

○ **Which technique results in greater cephalic tip rotation: interrupted or complete strip?**

Interrupted strip.

○ **How much cartilage should be preserved during a complete strip procedure?**

At least a 4–5 mm strip or 75% of the original cartilage volume.

○ **What techniques can be used to augment the effects of the complete strip, without sacrificing tip projection?**

Medial triangle excision, alternating incomplete incisions, crosshatching, gentle morselization, and transdomal suture narrowing.

○ **What are the various interrupted strip techniques?**

Lateral division, medial division, multiple vertical interrupting cuts, both medial and lateral division with a resection of a lateral segment, and rotation of a segment of lateral crus into medial crus.

○ **Which of these techniques is best for thick-skinned patients with abundant soft tissue and a wide, underprojected tip?**

Rotation of a segment of lateral crus into the medial crus.

○ **Which technique is ideal for patients with an overprojected tip due to overdeveloped alar cartilages?**

Medial and lateral division with resection of lateral segment.

○ **What are the advantages of lateral interruption techniques?**

Reduced likelihood of uneven tip-defining points becoming evident months after surgery; faster symmetrical healing; less loss of projection; avoidance of notching and pinching.

○ **What are the advantages and disadvantages of medial interruption techniques?**

Useful in more extreme anatomic situations to normalize tip projection but almost always result in a moderate to major loss of tip projection and have the potential for notching and pinching.

○ **What are the major adjunctive procedures for tip rotation?**

Caudal septal shortening, upper lateral cartilage shortening, high septal transfixion with septal shortening, and reduction of convex caudal medial crura.

○ **Which of these is preferred when the anatomy of the tip–infratip lobule and related structures is ideal?**

High septal transfixion with septal shortening.

○ **What are the minor adjunctive procedures for tip rotation?**

Complete transfixion incision, wide skin sleeve undermining, excision of excessive vestibular skin, proper tip taping, plumping grafts, columellar strut, division of the septi depressor muscle.

○ **What are the risk factors for developing bossae or horns after rhinoplasty?**

Thin skin, strong cartilages, and bifidity.

○ **What maneuver can be done to help prevent this complication?**

Transdomal suture to narrow the tip.

○ **What can be done for the patient whose lateral crura are concave?**

Dissect lateral crura completely free and reverse them 180 degrees.

○ **What is the Goldman technique for increasing tip projection?**

Interrupted strip; borrowed cartilage from the lateral crus is sutured into the medial crus, resulting in elongation of the medial crura.

○ **What techniques can be used to decrease tip projection?**

Sacrifice of major tip support mechanisms, reduction of a large nasal spine, resection of a small amount of cartilage from the lateral alar crus, softening the domes by serial crosshatching, reduction of overdeveloped cartilaginous dorsum.

○ **How do chin implants used in women differ from those used in men?**

More oval in women, squarer and larger in men.

○ **Where should the chin implant lie in relation to the lower incisors?**

The anterior surface should not lie beyond the labial surface of the lower incisors.

○ **What is the significance of the labiomental fold in chin implantation?**

If the fold is high, implantation can enlarge the entire lower face.

○ **What is the average gain in soft-tissue projection after implant placement?**

70% of the size of the implant.

○ **Why is the gain reduced?**

Implant settling, bone resorption, and soft-tissue compression.

○ **What are the advantages and disadvantages of the intraoral approach to chin implantation?**

No visible scars; increased potential for contamination; suture line irritation; requires larger incision than the external approach; unable to stabilize the implant internally.

○ **How is infection managed after chin implantation?**

A 10-day course of antibiotics is given, and if the infection does not resolve, the implant should be removed. If a microporous implant is used, the implant is removed without delay.

○ **What should be done if bony resorption occurs under the implant?**

Nothing.

○ **How much time should be allotted before removing an implant due to improper size?**

At least 3 months.

○ **In which patients are sliding genioplasty indicated?**

In patients with excess or insufficient vertical mandibular height, extreme microgenia, hemifacial atrophy, or mandibular asymmetry and in those who fail alloplastic chin augmentation.

○ **What is the most common complication of submental liposuction?**

Excessive submental wrinkling.

○ **What is the most likely cause of dimpling of the skin following liposuction of the jowls?**

Directing the opening of the extractor toward the skin.

○ **What is a V-Y advancement flap?**

Closure of a rectangular defect by incising an adjacent triangle of tissue and advancing it into the defect.

○ **What is the major vascular pedicle for the platysma myocutaneous flap?**

Submental branch of the facial artery.

○ **Which musculocutaneous flap has the largest area of skin available for transfer to the head and neck?**

Latissimus dorsi.

○ **What is the primary blood supply of the deltopectoral, temporal, forehead, and nape of neck cutaneous flaps?**

Deltopectoral—Internal mammary arteries.
Temporal—Superficial temporal artery.
Forehead—Supraorbital and supratrochlear arteries.
Nape of neck—Random (postauricular, occipital vertebral arteries).

○ **What is the primary blood supply of the pectoralis major muscle (PMM), trapezius, latissimus dorsi, and sternocleidomastoid myocutaneous (SCM) flaps?**

PMM—Thoracoacromial, lateral thoracic arteries.
Trapezius—Occipital or transverse cervical arteries.
Latissimus dorsi—Thoracodorsal artery.
SCM—Random (occipital, superior thyroid, transverse cervical arteries).

○ **What is the primary blood supply to the temporalis muscle flap?**

Deep temporal artery.

○ **Where should the medial incision be placed when raising the pectoralis major flap?**

Lateral to the perforating branches of the internal mammary artery to preserve the blood supply of a deltopectoral flap should it be needed in the future.

○   **Why should a rhomboid flap not be used to close a scalp defect?**

Causes improper orientation of the hair.

○   **What flaps are ideal for reconstruction of extensive scalp defects?**

Free latissimus dorsi surfaced with nonmeshed split-thickness skin graft; if entire scalp is involved, latissimus dorsi with serratus anterior.

○   **What is the best material for dural reconstruction?**

Fascia lata.

○   **What if the skull is involved?**

Can use a split calvarial, split rib, or methyl methacrylate plus latissimus dorsi flap.

○   **How can extensive midface defects involving the orbit and/or maxilla be reconstructed?**

With a prosthesis or latissimus dorsi flap with multiple skin paddles.

○   **What is the major limit of microsurgical reconstruction in this area?**

Difficult to restore normal contour.

○   **What if the skull base is involved?**

Reconstruction requires microsurgery with a latissimus dorsi, rectus abdominus, or free omental flap.

○   **What is the optimal flap for oral cavity soft tissue defects?**

Radial forearm free flap (RFFF).

○   **What are the best flaps for through-and-through cheek or oral cavity defects?**

Folded RFFF or double paddle scapula flap.

○   **What is the optimal flap for reconstruction of anterior mandibular defects?**

Fibular free flap (FFF).

○   **What is the primary blood supply to the FFF?**

Peroneal artery.

○   **Between which muscles does the peroneal artery run?**

Tibialis posterior and soleus muscles.

○   **On average, how much skin is perfused by the peroneal artery in the FFF?**

Approximately 10 × 21 cm.

○ **What is the role of angiography prior to fibula free flap?**

Necessary to confirm the presence of the peroneal artery and to confirm that it is free of disease and not the dominant source of blood supply to the distal leg.

○ **Why is the FFF optimal for reconstruction of mandibular defects?**

It provides enough length to reconstruct any size defect, can be harvested in the supine position and in tandem with tumor resection, has low donor site morbidity, and provides soft tissue for intraoral defects.

○ **What should be incorporated into the flap to promote viability of the skin paddle?**

A small cuff of soleus and flexor hallucis longus muscle.

○ **Where should the vascular pedicle lie on the new mandible?**

As close as possible to the new mandibular angle.

○ **To which vessels can the peroneal artery be anastomosed?**

Facial or external carotid artery.

○ **What is the purpose of IMF after FFF placement?**

To minimize movement near the vascular pedicle.

○ **If IMF is used, when is it removed?**

2 weeks postoperatively.

○ **What factors are associated with decreased skin paddle survival?**

Short skin island, short bone graft, use of the skin paddle intraorally.

○ **Which types of osseous free flaps allow enosseous dental implants?**

Iliac crest, scapula, fibula, and radius.

○ **What vessels is the iliac crest free flap based on?**

Deep circumflex iliac vessels.

○ **What is the optimal flap for reconstruction of pharyngoesophageal defects?**

Tubed RFFF or free jejunal (RFFF is better for base of tongue or oropharynx, free jejunal flap is better for total pharyngoesophagectomies).

○ **Which of these has a potentially higher fistula rate?**

Tubed RFFF.

○ **What vessels is the rectus abdominus free flap based on?**

Deep inferior epigastric vessels.

○ **What tissues are included in the posterior thigh fasciocutaneous flap?**

The fascia lata, subcutaneous tissue, and the descending branch of the inferior gluteal artery.

○ **The greater omentum axial flap is based on what vessels?**

Either the right or the left gastroepiploic artery.

○ **What are the reconstructive options when the mandibular condyle must be removed during tumor resection?**

Incompletely reconstruct the ramus so that it does not extend as high as the glenoid fossa.
Attach a prosthetic condyle to the flap.
Shape the end of the flap to simulate the condyle.
Use the resected condyle as a nonvascularized graft mounted onto the end of the flap with a miniplate.

○ **Which method is optimal?**

Autologous condyle transplantation as it preserves occlusion, TMJ function, and vertical facial height without increasing morbidity.

○ **What must be done prior to autologous condyle transplantation?**

Scrapings of the marrow cavity at the cut end should be sent for frozen section to confirm that it is free of tumor.

○ **What problems can occur if a lateral mandibular defect is not reconstructed?**

Contour deformity of the lateral lower 1/3 of the face, displacement of residual mandible toward the side of the defect, malocclusion.

○ **What are THORPs?**

Titanium hollow screw reconstruction plates.

○ **What are AOs?**

Titanium or steel fixation plates that are more malleable than THORPs.

○ **What is the most common complication of segmental mandibulectomy defect reconstruction with plates?**

Plate exposure.

○ **What factors significantly increase the risk of plate exposure?**

Radiation therapy and extensive soft-tissue resection.

○ **What is the primary advantage of using a soft tissue free flap over a pectoralis major flap in conjunction with a mandibular plate?**

Free flap results in a much lower rate of plate exposure.

○ **For full-thickness defects of the eyelid that cannot be closed primarily, what technique is attempted prior to using any flaps?**

Lateral cantholysis.

○ **What is the primary complication of the temporal advancement flap for reconstruction of the anterior lamella of the eyelid?**

Lateral canthal droop.

○ **What technique is ideal for reconstruction of posterior lamellar defects of the upper lateral eyelid?**

Tarsal rotation flap.

○ **What technique is ideal for reconstruction of large posterior lamella defects of the lower eyelid?**

Hughes tarsoconjunctival flap.

○ **Where should dissection of the tarsoconjunctival flap begin in relation to the eyelid margin?**

3–4 mm superior to the lid margin.

○ **What is the primary disadvantage of this procedure?**

Requires 6–8 weeks of ocular occlusion.

○ **True/False: Auricular cartilage grafts can be used to reconstruct the posterior lamella of the lower eyelid but should not be used in the upper eyelid.**

True: Placement in the upper lid can cause corneal abrasions.

○ **What four composite grafts can provide both rigidity and a mucosal surface for eyelid reconstruction?**

Eyelid margin graft, tarsoconjunctival graft, nasal chondromucosal graft, and hard palate mucoperiosteal graft.

○ **What is the primary advantage of the eyelid margin graft?**

Eyelash replacement.

○ **What technique is ideal for repair of large full-thickness defects of the upper lid?**

Cutler Beard or Bridge procedure.

○ **What should be done if the distal portion of the canaliculus is resected?**

The cut end should be marsupialized and stented for at least 3 weeks.

○ **Generally, what size defects of the lower lip can be closed primarily?**

<1/2 the lip.

○ **Which rotation flap is best suited for lateral defects of the lower lip?**

Estlander flap.

○ **What is the primary advantage of the Karapandzic circumoral rotation flap?**

Orbicularis oris muscle is preserved.

○ **What are the best reconstructive options for total lip defects?**

RFFF, groin flap, or scapular flap.

○ **What is the best flap for defects of the oral commissure?**

Estlander flap.

○ **What is the primary complication of this flap?**

Microstomia.

○ **What is the best method of reconstruction for defects between 1/2 and 2/3 of the lower lip, not involving the oral commissure?**

Abbe–Sabattini flap.

○ **How wide should the Abbe–Sabattini flap be?**

Half the width of the defect.

○ **What are the disadvantages of the Abbe–Sabattini flap?**

Two-staged procedure, risk of patient injuring the flap by opening the mouth too widely, and risk of microstomia.

○ **What is the best method of reconstruction for defects involving 2/3 or more of the lower lip?**

If centered in the midline, the Webster modification of the Bernard-Burrow repair.

○ **How wide are the Burrow's triangles designed?**

Bases are equal in width to 1/2 of the lip defect.

○ **What is the best method of reconstruction for defects involving 2/3 or more of the upper lip?**

Burrow–Dieffenbach +/− Abbe–Sabattini flap.

○ **What are the five stages in the repair of third-degree microtia?**

I—Auricular reconstruction.
II—Lobule transposition.
III—Atresia repair.
IV—Tragal construction.
V—Auricular elevation.

○ **What is the ideal age for unilateral microtia correction?**

Age 6.

○ **What does the converse technique attempt to reconstruct during surgery for the prominent ear?**

Antihelix of the auricle.

○ **What is the basic method of the converse technique?**

The antihelix is created using an island of cartilage.

○ **What technique involves placing several horizontal mattress sutures along the scapha to create an antihelical sulcus?**

Mustarde technique.

○ **What is the most common complication of otoplasty?**

Inadequate correction.

○ **What is the most feared complication of otoplasty?**

Chondritis.

○ **What complication is caused by too much flexion of the midportion of the antihelix and inadequate flexion at the superior and inferior poles?**

Telephone ear.

○ **What problem can occur with overzealous tightening of the superior and inferior third of the ear?**

Reverse telephone ear.

○ **What is lip adhesion?**

A preliminary step in cleft lip repair where a complete cleft lip is converted into an incomplete cleft.

○ **What is the purpose of lip adhesion?**

To facilitate definitive repair by decreasing the tension across the wound.

○ **At what age is lip adhesion performed?**

2–4 weeks of age.

○ **What is the primary disadvantage of lip adhesion?**

Creates scar tissue that can interfere with definitive repair.

○ **What is the most important factor in the aesthetic outcome of lip reconstruction?**

Alignment of the vermillion border.

○ **When is a cleft lip normally repaired?**

When the child is 10 weeks old, weighs 10 lbs, and has a hemoglobin of 10 ("rule of 10s"); this is delayed 4 months if lip adhesion is first performed.

○ **What are the three techniques most often used for unilateral cleft lip repair?**

Straight line repair, Tennison triangular flap repair, and Millard rotation advancement flap.

○ **What are the key features of the Millard cleft lip repair?**

A medial rotation flap to align the vermillion, a triangular C flap to lengthen the columella, and an advancement flap to close the upper lip and nostril sill.

○ **In a Millard repair, which part of the lip is rotated and which is advanced?**

The medial segment is rotated inferiorly, and the lateral segment is then advanced medially.

○ **What are the major advantages of the Millard repair?**

It preserves cupid's bow and the philtral dimple, and by placing the tension of closure under the alar base, it reduces flare and promotes improved molding of the underlying alveolar process.

○ **At what age is cleft palate repair performed?**

>6 months.

○ **What is the most common repair for complete unilateral cleft palate?**

Two flap palatoplasty, described by Bardach and Slayer.

○ **What is the term for repair of the levator veli palatini muscle during cleft palate repair?**

Intravelar veloplasty.

○ **What are the two most common methods of secondary cleft palate repair?**

The V-Y advancement and the double reversing Z-plasty.

○ **Which is best for clefts extending into the hard palate?**

The V-Y advancement.

○ **For which types of clefts is the double reversing Z-plasty best?**

For narrow soft palate clefts and submucous clefts.

○ **What is the significance of the timing of palatal repair on midfacial growth and speech?**

Earlier repair is associated with better speech but midface retrusion; later repair is associated with worse speech but minimal midface retrusion. More evidence exists to support the importance of timing on speech than on midface retrusion.

○ **What muscle is primarily responsible for preventing velopharyngeal insufficiency (VPI)?**

Superior constrictor muscle.

○ **What percent of patients with cleft palate eventually require pharyngoplasty to reduce VPI?**
Up to 20%.

○ **At what age is pharyngoplasty typically performed?**
4 years.

○ **What are the indications for pharyngoplasty after cleft palate repair?**
Intractable VPI not responsive to speech therapy.

○ **What are the two techniques for pharyngoplasty?**
Superior-based pharyngeal flap and sphincter pharyngoplasty.

○ **When is alveolar bone grafting typically performed in patients with cleft palate?**
Between ages 9 and 11.

○ **When does midface retrusion present in children with cleft palate?**
In the teenage years when the growth spurt occurs.

○ **How is midface retrusion treated?**
Maxillary advancement through LeFort osteotomies.

○ **What is usually the last surgery performed in children with clefts?**
Rhinoplasty.

○ **What are the absolute indications for surgical repair of frontal sinus fractures?**
Fractures involving the nasofrontal duct and significantly displaced posterior table fractures with or without dural tear and CSF leak.

○ **What is the treatment for a nondisplaced posterior table fracture with a CSF leak?**
Bed rest with head elevation +/− lumbar drain; cranialization considered if not resolved after 5–7 days.

○ **What are the indications for frontal sinus obliteration in the presence of a fracture?**
Displaced posterior table fractures with involvement of the nasofrontal duct.

○ **When is cranialization required for treatment of frontal sinus fractures?**
Displaced posterior table fractures with a CSF leak or significantly comminuted posterior table fractures.

○ **What materials can be used to obliterate the frontal sinus?**
Fat, muscle, fascia, or cancellous bone; can also allow spontaneous osteogenesis after burring the inner cortices.

○ **What is the indication for surgical treatment of isolated anterior table fractures?**

Cosmetic deformity.

○ **When are bone grafts used in the repair of anterior table fractures?**

When gaps >4–5 mm are present.

○ **What is the general approach to repair LeFort III fractures?**

Begin stabilization at the cranium then work caudally.

○ **Your patient has a fracture of the condylar head and mandibular body and a comminuted midface fracture. How do you approach reconstruction?**

First ORIF the midface, then place the patient into MMF, then ORIF the mandibular body fracture.

○ **Your patient has a fracture of the mandibular body and a comminuted midface fracture. How do you approach reconstruction?**

First MMF, then ORIF the mandible, then ORIF the midface.

○ **What is the treatment of choice for an edentulous 40-year-old epileptic man who sustains a LeFort I fracture during a seizure?**

Direct wiring of the zygomaticomaxillary buttresses.

○ **How can one repair a floating palate when the anterior and lateral walls of the maxilla are severely comminuted?**

Replace the comminuted bone with a bone graft fixed to the alveolar ridge and infraorbital rim.

○ **What is the difference in the mechanism of healing between facial fractures repaired with MMF and fractures repaired with ORIF?**

With MMF, a callus, formed via micromovement of the fractured ends, bridges the fractured ends together; with ORIF, no callus is formed, and the fracture heals via direct bone growth.

○ **What is the preferred donor site for bone grafting in the repair of nasoethmoidal (NOE) fractures?**

Outer or inner table of the parietal skull.

○ **What is the "workhorse" for exposure of the nasoethmoidal region?**

Coronal approach.

○ **Where should the point of attachment of the medial canthal tendons be directed?**

Posterior and superior to the lacrimal fossa to avoid telecanthus and blunting of the medial canthal area.

○ **In cases of panfacial fractures, when should NOE fractures be repaired?**

Last.

○ **What is the most likely cause of cyclovertical diplopia following repair of a NOE fracture?**
Disruption of the trochlea.

○ **What are the indications for endoscopic optic nerve decompression after facial trauma?**
66% reduction in amplitude of the visual-evoked response, loss of red color vision, bony impingement on the optic canal, and afferent papillary defect.

○ **What are the potential complications of endoscopic optic nerve decompression?**
CSF leak, carotid artery injury, transection of the ophthalmic artery, and orbital fat herniation.

○ **What postorbital fracture visual acuity scores are associated with a return to normal acuity after treatment?**
20/400 or better.

○ **What is the most common cause of loss of vision after reduction of facial fractures?**
Increased intraorbital pressure, usually secondary to venous congestion.

○ **What are the contraindications to orbital exploration after orbital trauma?**
Injury to an only-seeing eye; presence of hyphema, globe injury, or retinal tear; and medical instability.

○ **What are the three approaches to the inferior orbital rim/orbital floor?**
Transconjunctival, subciliary, and rim incisions.

○ **Which approach to the inferior orbital rim involves cutting the capsulopalpebral fascia?**
Transconjunctival.

○ **What are the two transconjunctival approaches?**
Preseptal and retroseptal.

○ **Which of these involves an incision in the fornix directly into the orbital fat?**
Retroseptal.

○ **What are the advantages to the preseptal approach?**
Protection of the inferior oblique muscle and periorbita.

○ **What is the primary disadvantage to the preseptal approach?**
Slightly higher risk of lower-lid entropion.

○ **What are the disadvantages of the retroseptal approach?**
Increased risk of injury to the inferior oblique muscle and prolapse of orbital fat into the surgical field.

○   **What can be done to improve exposure with the transconjunctival approach?**

Lateral canthotomy with cantholysis.

○   **What are the advantages of the subciliary approach?**

More direct, requires less understanding of orbital anatomy, and provides more exposure than the transconjunctival approach.

○   **How far posterior should dissection proceed when placing a porous polyethylene implant for defects of the posterior convex orbital floor?**

4 cm.

○   **What is the most common complication after orbital reconstruction?**

Enophthalmos.

○   **When is diplopia likely to persist after orbital reconstruction?**

If diplopia occurs within 30 degrees of the primary position.

○   **What are the three approaches to zygomatic arch fractures?**

Direct percutaneous, temporal (Gillies), and hemicoronal approaches.

○   **What are the advantages of the Gillies approach?**

No visible scar, protects the temporal branch of the facial nerve, and allows bimanual reduction.

○   **What is the plane of dissection with the Gillies approach?**

Dissection is carried out between the temporalis muscle and its overlying fascia.

○   **What is the most appropriate approach for exposure of the inferior maxillary buttresses?**

Upper labial buccal sulcus incision.

○   **What are the indications for surgical exploration after ZMC injury?**

Visual compromise, EOM entrapment, globe displacement, significant orbital floor disruption, displaced or comminuted fractures.

○   **What are the three approaches to the frontozygomatic buttress?**

Hemicoronal, lateral brow, and the upper blepharoplasty incisions.

○   **When approaching the frontozygomatic buttress through the hemicoronal incision, how is the temporal branch of the facial nerve avoided?**

Dissection begins just superficial to the superficial layer of the deep temporal fascia; 2 cm above the zygomatic arch, the dissection is carried deep to the superficial layer of the deep temporal fascia.

○   **What is a potential complication of this approach?**

Damage to the temporal fat pad, resulting in temporal wasting.

○   **What are the advantages of using miniplates over wires in reducing fractures of the ZMC?**

Wires only stabilize in the x plane, whereas miniplates add stabilization in all three spatial planes (x, y, z); wires are difficult to place in free-floating pieces of bone; wires require exposure of the deep surface of the bone.

○   **Reduction of which buttresses is essential to restore upper facial width?**

Frontozygomatic buttresses.

○   **Reduction of which buttresses is essential to restore the midfacial length?**

Zygomaticomaxillary and nasomaxillary buttresses.

○   **What is the general approach for repair of panfacial fractures?**

Begin laterally, work medially, and correct NOE and nasal septal fractures last; frontal fractures should be repaired before midface fractures.

○   **Rigid fixation is based on what two means of stabilization?**

Compression and splinting.

○   **The "zone of tension" refers to which area of the mandible?**

Superior border of the mandible.

○   **The "zone of compression" refers to which area of the mandible?**

Inferior border of the mandible.

○   **What does "dynamic compression" refer to?**

Two-plate system (compression and tension plates).

○   **How is stabilization by splinting performed?**

Reconstruction plates with bicortical screws.

○   **When is stabilization by splinting performed?**

When compression is impossible (e.g., inadequate fracture surface area, atrophic edentulous fractures, comminuted fractures, and defect fractures).

○   **What are the indications for extraction of teeth in mandibular fracture lines?**

Teeth that are grossly mobile, have fractured roots, have advanced dental caries and periapical pathology, have soft-tissue pathology, or that hinder fracture reduction.

○ **Which mandible fractures require ORIF with bicortical screws?**

Complex open fractures that are displaced, comminuted, or infected.

○ **What is the indication for reduction of coronoid process fractures?**

Trismus secondary to impingement of the fractured fragment on the zygoma.

○ **What are the approaches to ORIF of condylar fractures?**

Submandibular or retromandibular (most common); intraoral; preauricular face lift incision.

○ **How is closed reduction achieved in edentulous patients?**

The patient's dentures are wired to his or her jaws using circummandibular and circumzygomatic wires or screws. Gunning splints are used if dentures are not available.

○ **What sort of plates should be used in the severely atrophic mandible?**

Large reconstruction plates.

○ **What sort of plates should be used with comminuted mandible fractures?**

Large reconstruction plates.

○ **What are the only plates that can bear the stress of mastication during healing?**

Eccentric dynamic compression plates.

○ **Why should compression plates be overcontoured by 3 degrees to 5 degrees?**

Compression at the buccal surface tends to produce spreading on the lingual side; overcontouring will overcome this.

○ **Where are inferiorly positioned plates placed?**

At the inferior border of the mandible to avoid the neurovascular bundle.

○ **What types of screws are used to secure superiorly positioned plates?**

Monocortical to prevent damage to tooth roots.

○ **When should lag screws be used to reduce a fracture?**

For an oblique fracture with an intact inner fragment where the length of the fracture is at least twice the thickness of the bone.

○ **What are miniplates?**

Lightweight, compression-neutral plates designed to be used with self-tapping screws (2.0 mm, 1.5 mm, or 1.3 mm).

○ **What do "microplates" refer to?**

1.0 mm screw applications.

○ **What are the most common causes of delayed healing and nonunion after repair of mandible fractures?**

Infection and noncompliance.

○ **What is the most common cause of infection after ORIF?**

Poor plating technique.

○ **What is the treatment for infected extraoral mandibular ORIF?**

Removal of the tooth and the failed plate, debridement of dead bone, placement of a large reconstruction plate, and primary grafting if inadequate bone contact exists.

○ **What material is used for grafting?**

Fresh autogenous particulate marrow.

○ **10 days after ORIF of a mandibular body fracture, your patient presents with an exposed plate and purulent drainage. The reduction is grossly intact. What do you do?**

Open wound, remove involved tooth if applicable; if hardware is loose, replace it with a new plate; if hardware is rigid, continue drainage, wound care.

○ **4 weeks after ORIF of a mandibular body fracture, your patient presents with an exposed plate and purulent drainage. The reduction is grossly intact. What do you do?**

Open wound, remove involved tooth if applicable, remove hardware, and assess union; if nonunion is present, most patients will heal with MMF; other option is plate and bone graft (external approach).

○ **What is the most common complication of segmental mandibulectomy defect reconstruction with plates?**

Plate exposure.

○ **True/False: After mental nerve injury, sensation usually returns even without repair.**

True.

○ **What problem may arise in the edentulous, denture-wearing patient after mandible fracture with mental nerve disruption?**

Patients who wear a complete mandibular denture require gingival sensation; in the presence of bilateral mental nerve paresthesia, it may be impossible for the patient to tolerate a mandibular denture.

○ **After MMF for a condylar fracture, your patient complains of deviation of his jaw on opening. What should be done?**

The patient should look in the mirror while opening the jaw and practice forcing himself to open without deviation. The deviation can be overcome with these exercises.

○ **A patient presents to you with TMJ ankylosis after repair of a condylar fracture. What should be done?**

Surgical correction (interpositional arthroplasty, costochondral grafting, total joint prosthesis) followed by vigorous physical therapy.

○ **What is the typical long-term interincisal opening after surgical correction of TMJ ankylosis?**

25–28 mm.

○ **What is brisement force?**

Forced jaw opening under anesthesia; usually successful for treatment of trismus that does not respond to physiotherapy.

○ **What can be done for trismus that does not respond to brisement force?**

Coronoidectomies.

○ **What would be the optimal treatment for a 25-year-old man with a LeFort I fracture, bilateral dislocated subcondylar fractures, and a comminuted left parasymphyseal fracture?**

ORIF of the parasymphyseal fracture, ORIF of one subcondylar fracture, and MMF for 3 weeks.

○ **When are serial explorations indicated after penetrating injuries to the face?**

For high-energy gunshot or rifle (>1200 ft/s) injuries, shotgun injuries, and high-energy avulsion injuries.

○ **After high-energy avulsion injuries to the face, when is reconstruction of missing bone and soft tissue initiated?**

When no further necrosis is seen at reexploration of the wound.

○ **What are the contraindications to primary closure of bites?**

Any human bite; animal bites seen after 5 hours of injury; all avulsion injuries from any animal bite.

Section VII   GENERAL TOPICS

CHAPTER 54 Rehabilitation

● ● ● AURAL HABILITATION ● ● ●

○ **How can one determine if maskers will be effective in the treatment of tinnitus?**

Measure the minimum masking level (MML) and loudness matching; if the MML is lower or equal to the loudness matching, maskers will likely be effective.

○ **What percent of patients with severe tinnitus are successfully treated with masking devices?**

58–64%.

○ **What type of masking device is recommended for patients with hearing loss?**

Behind-the-ear hearing aid.

○ **Why are in-the-ear hearing aids not recommended in patients with tinnitus?**

They can produce too much occlusion effect and amplification of the lower frequencies, resulting in exacerbation of tinnitus.

○ **What devices are used in the habituation technique for the treatment of tinnitus?**

Viennatone maskers.

○ **What is the habituation technique for the treatment of tinnitus?**

Binaural broad-band noise generators are worn for at least 6 hours everyday for at least 12 months.

○ **True/False: Cochlear implantation has been shown to relieve tinnitus in a large percentage of profoundly deaf individuals.**

True.

○ **Which patients are least likely to benefit from vestibular rehabilitation programs?**

Patients with fluctuating nonstable vestibular lesions such as Menière's disease; patients in whom no provocative maneuvers or postural control abnormalities are found on examination.

○ **A patient with Menière's disease is able to work, drive, and travel but must exert a great deal of effort to do so and is "barely making it." What functional level is he/she?**
4 (out of 6).

○ **What are the three general types of hearing aids?**
Analogue devices, digitally programmable systems, and digital signal processors.

○ **What is the *gain* of a hearing aid?**
Difference in the output of the instrument relative to its input.

○ **What is the *frequency response* of a hearing aid?**
The gain of the hearing aid across a range of frequencies.

○ **What is a linear amplification system?**
One in which the amplitude output is directly proportional to the signal input until saturation is reached.

○ **How do linear amplification systems limit output?**
Peak clipping.

○ **What is a nonlinear amplification system?**
The ratio of input to output is <1 (compression).

○ **Which patients benefit most from nonlinear amplification systems?**
Those with a small range between their threshold for hearing and their loudness discomfort level (LDL).

○ **What are the three categories of compression?**
Compression limiting, wide dynamic range compression, and automatic volume control.

○ **Which of these is most appropriate for patients with substantially reduced dynamic ranges?**
Wide dynamic range compression.

○ **What is the basic function of assisted listening devices?**
To improve the signal-to-noise ratio at ear level by 15–20 dB in moderate noise and reverberation.

○ **What are the different types of assisted listening devices?**
FM systems, soundfield systems, infrared systems.

○ **What are the components of a cochlear implant?**
Implantable stimulator, headpiece and transmitter, and speech processor.

○ **What are the basic steps of sound processing performed by cochlear implants?**

Amplification, compression, filtering, and encoding.

○ **What are the criteria for cochlear implantation in postlingual deaf adults?**

Severe to profound bilateral sensorineural hearing loss (SNHL); properly aided sentence recognition score (HINT) <40%; psychological and motivational suitability; no medical contraindications to surgery with intact cochlea and auditory nerve.

○ **What are the criteria for cochlear implantation in prelingual deaf adults?**

Profound bilateral SNHL; minimal benefit from properly fitted hearing aids; psychological and motivational suitability; no medical contraindications to surgery with intact cochlea and auditory nerve.

○ **What are the criteria for pediatric cochlear implantation?**

In both prelingual and postlingual children, bilateral severe to profound SNHL (only profound hearing loss in children <2); properly aided open-set word recognition score <20–30% in children capable of testing; lack of auditory development with a proper binaural hearing aid trial documented by testing or parental questionnaire (for very young children); no medical contraindication with intact cochlea and auditory nerve.

○ **A 3-year-old child with cerebral palsy and bilateral severe SNHL meets the above criteria. Is he/she eligible for cochlear implantation?**

Yes.

○ **What factor is most predictive of enhanced ability to understand speech with a cochlear implant?**

Age at onset of deafness.

○ **What is the critical period for stimulating the auditory system?**

0–3 years of age.

○ **How do prelingually deafened children with cochlear implants compare with those with multichannel tactile aids in open-set word recognition skills?**

Those with cochlear implants do better.

○ **True/False: Speech perception of prelingually deafened children who have had cochlear implants for 5 years is likely to be equal to or better than postlingually deafened patients.**

True.

○ **What is the youngest age approved by the FDA for cochlear implantation?**

12 months.

○ **After cochlear implantation, children have better outcomes in which type of learning environment: total communication or oral education?**

Oral education.

• • • SWALLOWING REHABILITATION • • •

○ **What is the supraglottic swallow?**

Patient inhales, takes food into mouth, performs Valsalva to close the glottis, coughs to clear debris from the glottis, swallows, and then exhales.

○ **Why are patients prone to aspiration after supraglottic laryngectomy?**

Secondary to loss of epiglottis and closure of false cords, to decrease in laryngeal elevation and loss of afferent stimulation to the vocal cords with tracheostomy, and to decrease in sensation from loss of superior laryngeal nerves during tumor resection.

○ **What is the purpose of the "chin-tuck" when swallowing?**

To decrease the speed of the bolus passage.

○ **What device can be used to decrease nasal regurgitation in patients who have a defect in their palate?**

Palatal obturator.

○ **What utensil can be used to help move food to the back of the tongue in patients who have had a glossectomy?**

Glossectomy feeding spoon.

○ **In which direction should a hemiparetic patient turn their neck to assist with swallowing?**

Toward the hemiparetic side.

○ **What exercises have been shown to help improve swallowing function?**

Isotonic/isometric neck exercises where the patient lies on his/her back and lifts the head and isometric resistance tongue exercises.

• • • VOCAL/SPEECH/LANGUAGE THERAPY • • •

○ **After 3 months of voice therapy, what percent of benign vocal cord lesions will reduce in size or resolve?**

Approximately 45% will reduce in size and 10% will completely resolve.

○ **What percent of patients with glottic insufficiency will attain complete closure after voice therapy?**

20%.

○ **What are the three options for speech production after total laryngectomy?**

Esophageal speech, tracheoesophageal puncture (TEP), and electrolarynx.

○   **What percent of laryngectomy patients who fail voice restoration following TEP suffer from cricopharyngeal spasm?**

12%.

○   **What is the best imaging study to differentiate between cricopharyngeal spasm and stricture in patients who fail voice restoration following TEP?**

Contrast videofluoroscopy.

CHAPTER 55 Syndromes

● ● ● NAME THE SYNDROME ● ● ●

○ **Epicanthal folds, macroglossia, short neck, occipitoatlantoaxial instability:**
Down syndrome.

○ **Short, webbed neck, congenital hearing loss, cervical and/or thoracic fusion:**
Klippel–Feil syndrome.

○ **Craniosynostosis, beak nose, stapedial fixation, hypoplastic midface with relative mandibular prognathism, syndactyly, cervical fusion, foramen magnum stenosis:**
Apert's syndrome (acrocephalosyndactyly).

○ **Craniosynostosis, maxillary hypoplasia, shallow orbits, proptosis, cervical fusion:**
Crouzon's syndrome (craniofacial dysostosis).

○ **Pterygium colli, epicanthal folds, cervical cystic hygromas, cervical hypoplasia:**
Turner's syndrome.

○ **Hemifacial microsomia, epibulbar dermoids, colobomas, microtia, micrognathia, cleft lip/palate, facial nerve anomalies:**
Goldenhar's syndrome (oculo-auriculo-vertebral spectrum).

○ **Tracheoesophageal fistula with esophageal atresia, cervical segmentation defects, imperforate anus:**
VATER syndrome.

○ **Klippel–Feil anomaly with SNHL, VI nerve palsy, retracted globe, fused ribs:**
Wildervanck syndrome (cervico-oculo-acoustic).

○ **Large calvaria with frontal bossing, low nasal bridge, midface hypoplasia, congenital hearing loss:**
Achondroplasia.

○ **Midface retrusion, depressed and broad nasal bridge, congenital joint dislocations, congenital hearing loss, cervical instability:**
Larsen's syndrome.

○ **Coarse facial features, prominent frontal bones, mandibular prognathism, vertebral anomalies:**
Mucopolysaccharidoses.

○ **Nevoid basal cell carcinomas, odontogenic keratocysts, palmar pits, bifid ribs:**
Gorlin.

○ **Congenital hearing loss, blue sclerae, scoliosis:**
Osteogenesis imperfecta.

○ **Hyperextensible skin, joint hypermobility, easy bruising, cervical ligament instability:**
Ehlers–Danlos syndrome.

○ **Microcephaly, short palpebral fissures, epicanthal folds, long and smooth philtrum, thin upper lip vermilion border, congenital hearing loss, midface hypoplasia, C2-C3 fusion:**
Fetal alcohol syndrome.

○ **Cardiac malformations, hypernasal speech, clefting of the secondary palate, slender hands, learning disabilities:**
Velocardiofacial syndrome.

○ **White forelock, hearing loss, iridial chromic heterogeneity, dystopia of medial canthi:**
Waardenburg's syndrome.

○ **Uveitis, parotid enlargement, VIIth nerve paralysis:**
Heerfordt's syndrome.

○ **Cleft palate, micrognathia, glossoptosis:**
Pierre Robin sequence.

○ **Multiple telangiectasias of the skin and mucous membranes:**
Osler–Weber–Rendu syndrome (hereditary hemorrhagic telangiectasia).

○ **Multiple cavernous hemangiomas, dyschondroplasia, and propensity for development of chondrosarcoma:**
Maffucci syndrome.

○ **Hemangiomas of the cerebellum and retina and cysts of the pancreas and kidney:**
Von Hippel–Lindau disease.

○ **Port-wine stain, AV fistula, extremity angiomatosis, and skeletal hypertrophy:**

Klippel–Trenaunay–Weber syndrome.

○ **Multiple blue, compressible, cutaneous angiomas, and visceral angiomatosis:**

Blue rubber bleb nevus syndrome.

○ **What other syndromes is blue rubber bleb nevus syndrome associated with?**

Maffucci's and Klippel–Trenaunay–Weber syndromes.

○ **Facial port-wine stain, macroglossia, hypertrophy of pancreatic islet cells with hyperinsulinemia and hypoglycemia, and hypertrophy of the renal medulla and liver:**

Beckwith–Wiedemann syndrome.

○ **Paralysis of IX, X, and XI from a lesion in the jugular foramen:**

Vernet's syndrome.

○ **Ipsilateral tongue paralysis and fasciculations along with manifestations of Vernet's syndrome secondary to a lesion in the jugular foramen extending below the skull base:**

Collet's syndrome.

○ **Sympathetic trunk compromise in addition to IX–XII paralysis secondary to a lesion extending out of the jugular foramen:**

Villaret's syndrome.

○ **What are the characteristics of Crouzon's syndrome?**

Hypoplasia of the orbits, zygomas and maxilla, and variable craniosynostoses.

○ **What is the most frequently involved cranial suture in Crouzon's syndrome?**

The coronal suture.

○ **What are the differences between Apert's syndrome and Crouzon's syndrome?**

Children with Apert's syndrome also have syndactyly of the hands, a significant incidence of cleft palate and more serious facial deformities.

○ **Treacher Collins syndrome (mandibulofacial dysostosis) is characterized by hypoplasia of what embryologic structures?**

Those derived from the first and second brachial arches.

○ **What syndromes are associated with well-differentiated thyroid carcinoma in children?**

Gardner's syndrome and Cowden syndrome.

CHAPTER 56 Bullet Review

○ A 45-year-old man presents with a neck mass anterior to the sternocleidomastoid muscle. The mass is mobile laterally but not vertically. T1 MRI shows a soft tissue mass at the level of the carotid bifurcation that displaces the internal carotid artery posteriorly and the external carotid artery anteriorly. The mass enhances intensely and homogenously with gadolinium. What is the tumor?

Carotid body tumor.

○ Where are most esophageal foreign bodies found?

Just below the cricopharyngeus muscle.

○ A 3-year-old sustains bilateral subcondylar fractures of the mandible. Occlusion is normal and radiological studies demonstrate minimal displacement. What is the recommended management?

A soft diet and physical therapy aimed at maintaining range of motion.

○ What is the most common cause of massive hemoptysis (>600 mL of blood in 24 hours)?

Tuberculosis.

○ An 8-year-old boy has a draining ear filled with friable tissue. CT scan demonstrates a punched out lytic lesion of the temporal bone. Biopsies show only lipid-laden histiocytes. What is the most likely diagnosis?

Histiocytosis X.

○ What fungus produces a granulomatous tissue reaction and can cause the triad of pneumonitis, erythema nodosum, and arthralgias known as valley fever?

Coccidioidomycosis.

○ What is the most common cause of vertigo in a child?

Otitis media.

○ A patient with HIV presents with gingival pain and a foul mouth odor. Physical examination reveals fever and cervical lymphadenopathy; examination of his oral cavity is shown below. What is the most likely diagnosis?

Reproduced, with permission, from Knoop KJ, Stack LB, Storrow AB, Thurman RJ (eds). *The Atlas of Emergency Medicine*, 3rd edn. New York: McGraw-Hill, 2009.

Acute necrotizing ulcerative gingivitis, also known as trench mouth or Vincent's disease. The punched-out ulcerations of the interdental papillae are pathognomonic.

○ A patient with a frontal sinusitis presents with a large forehead abscess. What is the most likely diagnosis?

Pott's puffy tumor.

○ What physical features constitute the Pierre-Robin sequence?

Glossoptosis, micrognathia, and cleft palate.

○ An ill-appearing patient presents with a fever of 103°F, bilateral chemosis, third nerve palsy, and sinusitis. What is the most likely diagnosis?

Cavernous sinus thrombosis.

○ Retropharyngeal abscess is most common in what age group?

6 months to 3 years (retropharyngeal lymph nodes regress in size after the age of 3).

○ What is a ranula?

A mucous retention cyst involving the sublingual gland in the floor of the mouth characterized by a bluish surface.

○ A 48-year-old man presents with a high fever, trismus, dysphagia, and swelling inferior to the mandible in the lateral neck. What is the most likely diagnosis?

Parapharyngeal space abscess.

○ **True/False: A patient can lose more of the upper lip than the lower lip without cosmetic problems.**

False: Up to one-third of the lower lip can be avulsed or debrided and the patient may still have an acceptable cosmetic appearance. The upper lip is less forgiving due to the relationship with the columella, alar bases, and philtrum.

○ **What are the components of the CHARGE sequence?**

Coloboma, heart defects, choanal atresia, retarded growth, genital hypoplasia, and ear anomalies.

○ **What is scrofula?**

Tuberculous or nontuberculous cervical adenopathy.

○ **What percent of parotid and submandibular gland calculi are radiopaque on CT scan?**

10% and 90%, respectively.

○ **In which Le Fort fracture is CSF rhinorrhea most common?**

III.

○ **What is the treatment of choice for bullous myringitis?**

Erythromycin.

○ **The incidence of stones is highest in which salivary gland?**

The submandibular gland.

○ **What organism causes Lemierre's syndrome?**

Fusobacterium necrophorum.

○ **A toddler sustains an electrical injury to the commissure of his mouth after biting through an electrical cord from a floor lamp. What postinjury warning should be given to the parents?**

The labial artery may hemorrhage if the overlying soft tissue of the commissure breaks down. The parents should be instructed to hold digital pressure on the lip with their thumb and index finger to control the bleeding and seek help immediately.

○ **Fourth and sixth arch derivatives are innervated by which nerves?**

Superior laryngeal nerve and recurrent laryngeal nerve, respectively.

○ **Nystagmus is defined by which component?**

Fast component.

○ **Which syndromes are associated with hearing loss and renal abnormalities?**

Alport, Branchiootorenal, Fanconi anemia, Turner, and Weil.

○ **A 6-year-old boy is referred because of hearing loss. Audiometric studies reveal a 40-dB conductive hearing loss in the left ear. He is also noted to have downward sloping palpebral fissures, depressed cheek bones, deformed pinnas, receding chin, and a large *fishmouth*. What is the most likely diagnosis?**

Treacher Collins syndrome.

○ **A 32-year-old sailor presents with a 6-month history of vertigo. On evaluation, he has rotary nystagmus, scanning speech, an intention tremor, and bilateral intranuclear ophthalmoplegia. What is the most likely diagnosis?**

Multiple sclerosis.

○ **An 88-year-old white man presents with a painless mass just below his ear that has been slowly enlarging over 2–3 years. Pathology shows round, plump, granular eosinophilic cells with small indented nuclei. What is the most likely diagnosis?**

Warthin's tumor.

○ **Where would you expect to find the parathyroid glands in a 10-year-old patient with a lingual thyroid gland?**

In the tracheoesophageal groove.

○ **A 3-year-old boy presents with a midline anterior neck mass just below the hyoid bone that moves with deglutition and tongue protrusion. What is believed to be the cause of this congenital mass?**

Failure of complete obliteration of the thyroglossal duct.

○ **An infant presents with coughing, choking, and cyanosis during feeding. This clinical triad suggests what process?**

A tracheoesophageal fistula.

○ **What is the minimum systolic arterial pressure required to maintain cerebral perfusion?**

50 mm Hg.

○ **What diagnosis must be investigated in a patient presenting with pulsating exophthalmos?**

Carotid-cavernous fistula.

○ **What are the disadvantages of using technetium scans to monitor therapy for necrotizing otitis externa?**

It reflects osteoblastic activity and bone remodeling but is not specific for osteomyelitis. It also has poor spatial resolution and may remain positive long after clinical resolution.

○ **Why is facial electroneurography (ENoG) an unreliable prognostic indicator more than 3 weeks after the onset of facial paralysis?**

Asynchronous discharge from regenerating nerve fibers can give a false-positive or false-negative report of nerve status.

○ **Bilateral facial paralysis associated with progressive ascending motor neuropathy of the lower extremities and elevated CSF protein is characteristic of what clinical entity?**

Guillain–Barré syndrome.

○ **How would you grade facial nerve function in a patient with facial asymmetry at rest, incomplete eye closure, and minimal motion of the mouth with maximal effort?**

House Grade V.

○ **In the tonotopic organization of the cochlea, where are the low frequencies located?**

At the cochlear apex.

○ **Recurrent facial paralysis, facial edema, furrowed tongue, and cheilitis are consistent with what diagnosis?**

Melkersson–Rosenthal syndrome.

○ **True/False: A narrow internal auditory canal is a contraindication for cochlear implantation.**

True.

○ **In a child with bilateral congenital aural atresia, how is normal sensorineural hearing confirmed in the ear to be operated on first?**

Detection of an ipsilateral wave I on bone conduction ABR.

○ **True/False: Most acoustic neuromas are inherited on chromosome 22.**

False.

○ **What is the most common tumor of the middle ear?**

Glomus tumor.

○ **What is the most common site of origin of glomus tympanicum tumors?**

Jacobson's nerve.

○ **What is the primary treatment for erysipelas involving the ear?**

Oral or intravenous antistreptococcal antibiotics.

○ **What do neurofibromatosis, tuberous sclerosis, and Von Hippel–Lindau disease have in common?**

These are phakomatoses, a group of hereditary syndromes with neural, ocular, and cutaneous manifestations.

○ **What is the most common type of tracheoesophageal fistula?**

A blind-ending proximal esophageal pouch with a fistula from the lower esophagus to the trachea (85%).

○   **A 3-year-old boy presents with a firm neck mass. Examination reveals Horner's syndrome. What is the most likely diagnosis?**

Neuroblastoma.

○   **A 4-month-old female child has had a progressive barking cough and inspiratory stridor for 2 months. Examination reveals a raised, bright red lesion on her back that has been gradually enlarging. High kilovoltage X-rays of her neck demonstrate asymmetric narrowing of the subglottic region. What is the most likely diagnosis?**

Subglottic hemangioma.

○   **A 9-year-old boy presents with headaches and a rock-hard left posterior triangle mass. Examination is significant for mouth breathing and bilateral serous otitis media. Fine needle aspiration of the neck mass reveals poorly differentiated malignant cells. What is the most likely source of the tumor?**

The nasopharynx.

○   **A 7-year-old girl presents for evaluation of florid warty lesions growing from both tonsils. Biopsy demonstrates well-differentiated, nonkeratinizing squamous epithelium growing over a fibrovascular stalk. What is the most likely diagnosis?**

Papillomatosis.

○   **What etiology must be considered in the above patient?**

Sexual abuse.

○   **An 11-year-old underwent excisional biopsy of a midline cyst adjacent to the hyoid bone. He continues to experience drainage and breakdown of his surgical wound. What is the treatment of choice?**

A Sistrunk procedure, the definitive procedure for thyroglossal duct cysts.

○   **Which autoimmune disease causes both sensorineural hearing loss and interstitial keratitis?**

Cogan's syndrome.

○   **What organism is most commonly involved in bacterial tracheitis?**

Staphylococcus aureus.

○   **What is the most common cause of primary hypercalcemia?**

Parathyroid adenoma.

○   **Six days after parotidectomy, your patient develops a fluid collection at the angle of the mandible. What test would be most helpful in determining the etiology of the fluid?**

Amylase (to differentiate between sialocele and seroma).

○   **From which pharyngeal pouch is the tympanic membrane derived from?**

First.

○   **True/False: Vancomycin does not cross the blood–brain barrier.**
True.

○   **True/False: Cephalosporins are contraindicated in patients with a history of anaphylaxis to penicillin.**
True.

○   **What is the drug of choice for *pseudomembranous enterocolitis*?**
Metronidazole (less expensive than oral vancomycin).

○   **What is the most common complication of acute mastoiditis?**
Subperiosteal abscess.

○   **What is the most common presenting symptom in patients with Zenker's diverticulum?**
Dysphagia.

○   **What benign skin lesion capable of undergoing malignant transformation is characterized by irregular scattering of epidermal melanocytes with deepened rete ridges?**
Lentigo maligna.

○   **Two months after autograft hair transplantation, all of the hair falls out. What do you tell your patient?**
New hair should start to grow about 10–16 weeks after surgery.

○   **Which organ in the head and neck is most sensitive to radiation?**
The lens.

○   **What is the most common complication of recurrent cholesteatoma?**
Labyrinthine fistula.

○   **What is the primary blood supply to the trapezius muscle?**
Transverse cervical artery.

○   **What is the treatment of choice for granular cell tumor of the larynx?**
Endoscopic excision.

○   **What is the initial treatment for a patient with suspected air embolism?**
Placement of the patient in the left lateral decubitus position and Trendelenburg.

○   **What is the most common cause of a widened dorsum after rhinoplasty?**
Greenstick fractures from osteotomies.

○ **What is the most common reason for rhinoplasty revision?**
"Polly Beak" deformity or supratip swelling.

○ **What is the most common complication of blepharoplasty?**
Ectropion.

○ **What is the most common complication of rhytidectomy?**
Hematoma.

○ **What is the most common complication of the phenol peel?**
Cardiotoxicity.

○ **What precautions should be taken to prevent cardiotoxicity during phenol peel?**
IV fluid hydration and treatment of the face in separate units, 30 minutes apart.

○ **What are the most common complications of dermabrasion?**
Milia and hypopigmentation.

○ **What is the most common complication of tissue expanders?**
Implant exposure.

○ **What is the most common cause of flap failure?**
Venous thrombosis.

○ **When is arterial thrombosis most likely to occur?**
First 72 hours.

○ **What is the initial treatment for any free flap that appears to be failing?**
Immediate reexploration.

○ **What is the significance of time to reexploration and flap survival?**
If flaps are reperfused in 1–4 hours, 100% survival is likely. If reperfusion is established by 8 hours, 80% survival is likely. If reperfusion is not reestablished by 12 hours, flap survival is unlikely.

○ **Where is the defect through which a nasal dermoid protrudes?**
Foramen cecum.

○ **What is the diagnosis and treatment for a patient presenting with nasal obstruction and progressive destruction of the septal wall who is negative for cytoplasmic antineutrophil cytoplasmic antibody (c-ANCA)?**
Lethal midline granuloma; radiation.

○ **What is the basic structure of IgA?**

Dimer.

○ **What disorder is characterized by deficiency of C1q esterase inhibitor?**

Angioneurotic edema.

○ **What happens if Jacobson's nerve is divided?**

Loss of parasympathetic stimulation to the parotid gland.

○ **What cell bodies are contained within the geniculate ganglion?**

Cell bodies of somatic and visceral afferents of the mucous membranes of the nose, palate, and pharynx through the greater superficial petrosal nerve.

○ **Which part of the facial nerve would be divided if lacrimation and the stapedial reflex are preserved, but movement of the muscles of facial expression and taste to the anterior 2/3 of the tongue are absent?**

Tympanic.

○ **What part of the nerve unit is affected by Wallerian degeneration?**

Distal axon to the motor end plate and proximal axon to the first node of Ranvier.

○ **What is the function of vitamin C?**

Hydroxylation of proline and lysine.

○ **What two congenital malformations of the cochlea are contraindications to a cochlear implant?**

Michel aplasia and small internal auditory canal syndrome.

○ **What is the treatment for alar retraction of >2 mm?**

Auricular microcomposite graft.

○ **What is the most common cause of voice failures after TEP?**

Pharyngoesophageal spasm.

○ **What is class I occlusion?**

Mesiobuccal cusp of the maxillary 1st molar is in occlusion with the buccal groove of the mandibular 1st molar.

○ **After a knife wound to the cheek just inferior to the medial canthus, the patient has buccal branch paralysis. How is this managed?**

Observation; exploration is not warranted if the injury occurs medial to the lateral canthus.

○   **What complication is seen more often with cricothyroidotomy than tracheotomy?**
Subglottic stenosis.

○   **What is the mechanism of action of botulinum A toxin?**
Inhibition of the release of acetylcholine at the presynaptic nerve terminal.

○   **What is the most feared complication of septal hematoma?**
Saddle nose deformity.

○   **What muscles create vertical glabellar rhytids?**
Corrugator supercilii muscles.

○   **What is the anterior limit of the hiatus semilunaris?**
Uncinate process.

○   **What is rollover?**
A decrease in speech discrimination at high intensities suggestive of a retrocochlear lesion.

○   **What is the incidence of sterile tympanocentesis specimens in the presence of apparently active disease?**
20–30%.

○   **What is Griesinger's sign?**
Edema and tenderness over the mastoid cortex associated with thrombosis of the mastoid emissary vein secondary to lateral sinus thrombosis.

○   **What is the most common cause of chronic cervical adenopathy in children and adolescents?**
Cat-scratch disease.

○   **What is the etiology of a nasal dermal sinus?**
Defective obliteration of the dural projection through the foramen cecum and entrapment of epithelium as the dural tract resorbs.

○   **What is the blood supply to the sternocleidomastoid flap?**
Occipital artery, superior thyroid artery, transverse cervical artery, inferior thyroid artery.

○   **Where is verrucous carcinoma most likely to arise?**
Buccal mucosa.

○   **What is another name for papillary cystadenoma lymphomatosum?**
Warthin's tumor.

○ **What do biopsy specimens of rhinoscleroma show?**

Mikulicz cells, histiocytes, and Russell bodies.

○ **What bacterium is associated with rhinophyma?**

Demodex follicularis.

○ **Where is tuberculosis of the larynx most commonly found?**

Interarytenoid area and laryngeal surface of the epiglottis.

○ **What tumors are physaliferous cells seen in?**

Chordomas.

○ **What is the most common benign tumor of the esophagus?**

Leiomyoma.

○ **How long does it take for the dermis to normalize after chemical face peeling?**

10 months.

○ **True/False: Children are more likely than adults to form hypertrophic scars.**

True.

○ **Which nevi have the propensity for malignant degeneration?**

Junctional nevi.

○ **What finding on biopsy specimen distinguishes Sjögren's syndrome from lymphoma?**

Myoepithelial cells are only seen in Sjögren's syndrome.

○ **Acute, branching, septate hyphae are characteristic of which fungus?**

Aspergillus fumigatus.

○ **Which mandibular cyst forms around impacted molars?**

Dentigerous cysts.

○ **For which penetrating cervical injuries is angiography indicated in almost all cases?**

Injuries involving zone 1 or 3.

○ **What is a hamartoma?**

Circumscribed overgrowth of tissues, normally present in that part of the body.

○ **What laboratory values are abnormal in patients with von Willebrand's disease?**

Bleeding time and PTT.

○ **Where are the cell bodies of special visceral afferent nerves from taste buds in the anterior 2/3 of the tongue?**

Geniculate ganglion.

○ **Between what structures does a Killian-Jamieson dehiscence occur?**

Cricopharyngeus and circular fibers of the esophagus.

○ **What is the preferred method of hand hygiene as recommended by the CDC and WHO?**

Alcohol-based hand rub except when hands are visibly soiled or after caring for patients with infectious diarrhea, in which soap and water should be used.

○ **True/False:** *Clostridium difficile* **spores are killed using alcohol-based hand rubs.**

False: The best way to remove the spores from the hands is through hand washing and from surfaces is with bleach.

○ **Why is it important to wear a face mask when inserting a catheter or injecting material into the epidural or subdural space?**

Failure to wear face masks during these procedures has resulted in the development of bacterial meningitis in patients undergoing these procedures.

○ **According to the Spaulding classification system, what level of disinfection must be used on endoscopes?**

Endoscopes are considered "semi-critical" and require high-level disinfection prior to reuse.

○ **What is the blood supply to the cerebellum?**

Superior cerebellar artery, anterior inferior cerebellar artery and posterior inferior cerebellar artery.

○ **What is the most common hereditary cerebellar syndrome?**

FXTAS (Fragile X Tremor Ataxia Syndrome).

BIBLIOGRAPHY

Adler SC, Rousso D. Evaluation of past and present hair replacement techniques. *Arch Facial Plast Surg.* 1999;1:266-271.

Alberico RA et al. Imaging in head and neck oncology. *Surg Oncol Clin N Am.* 2004;13(1):13-35.

Albert B. Management of the complications of mandibular fracture treatment. *Op Tech Plast Reconstr Surg.* 1998;5:325-333.

Ali MK, Streitmann MJ. Excision of rhinophyma with the carbon dioxide laser: A ten-year experience. *Ann Otol Rhinol Laryngol.* 1997;106:952-955.

Anderson JE. *Grant's Atlas of Anatomy,* 8th ed. Baltimore: Williams & Wilkins, 1983.

Anson BJ et al. Surgical anatomy of the facial nerve. *Arch Otolaryngol.* 1972;97:201-213.

Antonelli PJ et al. Diagnostic yield of high-resolution computed tomography for pediatric sensorineural hearing loss. *Laryngoscope.* 1999;109:1642-1647.

Asakage T et al. Tumor thickness predicts cervical metastasis in patients with Stage I/II carcinoma of the tongue. *Cancer.* 1998;82:1443-1448.

Bailey BJ (ed.). *Head and Neck Surgery—Otolaryngology.* Philadelphia: J.B. Lippincott Co., 1993.

Backous DD et al. Trauma to the external auditory canal and temporal bone. *Otolaryngol Clin North Am.* 1996;29:853-866.

Bauer CA, Coker NJ. Update on facial nerve disorders. *Otolaryngol Clin North Am.* 1996;29:445-454.

Bayles SW et al. Mandibular fracture and associated cervical spine fracture, a rare and predictable injury. *Arch Otolaryngol Head Neck Surg.* 1997;123:1304-1307.

Beekhuis GJ. Blepharoplasty. *Otolaryngol Clin North Am.* 1982;15:179-193.

Benninger MS et al. Adult chronic rhinosinusitis: Definitions, diagnosis, epidemiology, and pathophysiology. *Otolaryngol Head Neck Surg.* 2003;129:S1-S32.

Beppu M et al. The osteocutaneous fibula flap: An anatomic study. *J Reconstr Microsurg.* 1992;8:215-223.

Bernstein L, Nelson RH. Surgical anatomy of the extraparotid distribution of the facial nerve. *Arch Otolaryngol.* 1984;110:177-182.

Bhupendra CK et al. Management of complex orbital fractures. *Facial Plastic Surg.* 1998;14:83-103.

Biavati MJ et al. Predictive factors for respiratory complications after tonsillectomy and adenoidectomy in children. *Arch Otolaryngol Head Neck Surg.* 1997;123:517-521.

Blackwell KE et al. Lateral mandibular reconstruction using soft-tissue free flaps and plates. *Arch Otolaryngol Head Neck Surg.* 1996;122:672-678.

Boyd JB. Use of reconstruction plates in conjunction with soft-tissue free flaps for oromandibular reconstruction. *Clin Plast Surg.* 1994;21:77.

Brackmann PE (ed.). *Otologic Surgery.* Philadelphia: WB Saunders, 1994.

Burt JD, Byrd HS. Cleft lip: Unilateral primary deformities. *Plast Reconstr Surg.* 2000;105:1043-1055.

Byers RM et al. Can we detect or predict the presence of occult nodal metastases in patients with squamous carcinoma of the oral tongue? *Head Neck.* 1998;20:139-144.

Byers RM et al. Frequency and therapeutic implications of 'skip metastases' in the neck from squamous carcinoma of the oral tongue. *Head Neck.* 1997;19:14-19.

Chang CY, Cass SP. Management of facial nerve injury due to temporal bone trauma. *Am J Otol.* 1999;20:96-113.

Chow JM et al. Radiotherapy or surgery for subclinical cervical node metastases. *Arch Otolaryngol Head Neck Surg.* 1989;115:981-984.

Chow SM. Side effects of high-dose radioactive iodine for ablation or treatment of differentiated thyroid cancer. *J HK Coll Radiol.* 2005;8:127-135.

Clark N et al. High-energy ballistic and avulsive facial injuries: Classification, patterns, and an algorithm for primary reconstruction. *J Plastic Reconstr Surg.* 1996;98:583-601.

Cotton RT. Pediatric laryngotracheal reconstruction. *Op Tech Otolaryngol Head Neck Surg.* 1992;3:165-172.

Cotton RT et al. Pediatric laryngotracheal reconstruction with cartilage grafts and endotracheal tube stenting: The single stage approach. *Laryngoscope.* 1995;105:818-821.

Cotton RT et al. Four-quadrant cricoid cartilage division in laryngotracheal reconstruction. *Arch Otolaryngol Head Neck Surg.* 1992;118:1023-1027.

Debry C et al. Drainage after thyroid surgery: A prospective randomized study. *J Laryngol Otol.* 1999;113:49-51.

Derkay CS et al. Management of children with von Willebrand disease undergoing adenotonsillectomy. *Am J Otolaryngol.* 1996;17:172-177.

Dettelbach MA et al. Effect of the Passy-Muir valve on aspiration in patients with tracheostomy. *Head Neck.* 1995;17:297-300.

Dorn MT et al. Pathologic quiz case 1. *Arch Otolaryngol Head Neck Surg.* 1999;125:694-697.

Doyle PW, Woodham JD. Evaluation of the microbiology of chronic ethmoid sinusitis. *J Clin Microbiol.* 1991;29:2396-2400.

Dyer RK, McElveen JT. The patulous Eustachian tube: Management options. *Otolaryngol Head Neck Surg.* 1991;105:832-835.

Eckel HE. Endoscopic laser resection of supraglottic carcinoma. *Otolaryngol Head Neck Surg.* 1997;117:681-687.

Eden BV et al. Esthesioneuroblastoma. *Cancer.* 1994;73:2556-2562.

Eliashar R et al. Can topical mitomycin prevent laryngotracheal stenosis? *Laryngoscope.* 1999;109:1594-1600.

Fauci AS, Braunwald E, Kasper DL, Hauser SL, Longo DL, Jameson JL, Loscalzo J. "Chapter 5. Principles of Clinical Pharmacology" (Chapter). In: Fauci AS, Braunwald E, Kasper DL, Hauser SL, Longo DL, Jameson JL, Loscalzo J. *Harrison's Principles of Internal Medicine,* 17th edn. Available at: http://www.accessmedicine.com/content.aspx?aID=9092427.

Ferguson BJ. Definitions of fungal rhinosinusitis. *Otolaryngol Clin North Am.* 2000;33:227-235.

Fedok FG. Comprehensive management of nasoethmoid-orbital injuries. *J Craniomaxillofac Trauma.* 1995;1:36-48.

Fick DM, Cooper JW, Wade WE, Waller JL, Maclean JR, Beers MH. Updating the Beers criteria for potentially inappropriate medication use in older adults: Results of a US consensus panel of experts. *Arch Intern Med.* 2003;163:2716-2724.

Fischbein NJ, Ong KC. "Chapter 3. Radiology" (Chapter). In: Lalwani AK. *CURRENT Diagnosis & Treatment in Otolaryngology—Head & Neck Surgery,* 2nd edn. Available at: http://www.accessmedicine.com/content.aspx?aID=2825206.

Fitzgerald PA. "Chapter 26. Endocrine Disorders" (Chapter). In: McPhee SJ, Papadakis MA. *CURRENT Medical Diagnosis & Treatment 2011.* Available at: http://www.accessmedicine.com/content.aspx?aID=14198.

Franceschi D et al. Improved survival in the treatment of squamous carcinoma of the oral tongue. *Am J of Surg.* 1993;166:360-365.

Gacek RR et al. Adult spontaneous cerebrospinal fluid otorrhea: Diagnosis and management. *Am J Otol.* 1999;20:770-776.

Gantz BJ et al. Surgical management of Bell's palsy. *Laryngoscope.* 1999;109:1177-1188.

Gardner DG, Shoback D. *Greenspan's Basic & Clinical Endocrinology, 8th edn.* New York: McGraw-Hill, 2007.

Geiger DG, Thompson NW. Thyroid tumors in children. *Otolaryngol Clin North Am.* 1996;29:711-720.

Gerber ME et al. Selected risk factors in pediatric adenotonsillectomy. *Arch Otolaryngol Head Neck Surg.* 1996;122:811-814.

Gluth MB, Driscoll CL, Lalwani AK. "Chapter 70. Cochlear Implants" (Chapter). In: Lalwani AK. *CURRENT Diagnosis & Treatment in Otolaryngology—Head & Neck Surgery,* 2nd edn. Available at: http://www.accessmedicine.com/content.aspx?aID=2832806.

Goodman AG, Rall TW, Nies AS, Taylor P. *Goodman and Gilman's the Pharmacological Basis of Therapeutics,* 8th edn. New York: Pergamon Press, 1990.

Gormley PK et al. Congenital vascular anomalies and persistent respiratory symptoms in children. *Int J Pediatr Otolaryngol.* 1999;51: 23-31.

Gosain AK et al. Surgical anatomy of the SMAS: A reinvestigation. *Plast Reconstr Surg.* 1993;92:1254-1263.

Greenfield LJ. *Scientific Principles and Practice,* 2nd edn. Baltimore: Lippincott-Raven, 1997.

Gress H et al. Indications and diagnostic sensitivity of CT and MRI in the otorhinolaryngology field. *HNO.* 2002;50(7):611025.

Grillo HC et al. Laryngotracheal resection and reconstruction for subglottic stenosis. *Ann Thorac Surg.* 1992;53:54-63.

Haberkamp TJ, Tanyeri HM. Management of idiopathic sudden sensorineural hearing loss. *Am J Otol.* 1999;20:587-595.

Haddadin KJ et al. Improved survival for patients with clinically T1/T2, N0 tongue tumors undergoing a prophylactic neck dissection. *Head Neck.* 1999;21:517-525.

Har-El G et al. Resection of tracheal stenosis with end-to-end anastomosis. *Ann Otol Rhinol Laryngol.* 1992;102:670-674.

Harrison LB et al. Long term results of primary radiotherapy with/without neck dissection for squamous cell cancer of the base of tongue. *Head Neck.* 1998;20:669-673.

Hemmila MR, Wahl WL. "Chapter 13. Management of the Injured Patient" (Chapter). In: Doherty GM. *CURRENT Diagnosis & Treatment: Surgery,* 13th edn. Available at: http://www.accessmedicine.com/content.aspx?aID=5212736.

Hidalgo DA. Condyle transplantation in free flap mandible reconstruction. *Plast Reconstr Surg.* 1994;93:770-781.

Hidalgo DA. Fibula free flap: A new method of mandible reconstruction. *Plast Reconstr Surg.* 1989;84:71-79.

Holinger PH. Clinical aspects of congenital anomalies of the larynx, trachea, bronchi and esophagus. *J Laryngol Otol.* 1961;75:1-44.

Houck JR, Medina JE. Management of cervical lymph nodes in squamous carcinomas of the head and neck. *Semin Surg Oncol.* 1995;11:228-239.

Hsu HE et al. Effect of pneumococcal conjugate vaccine on pneumoccocal meningitis. *N Engl J Med.* 2009;360:244.

Hsu J et al. Antimicrobial resistance in bacterial chronic sinusitis. *Am J Rhin.* 1998;12:243-248.

Isselbacher KJ. "On the Long-Term Use of Proton Pump Inhibitors" (Update). In: Fauci AS, Braunwald E, Kasper DL, Hauser SL, Longo DL, Jameson JL, Loscalzo J. *Harrison's Principles of Internal Medicine,* 17th edn. Available at: http://www.accessmedicine.com/updatesContent.aspx?aid=1001773.

Izdebski K. "Chapter 28. Clinical Voice Assessment: The Role & Value of the Phonatory Function Studies" (Chapter). In: Lalwani AK. *CURRENT Diagnosis & Treatment in Otolaryngology—Head & Neck Surgery,* 2nd edn. Available at: http://www.accessmedicine.com/content.aspx?aID=2827429.

James DG. Differential diagnosis of facial nerve palsy. *Sarcoidosis Vasc Diffuse Lung Dis.* 1997;14:115-120.

Johnson TM et al. The Rieger flap for nasal reconstruction. *Arch Otolaryngol Head Neck Surg.* 1995;121:634-637.

Kashima ML et al. Latex allergy: An update for the otolaryngologist. *Arch Otolaryngol Head Neck Surg.* 2001;127:442-446.

Koppula B, Rajendran JG. PET-CT in head and neck cancer. *Applied Radiology.* 2010;39:20-26.

Kroll SS et al. Costs and complications in mandibular reconstruction. *Ann Plast Surg.* 1992;29:341-347.

Kryger MH, Roth T, Dement WC. *Principles and Practice of Sleep Medicine,* 3rd ed. Philadelphia: WB Saunders, 2000.

Kuhn FA, Javer AR. Allergic fungal rhinosinusitis: Perioperative management, prevention of recurrence, and role of steroids and antifungal agents. *Otolaryngol Clin North Am.* 2000;33:419-431.

Kushner GM, Alpert B. Open reduction and internal fixation of acute mandibular fractures in adults. *Facial Plastic Surg.* 1998;14:11-21.

Kwee TC, Kwee RM. Combined FDG-PET/CT for the detection of unknown primary tumors: Systematic review and meta-analysis. *Eur Radiol.* 2009;19(3):731-44.

Lal G, Clark OH. "Management of Differentiated Thyroid Cancers—Updated Guidelines from the American Thyroid Association" (Update). In: Brunicardi FC, Andersen DK, Billiar TR, Dunn DL, Hunter JG, Matthews JB, Pollock RE. *Schwartz's Principles of Surgery,* 9th edn. Available at: http://www.accessmedicine.com/updatesContent.aspx?aid=1001701.

Larson DL, Sanger JR. Management of the mandible in oral cancer. *Semin Surg Oncol.* 1995;11:190-199.

Lee KJ. *Essential Otolaryngology,* 6th ed. Stamford, CT: Appleton & Lange, 1995.

Leipzig B, Hokanson JA. Treatment of cervical lymph nodes in carcinoma of the tongue. *Head Neck.* 1982;5:3-9.

Li KK et al. The importance of mandibular position in microvascular mandibular reconstruction. *Laryngoscope.* 1996;106:903-907.

Lindberg R. Distribution of cervical lymph node metastases from squamous cell carcinoma of the upper respiratory and digestive tracts. *Cancer.* 1972;29:1146-1149.

Lindner HH. The anatomy of the fasciae of the face and neck with particular reference to the spread and treatment of intraoral infections (Ludwig's) that have progressed into adjacent fascial spaces. *Ann Surg.* 1986;204:714.

Lippy WH et al. Far-advanced otosclerosis. *Am J Otol.* 1994;15:225-228.

Lobo E, Pellegrini F. "Chapter 4. Anesthesia for Head & Neck Surgery" (Chapter). In: Lalwani AK. *CURRENT Diagnosis & Treatment in Otolaryngology—Head & Neck Surgery,* 2nd edn. Available at: http://www.accessmedicine.com/content.aspx?aID=2823819.

Lutz CK et al. Supraglottic carcinoma: Patterns of recurrence. *Ann Otol Rhinol Laryngol.* 1990;99:12-17.

Manson PN et al. Subunit principles in midface fractures: The importance of sagittal buttresses, soft-tissue reductions, and sequencing treatment of segmental fractures. *Plast Reconstr Surg.* 1999;103:1287-1306.

Maran AGD et al. The parapharyngeal space. *J Laryngol Otol.* 1984;98:371-380.

McGraw-Wall B. Frontal sinus fractures. *Facial Plastic Surg.* 1998;14:59-66.

McGraw B, Cole R. Pediatric maxillofacial trauma: Age-related variations in injury. *Arch Otolaryngol Head Neck Surg.* 1990;116:41.

McGregor AD, MacDonald G. Routes of entry of squamous cell carcinoma to the mandible. *Head Neck.* 1998;10:294-301.

Meric-Bernstam, M.D., F.A.C.S. F, Pollock, M.D., Ph.D., F.A.C.S. RE. "Advances in Molecular Oncology" (update). In: Brunicardi FC, Andersen DK, Billiar TR, Dunn DL, Hunter JG, Matthews JB, Pollock RE, eds. *Schwartz's Principles of Surgery.* 9th ed. New York: McGraw-Hill. http://www.accessmedicine.com/updatesContent.aspx?aid=1001784. Accessed March 17, 2012.

Minor LB. Clinical manifestations of superior semicircular canal dehiscence. *Laryngoscope.* 2005;115:1717.

Minor LB. Intratympanic gentamicin for control of vertigo in Meniere's disease: Vestibular signs that specify completion of therapy. *Am J Otol.* 1999;20:209-219.

Monhian N et al. The role of soft-tissue implants in scar revision. *Facial Plast Surg Clin N Am.* 1998;6:183-190.

Montgomery WW. Suprahyoid release for tracheal anastomosis. *Arch Otolaryngol Head Neck Surg.* 1974;99:255-260.

Moscoso JF et al. Vascularized bone flaps in oromandibular reconstruction. *Arch Otolaryngol Head Neck Surg.* 1994;120:36-43.

Mueller RF et al. Congential non-syndromal sensorineural hearing impairment due to connexin 26 gene mutations-molecular and audiologic findings. *Int J Pediatr Otolarygnol.* 1999;50:3-13.

Myers JN et al. Squamous cell carcinoma of the tongue in young adults: Increasing incidence and factors that predict treatment outcomes. *Otolaryngol Head Neck Surg.* 2000;122:44-51.

Nelson RA. *Temporal Bone Surgical Dissection Manual,* 2nd edn. Palo Alto: House Ear Institute, 1991.

Nghiem P, Paulson K. Merkel Cell Carcinoma and a New Human Polyomavirus. In: Wolff K, Goldsmith LA, Katz SI, Gilchrest BA, Paller AS, Leffell DJ, eds. *Schwartz's Principles of Surgery.* 8th ed. New York: McGraw-Hill. http://www.accessmedicine.com/updatesContent.aspx?aid=1001402. Accessed March 17, 2012.

Nosan DK et al. Current perspective on temporal bone trauma. *Otolaryngol Head Neck Surg.*1997;117:67-71.

Onerci M et al. Atlantoaxial subluxation after tonsillectomy and adenoidectomy. *Otolaryngol Head Neck Surg.* 1997;116:271-273.

Paradise JL et al. Efficacy of tonsillectomy for recurrent throat infection in severely affected children. *New Engl J Med.* 1984;310:674-682.

Patti MG, Herbella FA, Korn M. "Chapter 35. Benign & Malignant Disorders of the Esophagus" (Chapter). In: Lalwani AK. *CURRENT Diagnosis & Treatment in Otolaryngology—Head & Neck Surgery,* 2nd edn. Available at: http://www.accessmedicine.com/content.aspx?aID=2828310.

Pauw BKH et al. Utricle, saccule, and cochlear duct in relation to stapedotomy. *Ann Otol Rhinol Laryngol.* 1991;100:966-970.

Persky MS, Lagmay VM. Treatment of the clinically negative neck in oral squamous cell carcinoma. *Laryngoscope.* 1999;109:1160-1164.

Piepergerdes JC et al. Keratosis obturans and external auditory canal cholesteatoma. *Laryngoscope.* 1980;90:383-391.

Pollock WF. Surgical anatomy of the thyroid and parathyroid glands. *Surg Clin N Am.* 1964;44:1161-1173.

Pou AM et al. Laryngeal framework surgery for the management of aspiration in high vagal lesions. *Am J Otolaryngol.* 1998;19:1-7.

Pransky SM et al. Intralesional cidofovir for recurrent respiratory papillomatosis in children. *Arch Otolaryngol Head Neck Surg.* 1999; 125:1143-1148.

Riechelmann J et al. Total, subtotal, and partial surgical removal of cervicofacial lymphangiomas. *Arch Otolaryngol Head Neck Surg.* 1999; 125:643-648.

Rohrich RJ, Zbar RIS. The evolution of the Hughes tarsoconjunctival flap for lower eyelid reconstruction. *Plast Reconstr Surg.* 1999; 104:518-522.

Rombeau JL, Caldwell M. *Clinical Nutrition, Enteral and Tube Feeding,* 2nd edn. Philadelphia: WB Saunders, 1990.

Rumbodt Z et al. Imaging in head and neck cancer. *Curr Treat Options Oncol.* 2006;7(1):23-24.

Sataloff RT. Office evaluation of dysphonia. *Otolaryngol Clin North Am.* 1992;25:843-855.

Satar B, Shah AR. "Chapter 5. Lasers in Head & Neck Surgery" (Chapter). In: Lalwani AK. *CURRENT Diagnosis & Treatment in Otolaryngology—Head & Neck Surgery,* 2nd edn. Available at: http://www.accessmedicine.com/content.aspx?aID=2824044.

Schaefer SD, Close LG. Acute management of laryngeal trauma. *Ann Otol Rhinol Laryngol.* 1998;98:104.

Schuknecht HF et al. Pathology of secondary malignant tumors of the temporal bone. *Ann Otol Rhinol Laryngol.* 1968;77:5-22.

Schusterman MA et al. Use of the AO plate for immediate mandibular reconstruction in cancer patients. *Plast Reconstr Surg.* 1991;88:588-593.

Schusterman MA et al. The osteocutaneous free fibula flap: Is the skin paddle reliable? *Plast Reconstr Surg.* 1992;90:787-793.

Schwartz SI. *Principles of Surgery,* 6th edn. New York: McGraw-Hill, 1994.

Schweinfurth JM, Koltai PJ. Pediatric mandibular fractures. *Facial Plast Surg.* 1998;14:43.

Secor CP et al. Auricular endochondral pseudocysts: Diagnosis and management. *Plast Reconstr Surg.* 1999;103:1451-1457.

Shah AR, Wise JB. Constantinides Minas, "Chapter 79. Facial Fillers & Implants" (Chapter). In: Lalwani AK. *CURRENT Diagnosis & Treatment in Otolaryngology—Head & Neck Surgery,* 2nd edn. Available at: http://www.accessmedicine.com/content.aspx?aID=2833611.

Shah JP et al. The patterns of cervical lymph node metastases from squamous carcinoma of the oral cavity. *Cancer.* 1990;66:109-113.

Shaha AR. Preoperative evaluation of the mandible in patients with carcinoma of the floor of mouth. *Head Neck.* 1991;13:398-402.

Sheehy JL. Diffuse exostoses and osteomata of the external auditory canal: A report of 100 operations. *Otolaryngol Head Neck Surg.* 1982; 90:337-342.

Sheehy JL, Brackmann DE. *Surgery of Chronic Otitis Media.* Otolaryngology, Vol 1, Chapter 20. Philadelphia: J.B. Lippincott Co, 1994.

Shorr N, Enzer Y. Considerations in aesthetic eyelid surgery. *J Dermatol Surg Oncol.* 1992;18:1081-1095.

Shridharani SM et al. Psychology of plastic and reconstructive surgery: A systemic clinical review. *Plast Reconstr Surg.* 2010;126:2243-51.

Shumrick KA, Smith TL. The anatomic basis for the design of forehead flaps in nasal reconstruction. *Arch Otolaryngol Head Neck Surg.* 1992;118:373-379.

Spira M. Otoplasty: What I do now—A 30-year perspective. *Plast Reconstr Surg.* 1999;104:834-840.

Stammberger HR, Kennedy DW. Paranasal sinuses: Anatomic terminology and nomenclature. *Ann Otol Rhinol Laryngol Suppl.* 1995;167:7-16.

Stoeckli SJ et al. Role of routine panendoscopy in cancer of the upper aerodigestive tract. *Otolaryngol Head Neck Surg.* 2001;124:208-212.

Strong EB, Sykes JM. Zygoma complex fractures. *Facial Plastic Surg.* 1998;14:105-115.

Stucker FJ et al. Management of animal and human bites in the head and neck. *Arch Otolaryngol Head Neck Surg.* 1990;116:789-793.

Stuzin JM et al. Anatomy of the frontal branch of the facial nerve: The significance of the temporal fat pad. *Plast Reconstr Surg.* 1989;83:265-271.

Stuzin JM et al. The relationship of the superficial and deep facial fascias: Relevance to rhytidectomy and aging. *Plast Reconstr Surg.* 1992;89:441-449.

Surana NK, Kasper DL. "Fidaxomicin: A New Treatment Option for *Clostridium difficile* Infections" (Update). In: Fauci AS, Braunwald E, Kasper DL, Hauser SL, Longo DL, Jameson JL, Loscalzo J. *Harrison's Principles of Internal Medicine*, 17th edn. Available at: http://www.accessmedicine.com/updatesContent.aspx?aid=1001761.

Tardy ME. *Rhinoplasty: The art and the science*. Philadelphia: WB Saunders, 1997.

Tatum SA, Kellman RM. Cranial bone grafting in maxillofacial trauma and reconstruction. *Facial Plastic Surg.* 1998;14:117-129.

Tharp ME, Shidnia H. Radiotherapy in the treatment of verrucous carcinoma of the head and neck. *Laryngoscope.* 1995;105:391-396.

Tom SG. "Chapter 3. Fluid and Electrolyte Management of the Surgical Patient" (Chapter). In: Brunicardi FC, Andersen DK, Billiar TR, Dunn DL, Hunter JG, Matthews JB, Pollock RE. *Schwartz's Principles of Surgery*, 9th edn. Available at: http://www.accessmedicine.com/content.aspx?aID=5011700.

Urban KG, Terris DJ. Percutaneous endoscopic gastrostomy (PEG): Indications and technique. *Op Tech Otolaryngol—Head Neck Surg.* 1997;8:77-84.

Urken ML et al. Functional evaluation following microvascular oromandibular reconstruction of the oral cancer patient: A comparative study of reconstructed and nonreconstructed patients. *Laryngoscope.* 1991;101:935-950.

Utley DS et al. The failing flap in facial plastic and reconstructive surgery: Role of the medicinal leech. *Laryngoscope.* 1998;108:1129-1136.

Vincent R et al. Malleus ankylosis: A clinical, audiometric, histologic, and surgical study of 123 cases. *Am J Otol.* 1999;20:717-725.

Wang Y. "Hot Topic: Update on the Role of Antibiotics in Children Less Than 2 Years of Age with Acute Otitis Media" (Update). In: Tintinalli JE, Stapczynski JS, Cline DM, Ma OJ, Cydulka RK, Meckler GD. *Tintinalli's Emergency Medicine: A Comprehensive Study Guide*, 7th edn. Available at: http://www.accessmedicine.com/updatesContent.aspx?aid=1001737.

Wagner HE, Seiler C. Recurrent laryngeal nerve palsy after thyroid gland surgery. *Br J Surg.* 1994;81:226-228.

Wiessler MC, Pillsbury HC. *Complications of Head and Neck Surgery*. New York: Thieme Medical Publishers, 1995.

Wolfensberger M, Dort JC. Endoscopic laser surgery for early glottic carcinoma: A clinical and experimental study. *Laryngoscope.* 1990;100:1100-1105.

Yousif NJ et al. The nasolabial fold: An anatomic and histologic reappraisal. *Plast Reconstr Surg.* 1994;93:60-65.